FOURTH EDITION

Math Basics

for the Health Care Professional

Michele Benjamin Lesmeister, MA

Renton Technical College
Renton, Washington

PEARSON

Boston   Columbus   Indianapolis   New York   San Francisco   Upper Saddle River
Amsterdam   Cape Town   Dubai   London   Madrid   Milan   Munich   Paris   Montréal   Toronto
Delhi   Mexico City   São Paulo   Sydney   Hong Kong   Seoul   Singapore   Taipei   Tokyo

Publisher: Julie Levin Alexander
Publisher's Assistant: Regina Bruno
Editor-in-Chief: Marlene McHugh Pratt
Executive Editor: Joan Gill
Developmental Editor: Jill Rembetski, iD8/TripleSSS
  Media Development, LLC
Editorial Project Manager: Melissa Kerian
Editorial Assistant: Stephanie Kiel
Director of Marketing: David Gesell
Marketing Manager: Katrin Beacom
Senior Marketing Coordinator: Alicia Wozniak
Marketing Specialist: Michael Sirinides
Managing Production Editor: Patrick Walsh
Production Liaison: Julie Boddorf

Production Editor: Michelle Dellinger
Senior Media Editor: Matt Norris
Media Project Manager: Lorena Cerisano
Manufacturing Manager: Lisa McDowell
Creative Director: Andrea Nix
Senior Art Director: Maria Guglielmo
Interior Designer: Wanda España
Cover Designer: Wanda España
Cover images: Attila Nemeth/Fotolia; Aleksandar
  Mijatovic/Fotolia; AfricaStudio/Fotolia;
  orchidflower/Fotolia
Composition: Integra Software Systems Ltd. Pvt.
Printing and Binding: Courier Kendallville
Cover Printer: Lehigh-Phoenix Color/Hagerstown

Credits and acknowledgments borrowed from other sources and reproduced, with permission, in this textbook appear on appropriate page within text.

Every effort has been made to provide accurate and current Internet information in this book. However, the Internet and information posted on it are constantly changing, so it is inevitable that some of the Internet addresses listed in this textbook will change.

Library of Congress Cataloging-in-Publication Data

Benjamin-Lesmeister, Michele.
  [Math basics for the healthcare professional]
  Math basics for the health care professional/Michelle Benjamin Lesmeister, MA.—Fourth edition.
    pages   cm
  Revised edition of: Math basics for the healthcare professional/Michele Benjamin Lesmeister. 2nd ed. 2005.
  Includes bibliographical references and index.
  ISBN-13: 978-0-13-310415-8
  ISBN-10: 0-13-310415-X
  1. Medicine—Mathematics.   2. Mathematics.   3. Medical sciences.   I. Title.
  R853.M3B46 2014
  610.1'5195—dc23
                    2013003786

10 9 8 7 6 5 4 3 2 1

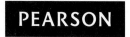

ISBN 13: 978-0-13-310415-8
ISBN 10:   0-13-310415-X

◆◆◆◆ Dedication

For Max and Theresa Benjamin—the masters of encouragement, perseverance, and inspiration.

Special appreciation to Albert Lesmeister, ever-supportive partner who truly understands why I teach and devote myself to education.

CONTENTS

PREFACE FOR EDUCATORS AND LEARNERS

Math Basics for the Health Care Professional was written to serve a large population of learners preparing for careers within health occupations as well as those working toward employment upgrades in the field. Suggested specific applications of this work text are high school vocational programs; adult education programs that prepare students for health fields; self-study by individuals preparing for workplace transitions, upgrades, or changes; pre-nursing studies; and in-house or on-the-job training programs and a general brush up for work in the health care professions. The work text was designed with student success in mind. The context is geared toward allied health students, and this contextualization helps students appreciate the value of learning math for success in their future health care careers.

The text begins with a comprehensive pre-test to gauge students' abilities and areas where remediation is required. The 14 units in the text cover the following topics: pre-algebra basics; the metric system; reading drug labels, medicine cups, syringes, and intravenous fluid administration bags; parenteral dosages; basic intravenous fluid administration; and basic dosage by body weight. Each unit provides a 15-question pre-test for additional practice in self-assessment, followed by a concept review and instruction, examples, practice problems, critical thinking questions, and a post-test. Students will find the answers to the odd-numbered practice problems in Appendix C. In addition, extra practice units are included in Appendix B, and Appendix A contains a comprehensive post-test.

◆◆◆◆ A Focus on Adult Learners

The materials in this work text have been successfully applied to help students prepare for a wide variety of health care training fields at a technical college. Students' feedback and input have played a prominent role in the design and sequencing of the content, teaching methods, and presentation. Thus, the text's organization is central to students' success. The students who have worked through these materials have been successful in their vocational training and workplace upgrading because they have reached a mastery level in the fundamental concepts, making them ready to learn the additional concepts and applications of their specific training areas.

This work text focuses on the needs of adult learners and features the following learner-based tools for success:

- Sequential skill building on basic math skills
- Ties between the application of the skill and each math concept
- Mnemonic devices to build memory of the basic skills
- A variety of practice opportunities with occupation-based examples and problems
- Mixed applications to build on basic skills and promote critical thinking
- Post-tests to promote confidence and skill building
- Critical thinking applications to increase application and skill building
- White space in the design for thinking and working through the problems

◆◆◆◆ New to this Edition

This fourth edition continues to provide a basic mathematics approach as well as dimensional analysis for all the application units. A new appendix focused exclusively on dimensional analysis provides students further instruction on and examples of this sometimes challenging concept. Another new appendix includes student resources, such as graphic organizers and other tools that provide additional support and strategies for learning and working in math.

The fourth edition of this work text has been updated to include the following features and changes:

- New, full-color design that includes more room for students to work out math problems
- Larger illustrations to help students visualize and solve problems
- Student learning objectives at the beginning of each unit
- Math Sense and Set-Up Hint features in every unit
- Pre-tests at the beginning of each unit
- Critical thinking problems at the end of each unit
- Professional Expertise tips at the end of each unit
- New appendix on dimensional analysis
- New appendix of student resources for learning math, including a math notetaker

 ## About the Author

Michele Benjamin Lesmeister has more than 35 years of experience teaching a wide variety of adults including second-language learners, industry experts, college preparatory students, public agency personnel, and other faculty. She embraces the attitude that all students can learn math. Furthermore, she believes that a student's success is often tied to the presentation of materials. Therefore, the colloquial quality of this text's explanations of math processes creates a can-do approach to and image of math. In health care, math is a necessary job skill; math proficiency, in turn, will lead to more job opportunities.

 ## Supplements

The Instructor's Resource Manual has reproducible tests that accompany the work text as a ready test bank on which instructors can rely. The unit tests (two per unit) ask the student to perform math calculations similar to those in the units. These unit tests each require 25 answers; thus, the tests do not overwhelm the student, but promote self-reliance and confidence building in math.

Two post-tests, which ask students to supply a total of 50 answers, are included.

MyMathLab (access code required) is a comprehensive online program that gives the student the opportunity to test their understanding of information and concepts to see how well the student knows the material. From the test results, MyMathLab builds a self-paced, personalized study plan unique to the student's needs. The student can work through the program until the study plan is complete and the student has mastered the content. MyMathLab is available as a standalone program or with an embedded e-text.

TestGen allow instructors to design customized quizzes and exams. The TestGen wizard guides instructors through the steps to create a simple test with drag-and-drop or point-and-click transfer. Instructors can select test questions either manually or randomly and use online spellchecking and other tools to quickly polish the test content and presentation. Instructors can save the test in a variety of formats both locally and on a network, print up to 25 variations of a single test, and publish the tests in an online course.

PowerPoint lectures contain key discussion points, along with color images, for each chapter. This feature provides dynamic, fully designed, integrated lectures that are ready to use and allows instructors to customize the materials to meet their specific course needs. These ready-made lectures will save instructors time and ease the transition into use of this resource.

REVIEWERS

I would like to thank the reviewers of this book for their suggestions, comments, and encouragement, all of which are greatly appreciated. These reviewers include:

Michele Bach, MS
Kansas City Community College
Kansas City, Kansas

Jennifer M. L. Bunker, BA ESE-Ed
ATA Career Education
Spring Hill, Florida

Robert E. Fanger, BS HCM, MS Ed
Del Mar College
Corpus Christi, Texas

Thomas D. Flaherty, Jr., BS, MEE, EdD
Quinsigamond Community College
Worcester, Massachusetts

Sally L. Haith-Glenn, RMA, AHI, MBA-HCM
Virginia College
Greensboro, North Carolina

Liz Hoffman MA Ed, CMA (AAMA), CPT (ASPT)
Baker College
Clinton Township, Michigan

Kim Ingram, MA, CRC
Houston Community College
Houston, Texas

Pilar Perez-Jackson, BA, CPhT
Sanford-Brown Institute
Iselin, New Jersey

Helen Reid, EdD, MSN, RN, CNE
Trinity Valley Community College
Kaufman, Texas

Paula Denise Silver, BS Biology, PharmD
ECPI University
Newport News, Virginia

Richard Witt, R Ph
Allegany College of Maryland
Cumberland, Maryland

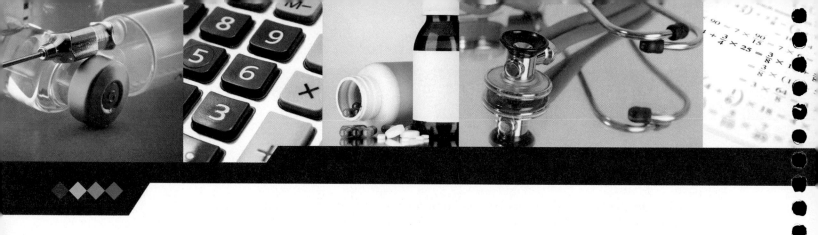

HEALTH OCCUPATIONS MATRIX OF MATH SKILLS AND PRE-TEST

Each health care field has its own emphasis on and requirements for math skills. Many successful adults search out materials that serve their immediate learning needs because their studies are just one part of their busy days. This workbook has been designed to help you measure your readiness for additional math training in and for your specific field.

To assist individuals new to health occupations, a matrix of skills has been developed to answer the question: What math do I need to know to be a _____? Refer to the matrix to obtain a general idea of the math skills necessary for your program preparation or workplace upgrade. These skills will form the core of your math abilities, and you will build on them in more specific ways within your specific field of study.

Once you understand what math skills you need for success in the program, you are ready to take the self-assessment. This tool is divided into categories that match the workbook's content to help you work independently or with your classmates; it also allows you to begin at your own comfort or skill level. The idea behind the self-assessment is to provide enough review and practice so that you are able to solve the problems for your program accurately and efficiently. Use the scoring sheet to prepare an individualized study plan for yourself or as a sheet to refer to when these units are covered to ensure that you have mastered the material.

By completing this workbook, you will be ready for the specific math training that you will receive in your program of study or in the workplace.

A final word about calculators: Calculators are wonderful tools. However, calculator use may be limited to certain class situations, and calculator use may or may not be allowed on exams. For these reasons, mental math is a valuable skill to review. When you put your calculator away before you work through these materials, two things will result: Your proficiency will increase, and your self-confidence will soar as you become an efficient math problem solver.

MATRIX OF SKILLS

	Certified nursing assistant	Hospital nursing assistant	Massage therapist	Dental assistant	Pharmacy technician	Surgical technologist	Medical assistant	Licensed practical nurse	Registered nurse	Medical lab technician	Your program
Practice Pre-Test	X	X	X	X	X	X	X	X	X	X	
Unit 1: Whole Number Review	X	X	X	X	X	X	X	X	X	X	
Unit 2: Fractions	X	X	X	X	X	X	X	X	X	X	
Unit 3: Decimals	X	X	X	X	X	X	X	X	X	X	
Unit 4: Ratio and Proportion	X	X	X	X	X	X	X	X	X	X	
Unit 5: Percents	X	X	X	X	X	X	X	X	X	X	
Unit 6: Combined Applications	X	X	X	X	X	X	X	X	X	X	
Unit 7: Pre-Algebra Basics	X	X	X	X	X	X	X	X	X	X	
Unit 8: The Metric System	X	X	X	X	X	X	X	X	X		
Unit 9: Reading Drug Labels, Medicine Cups, Syringes, and Intravenous Fluid Administration Bags	X	X	X	X	X	X	X	X	X	X	
Unit 10: Apothecary Measurement and Conversion					X		X	X	X		
Unit 11: Dosage Calculations					X		X	X	X		
Unit 12: Parenteral Dosage					X		X	X	X		
Unit 13: The Basics of Intravenous Fluid Administration					X		X	X	X		
Unit 14: Basic Dosage by Body Weight					X		X	X	X		
Practice Post-Test	X	X	X	X	X	X	X	X	X		

The Math for Health Care Professionals Pre-Test is provided on the next several pages. The pre-test is designed to highlight the major points in each of the 14 units. Some of these skills may be familiar to you, while others may be new topics that you'll need to study.

◆◆◆◆ Math for Health Care Professionals Pre-Test

Whole Number Skills

1. Find the mean of the set of numbers: 16, 10, 5, 9, 10, 7, 3, 20 _____

2. 609 + _____ + 37 = 812

3. 1,876 − 618 = _____

4. 34 × 97 = _____

5. $26\overline{)324}$ = _____

6. The heights of Michele's family members are 67 inches, 81 inches, 69 inches, 70 inches, and 68 inches. Find the range in height of Michele's family members. _____

7. Convert from 3:15 P.M. standard time to Universal time. _____

Fraction Skills

8. Order the fractions from smallest to largest: $\dfrac{7}{8}, \dfrac{5}{6}, \dfrac{1}{4}, \dfrac{3}{4}$ _____

9. $30\dfrac{3}{5} + 12 + 3\dfrac{5}{6} =$ _____

10. $46\dfrac{1}{3} - 8\dfrac{7}{12} =$ _____

11. $3\dfrac{4}{5} \times \dfrac{3}{7} \times 5 =$ _____

12. $7\dfrac{1}{6} \div \dfrac{1}{2} =$ _____

13. Solve: $\dfrac{\frac{1}{20}}{\frac{1}{4}} =$ _____

Decimal Skills

14. Express as a fraction: 8.022 _____

15. Express as a decimal: $6\dfrac{7}{8}$ _____

16. 10.6 + 0.5 + 9 = _____

17. 59.3 − 5.65 = _____

18. 0.6 × 31.2 = _____

19. 228.06 ÷ 0.4 = _____

Ratio and Proportion Skills

20. A container holds 54 milliliters of medication. How many full 1.25 milliliter doses can be administered from this container? _____

21. Solve: $6 : 75 :: 2.5 : x$ $x =$ _____

22. Solve: $7 : x :: 42 : 200$ $x =$ _____ Write the answer as a mixed number.

23. Solve: $\dfrac{1}{4} : 8 :: x : 72$ $x =$ _____

24. Solve: $\dfrac{1}{50} : 5 :: \dfrac{10}{250} : x$ $x =$ _____

25. Simplify the ratio to its lowest terms: $2\dfrac{1}{2} : 3$ _____

Percent Skills

26. What is $11\dfrac{3}{4}\%$ of 55? _____ Round to the nearest tenth.

27. What percent is 22 of 144? _____ Round to the nearest hundredth.

28. 16% of 140 is what number? _____

29. The original price of a new nursing jacket is $42.50. There is a 15% discount. What is the new price for the nursing jacket before tax? Round the discounted amount, and then calculate the discount. _____

30. There are 5 grams of pure drug in 65 mL of solution. What is the percent strength of the solution? _____

Combined Applications Skills

31. $3\dfrac{1}{4}$ feet = _____ inches

32. _____ quarts = 12 pints

33. 15 pounds = _____ kilograms

34. _____ teaspoons = 30 milliliters

35. Convert 0.5% to a fraction. _____

36. Convert $3\dfrac{1}{2}$ to a percent. _____

37. Convert 18 to a percent. _____

38. Write 1.001 as a fraction. _____

39. Write 0.07% as a decimal. _____

Pre-Algebra Skills

40. $45 + (-10) =$ _____

41. $-12 - 42 =$ _____

42. $-63 \div 9 =$ _____

43. $-128 \times (-4) =$ _____

44. $32 + \sqrt{144} =$ _____

45. $(5^2 - 3^2) \div 5 =$ _____

Metric Measurement Skills

46. 129.45 micrograms = _____ milligrams

47. 94 grams = _____ kilogram. Round to the nearest tenth.

48. Complete the table for this drug label. If the information is not provided, write *Not shown*.

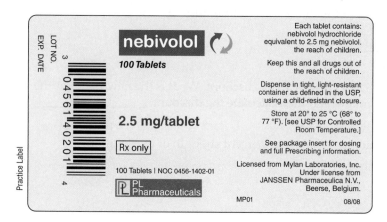

Generic name _____

Trade name _____

Manufacturer _____

National Drug Code (NDC) number _____

Lot number (control number) _____

Drug form _____

Dosage strength _____

Usual adult dose _____

Total amount in vial, packet, box _____

Prescription warning _____

Expiration date _____

49. The medical assistant was asked to dispense 14 milliliters of a liquid medication. Shade the medicine cup to indicate this dosage.

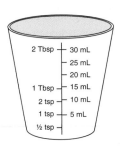

50. The physician has ordered an intramuscular (IM) injection of 1.8 milliliters. Shade the syringe to indicate this volume of medication.

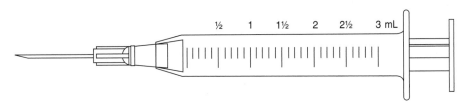

Apothecary Measurement Skills

51. fluid ounces 18 = _____ milliliters

52. 16 teaspoons = _____ milliliters

53. 3 pints = _____ milliliters

54. 0.5 milligrams = grain _____

55. grain $\dfrac{1}{300}$ = _____ milligrams

56. 3 grams = grains _____

57. $3\dfrac{1}{2}$ teaspoons = _____ milliliters

Oral Medication Skills

58. Desired: Aspirin 1.5 grams every 4 hours
Available: Aspirin 500 milligram scored tablets
Give: _____

59. The patient is prescribed Vistaril 20 milligrams orally every 6 hours for nausea relief. You have on hand Vistaril oral suspension 5 milligrams in 2.5 milliliters.
You administer _____.

Dosage Calculation Skills

60. Ordered: Zocor 40 milligrams
Have: Zocor 20 milligrams per tablet
Give: _____

61. The doctor has ordered Zyloprim 0.25 gram orally twice a day. On hand is Zyloprim 100 milligram scored tablets. The nurse should give _____.

62. The client receives an order for Augmentin 250 milligrams. The Augmentin label reads 125 milligrams in 5 milliliters. The client will be given _____.

Parenteral Dosage Skills

63. The physician orders megestrol acetate 800 milligrams per day. The megestrol acetate label reads oral suspension 40 milligrams per milliliter. Give _____.

64. Give Dilaudid 0.5 milligram IM from a vial that is labeled 4 milligrams per milliliter. Give _____. Round to the nearest hundredth.

65. Ordered: Atropine sulfate 0.5 milligram IM
Have: Atropine sulfate 0.3 milligram per milliliter
Give: _____. Round to the nearest hundredth.

66. The doctor prescribes heparin 3500 units sub-Q four times a day. You have heparin 2500 units per milliliter. You give _____.

67. Ordered: quinidine 0.4 grams orally every 4 hours. Quinidine is supplied in 200 milligram tablets. How many tablets will you give? _____

Calculating IV Dosage Skills

68. The patient with oliguria has an order for 75 milliliters of 0.9% Normal Saline (NS) over 2 hours. The drop factor is 15 drops per milliliter (gtts/mL). How many drops per minute should be given? _____

69. The nurse receives an order that reads 1200 milliliters 5% dextrose water (D_5W) intravenous (IV) at 150 milliliters per hour. The nurse should infuse for _____.

70. The nurse will administer an IV solution at 115 milliliters per hour for 12 hours. What will the total volume infused be? _____

Basic Dosage by Body Weight Skills

Perform the calculations to determine whether the following prescription is a therapeutic dosage for this child:
Ordered medication: ABC 5 milligrams orally every 12 hours for a child weighing 14 pounds. You have medication ABC 15 milligrams per milliliter. The recommended daily oral dosage for a child is 2.5 milligrams per kilogram per day in divided doses every 12 hours.

Medication ABC
Oral Solution
15 mg/mL

71. This child's weight is _____ kilograms.

72. What is the recommended dosage for this child? _____ milligrams per day

Weight:	34 pounds 6 ounces
Ordered dosage:	1.4 milligrams per kilogram per day
Recommended dosage from drug label:	3 milligrams every 8 hours

73. What is the daily dose? _____

74. What is the individual dose? _____

75. Does the ordered dose match the recommended dosage? _____

Answers to Pre-Test

1. 10

2. 166

3. 1,258

4. 3,298

5. 12.46 or 12 R 12 or $12\frac{6}{13}$

6. 14

7. 1515

8. $\frac{1}{4}, \frac{3}{4}, \frac{5}{6}, \frac{7}{8}$

9. $46\frac{13}{30}$

10. $37\frac{3}{4}$

11. $8\frac{1}{7}$

12. $14\frac{1}{3}$ or 14 R 1 or 14.33

13. $\frac{1}{5}$

14. $8\frac{11}{500}$

15. 6.875

16. 20.1

17. 53.65

18. 18.72

19. 570.15

20. 43

21. 31.25

22. $33\frac{1}{3}$

23. 2.25

24. 10

25. 5 : 6

26. 6.5

27. 15.28

28. 22.4

29. $36.12

30. 7.7%

31. 39

32. 6

33. 6.8

34. 6

35. $\frac{1}{200}$

36. 350%

37. 1800%

38. $1\frac{1}{1000}$

39. 0.0007

40. 35

41. −54

42. −7

43. 512

44. 44

45. 3.2 or $3\frac{1}{5}$

46. 0.12945

47. 0.1

48.

Generic name	nebivolol
Trade name	Not shown
Manufacturer	PL Pharmaceuticals, Inc.
National Drug Code (NDC) number	0456-1402-01
Lot number (control number)	Not shown
Drug form	Tablets
Dosage strength	2.5 milligrams
Usual adult dose	Not shown; see package insert
Total amount in vial, packet, box	100 tablets
Prescription warning	Rx only
Expiration date	Not shown

49. 14 milliliters of a liquid medication

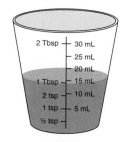

50. 1.8 milliliters Shade the syringe to indicate this volume of medication.

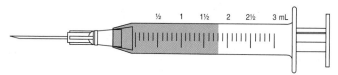

51. 540

52. 80

53. 1500

54. $\dfrac{1}{200}$

55. 0.2

56. 50

57. 17.5

58. 3 tablets

59. 10 milliliters

60. 2 tablets

61. $2\frac{1}{2}$ tablets

62. 10 milliliters

63. 20 milliliters

64. 0.13 milliliter

65. 1.67 milliliters

66. 1.4 milliliters

67. 2 tablets

68. 9 drops per minute

69. 8 hours

70. 1380 milliliters

71. 6.36

72. 15.9

73. 21.88 milligrams per day

74. 7.29 milligrams per dose

75. No, the physician should be contacted for clarification.

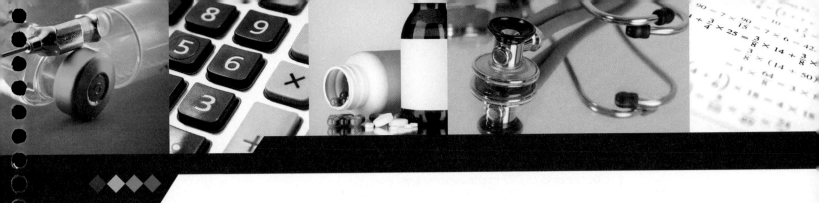

1 Whole Number Review

STUDENT LEARNING OUTCOMES

After completing the tasks in this unit, you will be able to:

1-1 Use symbols to complete a math statement

1-2 Write number statements

1-3 Find the sum of whole numbers

1-4 Subtract whole numbers

1-5 Multiply whole numbers

1-6 Factor whole numbers

1-7 Divide whole numbers

1-8 Solve for the unknown in whole number operations

1-9 Round to specific place value

1-10 Estimate using whole numbers

1-11 Calculate an arithmetic mean, median, mode, and range

1-12 Convert between Roman numerals and Arabic numerals

1-13 Convert between standard time and military time

1-14 Apply whole numbers to critical thinking exercises

◆◆◆◆ Overview

Mathematics is a key skill of health care workers. As a health care worker, you know that accuracy is important. Being competent in whole number concepts and addition, subtraction, multiplication, and division will form the basis for successful computations on the job. These basic skills form the foundation for the other daily math functions you will use in the workplace.

PRE-TEST

Complete the following math problems:

1. $48 + \underline{\hspace{1cm}} + 123 = 188$

2. $2{,}008 - 199 =$

3. $49 \times 127 =$

 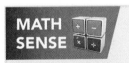

4. $1,530 \div 6 =$

5. Draw a factor tree for 324.

6. Round 15,875 to the nearest tens place.

7. Round 2,893 to the nearest hundreds.

8. Sally is a dental assistant who works a variable schedule. During the month of December, she has averaged the following weekly total hours of work: 28 hours, 32 hours, 24 hours, and 40 hours. What is the mean or the average number of hours she has worked each week during the month of December?

9. Find the median for the chemistry data set: 12, 37, 15, 19, 20, 42, 18, 6, 10

10. Patients at the Village Central Rehabilitation Center, Wing B, are the following ages: 18, 28, 47, 98, 81, 83, 87, 31, 38, 56, 76, 69. What is the range of patient ages for the residents in Wing B?

11. Write the Roman numeral for 28.

12. Convert 12:23 P.M. to Universal or military time.

13. Read the number: 108,273. The place value of the underlined digit is _____.

14. A dental assistant needs 192 hours of clinical practical work. The dental assistant has completed 89 hours; how many hours remain to fulfill the clinical requirement?

15. A patient's weight is fluctuating. The patient initially weighed 198 pounds, then he lost 13 pounds, only to gain another 7, and lose another 3. What is his new weight?

◆◆◆◆ Whole Numbers

REVIEW

What is a whole number? A **whole number** is a positive number. Whole numbers do not include a fraction or a decimal. We use whole numbers in our everyday lives to add calories, count medicine capsules, calculate wages, arrive at a total cost of a purchase, and measure our weight in pounds. Math is used in the health care setting, and whole numbers and the operations of addition, subtraction, multiplication, and division form the basis for excellence in health care math.

Practice 1

Brainstorm: List at least ten uses of whole numbers in the health care field.

1. _____

2. _____

3. _____

4. _____

5. _____

6. _____

7. _____

8. _____

9. _____

10. _____

We are surrounded by numbers in almost every aspect of our lives. Let's look at the prevalence of whole numbers in the context of health care.

Practice 2

Circle the whole numbers in the figures below and note what information is provided by these whole numbers:

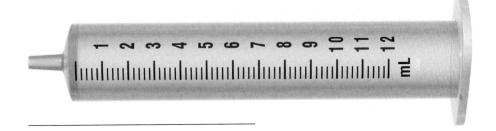

_____

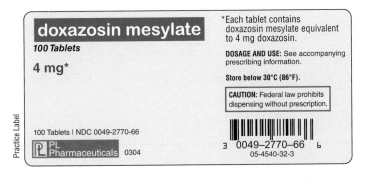

_____

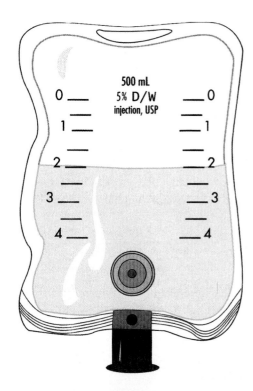

500 mL
5% D/W
injection, USP

0 — 0
1 — 1
2 — 2
3 — 3
4 — 4

_____

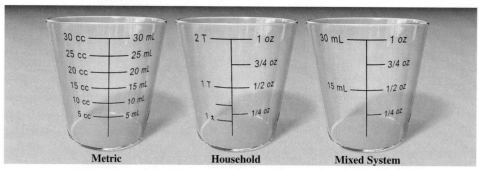

Metric   **Household**   **Mixed System**

_____

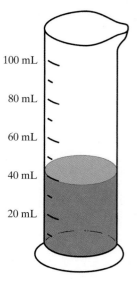

100 mL
80 mL
60 mL
40 mL
20 mL

_____

40 mL of 1:40
acetic acid (solution)

INTEGERS

Whole numbers and their opposites are called **integers**. For example, 7 and –7 are integers, and they are opposite numbers. We often use a number line to visualize integers and their relationships with other integers. The **number line** is a line labeled with the integers in increasing order from left to right. The number line extends in both directions:

Remember that any integer is always greater than the integer to its left. In negative numbers, the closer a negative number is to 0 on the number line, the larger the number is. For example, −3 is larger than −19 because −3 is closer to 0 on the number line than −19 is.

◆◆◆◆ Symbols and Number Statements

REVIEW

Symbols may be used to show the relationship among numbers. Symbols are important in creating math statements and relationships.

Symbol	Meaning	Example
=	is equal to	$1 + 7 = 8$
>	is greater than	$19 > 6$
<	is less than	$5 < 12$
≤	is equal to or less than	age ≤ 5
≥	is equal to or greater than	weight ≥ 110 pounds

A **number statement** or **simple equation** shows the relationship between numbers, operations, and/or symbols.

Practice 3

Use the symbols (=, >, <, ≤, and ≥) to complete the number statement.

1. 44 _____ 34

2. −5 _____ −17

3. 12 _____ −7

4. 12 P.M. _____ noon

5. Seven less than 4 _____ the numbers −5, −4, −3

6. $2.00 _____ 2 hundred pennies

7. 235 _____ 187

8. 2 nickels _____ a quarter

9. 245 _____ 78 + 34 + 3

10. One dollar + 2 quarters _____ $1.35

11. The numbers 0, 1, 2, are _____ the number 2

12. 3 _____ 4 ÷ 2

Practice 4

Write five number statements of your own:

1. _____

2. _____

3. _____

4. _____

5. _____

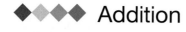 Addition

REVIEW

Addition involves finding a total, or sum, by combining two or more numbers. To add, line up numbers in a vertical column and add them to find the total. In addition problems, the total, or answer, is called the **sum**.

Practice 5

Find the sum of each problem.

1. $7 + 8 + 10 + 9 =$ _____

2. $21 + 47 =$ _____

3. $1,297 + 90 + 102 + 5 =$ _____

4. $916 + 897 =$ _____

5. $1,773 + 233 + 57 =$ _____

6. $9 + 245 + 32 =$ _____

7. $11 + 357 + 86 + 34 =$ _____

8. $24,578 + 9,075 =$ _____

9. $443 + 2,087 + 134 =$ _____

10. $910 + 3 + 125 =$ _____

Practice 6

Inventory is an important clerical function in the health care industry. Supply technicians, clerks, nursing assistants, or other staff will sometimes perform this work. Keeping accurate inventory reduces overstocking and helps avoid the problem of understocking medical supplies.

Find the sum of each addition problem.

1. The Golden Years Care Center performs an inventory monthly. Find the sum for each category.

Category	Sum
a. Examination gloves: 31 + 88 + 47 + two boxes of 50	_____
b. Thermometer covers: 281 + 304 + 17 + 109	_____
c. Medicine cups: 313 + 245 + 106 + 500 + 12	_____
d. Boxes of disposable syringes (50 per box): 2 + 6 + 9 + 3	_____

2. Intake and output totals require addition skills. Unlike household measurements, which are measured in cups, health care patient intake and output units are measured in milliliters (mL). Intake includes oral ingestion of fluids and semi-liquid food, intravenous feedings, and tubal feedings.
    Find the intake totals.

Type of Intake	Milliliters (mL)	Sum
a. Oral	120, 210, 150, 240	_____
b. Intravenous	250, 500	_____
c. Blood	500	_____
d.	Total Intake	_____

The intake sums would be charted in the patient's medical record.

3. Measuring output is important because it helps the health care worker ensure a patient's health and hydration. Output is measured in milliliters. Cubic centimeters were formerly used and may still appear on occasion; however, the metric units of milliliter or liter are the standard units of measure for volume today. Output includes liquid bowel movements or diarrhea, urine, emesis (vomiting), and gastric drainage. Find the output totals.

Type of Output	Milliliters (mL)	Sum
a. Diarrhea	100, 200	_____
b. Urine	330, 225, 105, 60	_____
c. Gastric Drainage	40, 35	_____
d. Blood/Emesis	110	_____
e.	Total Output	_____

4. Assuming you have recorded intake and output for the same patient in problems 2 and 3, has this patient had a greater intake or a greater output? _____

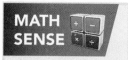

MATH SENSE

Fewer errors occur if the subtraction problem is set up vertically. Rewrite the problems.

◆◆◆◆ # Subtraction

REVIEW

Subtraction involves taking one number away from another number. To subtract, line up the numbers according to place value. Place value shows the ones, tens, hundreds, thousands, and so on, columns. Start with the right side of the math problem and work your way toward the left side, subtracting each column.

EXAMPLE

$$89 - 31 = \underline{\hspace{1cm}} \qquad 475 - 34 = \underline{\hspace{1cm}}$$

$$\begin{array}{r} 89 \\ -31 \\ \hline 58 \end{array} \qquad \begin{array}{r} 475 \\ -34 \\ \hline 441 \end{array}$$

SET-UP HINT

Keep track of borrowing by marking through the number in the column borrowed from and reducing the numbers involved by 1.

If a number cannot be subtracted from the number directly above it, then increase the value of the smaller number by borrowing 1 from the column to its immediate left. This is a two-step process: First, subtract 1 from the top number in the column directly to the left of the number that is too small. Then add 1 to the column that needs to be larger—the number to the immediate right. This process may be repeated as many times as needed to complete the subtraction.

EXAMPLE

$$\begin{array}{r} 3\,{}^7\!8\,{}^1\!1 \\ -65 \\ \hline 316 \end{array}$$

You can avoid making careless errors by taking a few seconds to use this check method. Box the number subtracted and the answer derived, and then add these boxed numbers together. Your answer should be the top number that you were subtracting from.

$$\begin{array}{r} 381 \\ \boxed{-65} \\ \hline \boxed{316} \end{array} \rightarrow \begin{array}{r} 316 \\ +65 \\ \hline 381 \end{array}$$

Thus, the answer is correct.

Practice 7

Answer the following subtraction problems.

1. $298 - 41 = $ _____

2. $584 - 189 = $ _____

3. $456 - 24 = $ _____

4. $7,547 - 2,289 = $ _____

5. $1,236 - 799 = $ _____

6. $1,575 - 896 = $ _____

7. $2,001 - 128 =$ _____

8. $10,300 - 497 =$ _____

9. $4,301 - 89 =$ _____

10. $8,934 - 2,987 =$ _____

Practice 8

Subtraction is used in inventory as well. Read the following applications and write your answers in the spaces provided.

1. At the beginning of the month, a dental office started with 2,258 latex examination gloves. On the last working day of the month, 784 remained. How many gloves did the dental office use during the month?

2. A dental office must keep an inventory of dental file labels at 2,000. Paula's inventory indicates 579 are on hand. How many labels does she need to order?

3. Labels come in boxes of 500. Use the answer from problem 2 to determine how many boxes of labels Paula should order to obtain the required 2,000 minimum inventory. Draw a sketch to help visualize this problem.

4. Patients see the dentist most often during the summer months. Dr. Brown has a total of 13,576 patient files. If he sees 8,768 of these patients during the summer, how many remain to be contacted for an appointment?

◆◆◆◆ Multiplication

Multiplication is repeated addition. For example: $5 \times 3 = 5 + 5 + 5 = 15$. Memorizing the multiplication tables is essential to sound mental math. If you are dependent on a calculator or have forgotten some of the tables, practice memorizing the multiplication tables using the chart shown in the Student Resources Appendix at the front of the text. It is important that you memorize the multiplication tables for the numbers 1 through 12 and also those for number 15. Students in health care use the number 15 frequently in dosage calculations, such as the conversions of medications from the apothecary system to metric and vice versa.

REVIEW

To multiply, line up the numbers according to place value. By putting the largest number at the top of the problem, you will avoid making careless errors.

EXAMPLE

$$2 \times 14 = \underline{\quad}$$

$$\begin{array}{r} \to 14 \\ \times\ 2 \\ \hline 28 \end{array}$$

$$\begin{array}{r} 178 \\ \times\ 23 \\ \hline 534 \\ 3560 \\ \hline 4{,}094 \end{array}$$

Move the second line of numbers one place to the left. Adding a zero keeps your numbers aligned.

Practice 9

Answer the following multiplication problems.

1. $\begin{array}{r} 58 \\ \times\ 8 \\ \hline \end{array}$

4. $\begin{array}{r} 50 \\ \times\ 9 \\ \hline \end{array}$

7. $\begin{array}{r} 512 \\ \times\ 24 \\ \hline \end{array}$

10. $\begin{array}{r} 803 \\ \times\ 17 \\ \hline \end{array}$

2. $\begin{array}{r} 92 \\ \times\ 23 \\ \hline \end{array}$

5. $\begin{array}{r} 1{,}020 \\ \times\ 98 \\ \hline \end{array}$

8. $\begin{array}{r} 927 \\ \times\ 35 \\ \hline \end{array}$

11. $\begin{array}{r} 346 \\ \times\ 12 \\ \hline \end{array}$

3. $\begin{array}{r} 1{,}306 \\ \times\ 18 \\ \hline \end{array}$

6. $\begin{array}{r} 189 \\ \times\ 27 \\ \hline \end{array}$

9. $\begin{array}{r} 5{,}791 \\ \times\ 16 \\ \hline \end{array}$

12. $\begin{array}{r} 9{,}004 \\ \times\ 73 \\ \hline \end{array}$

Practice 10

Use multiplication to answer the following word problems.

1. Last month a nurse worked fourteen 10-hour shifts and two 12-hour shifts. At $21 per hour, what was the nurse's total hourly income before deductions?

2. Health care facilities monitor all medications taken by their patients. Assume that the same dosage is given each time the medication is dispensed. What is the total daily dosage of each medication received?

Total medication received is as follows:

a.	Patient Bao	50 milligrams	4 times a day	_____ milligrams
b.	Patient Mary	25 milligrams	2 times a day	_____ milligrams
c.	Patient Luke	125 micrograms	3 times a day	_____ micrograms
d.	Patient Vang	375 micrograms	2 times a day	_____ micrograms

3. The radiology lab ordered 15 jackets for its staff. The jackets cost approximately $35 each. What is the estimated cost of this order?

◆◆◆◆ Prime Factorization

REVIEW

Sometimes in a math class, students are asked to use factor trees to illustrate the prime factors of a number. A **factor** is a number that divides exactly into another number. When two or more factors are multiplied, they form a **product**. A **prime factor** is a number that is the product of only "1" and itself. Knowing these terms will help you when you are reading math problems and on exams. We review prime factorization in this unit because it is a foundational skill that will help you complete other math functions. For example, factoring helps you figure out divisible numbers for division, arrive at common denominators, and find equivalent fractions. Furthermore, solutions are expressed in their simplest form, which means that you may need to rely on factors such as 10×4^2 in writing out the units in a solution.

$$
\begin{array}{c}
48 \\
\wedge \\
4 \quad 12 \\
\wedge \quad \wedge \\
2\ 2 \quad 4\ 3 \\
\wedge \\
2\ 2 \\
2 \times 2 \times 2 \times 2 \times 3 = 48 \\
\text{or} \quad 2^4 \cdot 3 = 48 \\
\text{or} \quad (2^4)(3) = 48
\end{array}
$$

For example: 4 (factor) $\times$ 12 (factor) = 48 (product)

The prime factors of 48 are 2 and 3. ($2 \times 2 \times 2 \times 2 \times 3$)

$$
\begin{array}{c}
48 \\
\wedge \\
3 \quad 16 \\
\wedge \\
4 \quad 4 \\
\wedge \quad \wedge \\
2\ 2 \quad 2\ 2 \\
3 \times 2 \times 2 \times 2 \times 2 = 48 \\
\text{or} \quad 3 \cdot 2^4 = 48 \\
\text{or} \quad (3)(2^4) = 48
\end{array}
$$

Note that $16 \times 3 = 48$.

The prime factors are still the same:

$2 \times 2 \times 2 \times 2 \times 3$.

The prime factors are always the same for any number.

Draw the factor trees for the following numbers and write the prime factors on the lines below.

124	75	92

1. _____   2. _____   3. _____

◆◆◆◆ Division

Division is the act of splitting numbers or amounts into equal parts or groups. To divide whole numbers, determine (a) what number is being divided into smaller portions; and (b) the size of the portions.

Division can appear in three different formats:

a. $27 \div 3 =$

b. Twenty-seven divided by three

c. $3\overline{)27}$

Setting up the problem correctly will help ensure finding the correct answer.

EXAMPLE

$$81 \quad \div \quad 3 = \underline{\quad}$$
$$\uparrow \qquad\qquad \uparrow$$
$$\text{dividend} \qquad \text{divisor}$$

means eighty-one divided by three or how many 3s are in 81.
The answer is the quotient.

$$
\begin{array}{r}
27 \leftarrow \text{quotient} \\
\text{divisor} \to 3\overline{)81} \leftarrow \text{dividend} \\
\underline{6} \\
21 \\
\underline{21} \\
0
\end{array}
$$

Practice 12

Practice the correct setup, but do not work the problems.

1. Divide 3,358 by 46.

2. 209 ÷ 63

3. Forty-nine divided by seventeen is what number?

4. What is 8,794 ÷ 42?

5. A person works a total of 2,044 hours a year. How many days does the person work if he works 8 hours a day?

Follow the steps below to complete all of your whole number division problems:

STEP 1:   Underline the number of places that the divisor can go into, and then write the number of times the divisor can go into the dividend on the quotient line. Place it directly above the underlined portion of the number. This keeps track of your process. Multiply the number by the divisor and place it below the underlined portion of the dividend. Then subtract the numbers.

EXAMPLE

$$
\begin{array}{r}
1 \\
34\overline{)5492} \\
-34 \\
\hline
20
\end{array}
$$

STEP 2:   Bring down the next number of the dividend. Use an arrow to keep the numbers aligned and also keep track of which numbers you have worked with. Then repeat step 1.

$$
\begin{array}{r}
161 \\
34\overline{)5492} \\
-34\!\downarrow \\
\hline
20
\end{array}
\qquad
\begin{array}{r}
161\ R\ 18 \\
34\overline{)5492} \\
-34\!\downarrow \\
\hline
209 \\
204\!\downarrow \\
\hline
52 \\
34 \\
\hline
18
\end{array}
$$

Repeat steps 1 and 2 until all the numbers of the dividend have been used. The number left over, or remaining, is called the remainder. Place it next to an *R* to the right of the quotient. In fractions, the remainder becomes a fraction; in whole numbers, it remains a whole number.

After bringing a number down from the dividend, you must place a number in the quotient. Zeros may be used as place holders. Follow the division steps as shown previously to solve the practice problems.

$$
\begin{array}{r}
106\ R\ 41 \\
75\overline{)7991} \\
-75\!\downarrow \\
\hline
49 \\
-0\!\downarrow \\
\hline
491 \\
-450 \\
\hline
41
\end{array}
$$

Practice 13

Use division to solve the following problems.

1. $8\overline{)932}$

2. $15\overline{)6789}$

3. $4\overline{)12345}$

4. $956 \div 66 =$

5. $6\overline{)5444}$

6. $53\overline{)5088}$

7. $15\overline{)23648}$

8. $1,254 \div 29 =$

9. $2\overline{)46882}$

10. $18\overline{)12564}$

11. $7\overline{)87543}$

12. $74,943 \div 271 =$

Practice 14

Use division to solve the following word problems.

1. Room rates vary by the services provided. At the local hospital, intensive care unit (ICU) rooms are $1,258 a day. Bob's overall room charge was $11,322. How many days was Bob in ICU?

2. Carbohydrates have 4 calories per gram. If a serving of soup has 368 calories of carbohydrates, how many grams of carbohydrates are in that serving?

3. A medical assistant subscribes to 14 magazines for the office. If the total subscription bill is $322, what is the average cost of each magazine subscription?

4. A pharmacy technician receives a shipment of 302 boxes of acetaminophen. This shipment needs to be returned to the supplier because the expiration date on the medicine would not allow sufficient time for the pharmacy to sell the medicine. If each case holds 36 individual boxes, how many cases must the pharmacy technician use to pack the medicine?

5. A surgical technologist made $39,744 last year. He is paid twice a month. What is the gross or total amount of each of his paychecks?

6. A licensed practical nurse gives 1,800 milligrams of an antibiotic over a 36-hour time period. If the dosage is given every 6 hours, how many milligrams are in each dose if each dose is the same amount?

7. Each gram of fat contains 9 calories. How many grams of fat are in 81 calories of fat in a piece of steak?

◆◆◆◆ Solving for the Unknown Number with Basic Mathematics

REVIEW

Sometimes number statements in math class ask for the unknown number. Looking for an unknown number is an aspect of algebra. To solve these problems, you must understand the relationship between the numbers.

For example, _____ $+ 12 = 75$

To find the unknown number, you must subtract 12 from 75. The answer, or unknown number, is 63.

Practice 15

Solve for the unknown number.

1. $49 +$ _____ $= 107$

2. _____ $+ 12 + 2 = 68$

3. $45 +$ _____ $= 63$

4. _____ $= 112 + 17$

5. _____ $+ 987 = 1,000$

Practice 16

Solve for the unknown number.

1. $47 - 12 =$ _____

2. $538 -$ _____ $= 125$

3. _____ $- 69 = 543$

4. $45 - 19 =$ _____

5. $12 =$ _____ $- 23$

Practice 17

Solve for the unknown number.

1. $52 \times 3 =$ _____

2. _____ $\times 31 = 279$

3. _____ $\times 23 = 1,334$

4. $125 \times$ _____ $= 500$

5. _____ $= 15 \times 5$

Practice 18

Solve for the unknown number.

1. 693 ÷ 3 = _____

2. _____ ÷ 16 = 4

3. 51 ÷ _____ = 17

4. 1,405 = _____ ÷ 5

5. 108 ÷ 6 = _____

◆

MATH SENSE

Rounding is used when an exact number is not necessary, as when taking inventory and ordering supplies: Round up to make a full case of a product when you are placing an order. If a full case has 36 boxes and you need to order 32 boxes, you will order 1 case or 36 boxes, so you have rounded up to the nearest case.

◆◆◆◆ Rounding

REVIEW

Whole numbers have place values. The number 3,195 has four specific place values:

3,   1   9   5
↑   ↑   ↑   ↑   (three thousand one hundred ninety-five)
thousand hundreds tens ones

By using the place values in a number, we can round the number to a particular and specific place unit. **Rounding** means reducing the digits in a number while keeping the value similar. Rounding is valuable because it helps to estimate supplies, inventory, and countable items to the nearest unit.

Rounding is accomplished in three steps.

EXAMPLE

Round 7,872 to the nearest hundred.

STEP 1: Locate the hundreds place and underline it.

$$7,\underline{8}72$$

STEP 2: Circle the number to the right of the underlined number.

$$7,\underline{8}\,⑦\,2$$

STEP 3: If the circled number is 5 or greater, add 1 to the underlined number and change the number(s) to the right of the underlined number to zero(s). If the number is 4 or less, round to the next number that is smaller. Use zeros as place holders for the digits.

$$7,\underline{8}\,⑦\,2$$
$$↓\ ↓$$
$$7,9\,0\,0$$

EXAMPLE

Round 3,445 to the nearest thousand.

STEP 1: Locate the thousands place and underline it.

$$\underline{3},445$$

STEP 2: Circle the number to the right of the underlined number.

$$\underline{3},④45$$

STEP 3: If the circled number is 5 or greater, add 1 to the underlined number and change the number(s) to the right of the underlined number to zero(s). If the number is 4 or less, round to the next number that is smaller. Use zeros as place holders for the digits.

So the final answer for 3,445, rounded to the thousands, is 3,000 because we use zeros as place holders since the 4 is less than 5. The zeros also retain the proper place values.

Rounding is used a great deal in health care. Rounding of whole numbers occurs in inventory, in packaging of supplies, and in daily activities.

Practice 19

1. Round to the nearest 10:

   a. 5,218 _____   **c.** 7,614 _____   **e.** 15,932 _____

   b. 792 _____   **d.** 1,925 _____   **f.** 99 _____

2. Round to the nearest 100:

   a. 4,578 _____   **c.** 1,293 _____   **e.** 35,292 _____

   b. 3,654 _____   **d.** 17,854 _____   **f.** 1,925 _____

3. Round to the nearest 1,000:

   a. 8,199 _____   **c.** 6,950 _____   **e.** 432,500 _____

   b. 14,987 _____   **d.** 12,932 _____   **f.** 2,987 _____

Additional rounding practice will be presented in Unit 3: Decimals.

◆◆◆◆ Estimation

REVIEW

Estimation is a method of coming up with a math answer that is general, not specific. When we estimate, we rely on rounding to help us get to this general answer. For example, with money, rounding is done to the nearest dollar. If an amount is 50 cents or more, *round* to the nearest dollar and drop the cent amount. If an amount is under 50 cents, *retain* the dollar amount and drop the cent amount.

EXAMPLE

Estimate Bob's expenses for his co-payment of his dental expenses for his two six-month checkups.

	Actual Expense	Estimated Expense
March	$65.85	$66
October	$59.10	$59

Add the estimated expenses of $66 + $59 = _____
The estimated annual total is $125.
So estimation is a skill that uses rounding to reach a general rather than a specific answer.

Practice 20

Use estimation to answer the following problems.

1. Find the sum using estimation to the nearest dollar:

   a. $72.90 + $15.45 + $120.99 _____

   b. $542.39 + $13.98 + $25.20 _____

   c. $23.45 + $32.29 + $56.65 _____

   d. $2,900.87 + $12.89 _____

2. Find the sum using estimation to the nearest hour:

   a. 1 hour 25 minutes + 2 hours 14 minutes + 5 hours 37 minutes _____

   b. 7 hours 8 minutes + 10 hours 34 minutes + 15 hours 45 minutes _____

   c. 3 hours 35 minutes + 22 hours 16 minutes + 9 hours 59 minutes _____

   d. 6 hours 39 minutes + 13 hours 18 minutes + 5 hours 2 minutes _____

◆◆◆◆   Basics of Statistical Analysis

The basics of statistical analysis include the topics of *mean* (average), *median, mode,* and *range*. Each of these topics deals with groups or subsets of numbers and their relationships to each other and to the set as a whole.

ARITHMETIC MEAN OR AVERAGE

REVIEW

The **arithmetic mean** is also called the **average**. An average is a number that represents a group of the same unit of measure. It provides a general number that represents this group of numbers as long as all the numbers are the same units. Averages are useful in health occupations because they provide general trends and information. You will use addition and division skills to compute averages.

To compute a mean or average, follow these two steps:

STEP 1: Add the individual units of measure.

STEP 2: Divide the sum of the units of measure by the number of individual units.

EXAMPLE

Mary Ann wanted to know the average score of her anatomy and physiology tests. Her scores were 92%, 79%, 100%, 89%, and 95%.

STEP 1: $92 + 79 + 100 + 89 + 95 = 455$

STEP 2: There were a total of 5 grades.

STEP 3: Divide 455 by 5.

Mary Ann's average score was 91%.

$$
\begin{array}{r}
91 \\
5\overline{)455} \\
45\downarrow \\
\hline
5 \\
5 \\
\hline
0
\end{array}
$$

Practice 21

Use addition and division to find the averages in the following word problems.

1. Deb needed to purchase new calendars for the examination rooms. Find the average if the calendars cost $11, $7, $10, $5, $10, $12, $8, and $9.

2. Certified nursing assistants work a varied number of hours every week at Village Nursing Home. The weekly hours are 32, 38, 40, 35, 40, 16, and 30. What is the average number of hours each assistant works?

3. The staff phone use during morning break is increasing. The director is considering adding additional phones and is researching the usage in minutes. Using the following data, compute the average length of each call: 7, 4, 3, 1, 2, 4, 5, 7, and 12.

4. A diabetic patient is counting calories. The patient adds up calories from portions of fruit: 90, 80, 60, 15, 40. What is the average caloric intake from each portion?

5. Beth was working hard to increase the amount of fruit and vegetables in her diet. She kept a log of servings: Monday, 8; Tuesday, 7; Wednesday, 6; Thursday, 5; Friday, 8; Saturday, 6; Sunday, 9. What is the mean daily intake of fruits and vegetables for Beth?

MEDIAN

REVIEW

The **median** is the middle number in a list of numbers that are arranged in order from the smallest to the largest. The median is a literal measure of the center of a data set, for half the data is below the median and half has values above the median. The median is useful in health care when we are looking at data or information that has a lot of variance or extreme values because the median helps group that information around the center number. One example is looking at data from a flu outbreak. The median would help generalize or center the data.

To determine the median, follow these steps:

STEP 1: Sort the list of numbers from smallest to largest.

STEP 2: Cross off one number from each end of the line of numbers until one number is reached in the middle.

EXAMPLE

Find the median of this set of numbers: 23, 54, 76, 34, 12.

STEP 1: Sort from smallest to largest.   12, 23, 34, 54, 76

STEP 2: Cross a number off from each end   ~~12~~, 23, 34, 54, ~~76~~
until the middle number is reached.   ~~12~~, ~~23~~, 34, ~~54~~, ~~76~~

Answer: 34 is the median.

If a list contains an even set of numbers, add the final two numbers and then divide by 2 to get the median. For example, consider the following set of numbers: 23, 54, 76, 34, 12, 36.

STEP 1: Sort from smallest to largest.   12, 23, 34, 36, 54, 76

STEP 2: Cross a number off from each end   ~~12~~, 23, 34, 36, 54, ~~76~~
until the last pair is reached.   ~~12~~, ~~23~~, 34, 36, ~~54~~, ~~76~~

STEP 3: Add the two remaining numbers.   34 + 36 = 70

STEP 4: Divide the answer by 2 to get the median.   70 ÷ 2 = 35

Answer: 35 is the median.

Note: The median may include a partial number such as $\frac{1}{2}$ or 0.5.

Practice 22

Find the median in the following word problems.

1. Bah's temperature fluctuated all day. Her temperature readings were 98, 99, 97, 101, and 100. What is her median temperature?

2. The young patients played a game. The scores for five games were 365, 251, 105, 280, and 198. What is the median of this set of scores?

3. The medical assistant was working on inventory. She wanted to figure out the median of the number of cases of protective sheeting that were used for the first six months of the year in the large medical practice.

Month	Number of Cases
January	26
February	22
March	31

Month	Number of Cases
April	28
May	26
June	19

What is the median for this set of data?

4. Azeb is an excellent student. She is curious about the median of her test scores in biology class. Her scores are 99, 100, 98, 97, and 100. Her median is _____.

5. The students were measuring tardiness to class by incidence each week. Look at the data set: 7, 8, 10, 10, 15, 12, 8, 7. What is the mean of this data set? _____

MODE

REVIEW

The **mode** is the "most popular" value or the most frequently occurring item in a set of numbers. To locate the mode of a series or listing of numbers, identify the number that occurs the most.

For example, look at the calories of Bob's snack food intake for a two-day period:

Bob's caloric intake of snacks by day

Saturday: 120, 120, 50, 78, 134, 187

Sunday: 220, 125, 90, 85, 120, 120

What is the mode of the calorie intake of Bob's snack intake over this two-day period?

The answer is 120. It occurs four times.

Practice 23

Find the mode in the following word problems.

1. Look at the pH values of the following data set: 14, 11, 23, 14, 8, 12. What is the mode for this data set?

2. Look at the prices of toothbrushes: $7.00, $4.00, $6.13, $3.00, $3.00, $1.00, $3.00. What is the mode of these toothbrush prices?

3. The color combinations preferred by new dental offices include: paint sample #24, paint sample #154, paint sample #654, paint sample #24, paint sample #154, paint sample #24, and paint sample #63. What is the mode?

4. Designer eyeglass frames cost a lot. This season's top-selling frame prices are $330, $199, $230, $400, $497, and $330. What is the mode of these eyeglass frame prices?

5. The Healthville Residence is having a problem with absenteeism during the summer months. The administrator wants to find out who is missing work the most. First add the days absent for each employee, and write the number in the "Total days absent" column. Compare the total days absent from work; what is the mode for the number of days absent for the summer months?

Employee	Days Absent in June	Days Absent in July	Days Absent in August	Total Days Absent
Verna	3	2	2	_____
Xuyen	4	4	3	_____
Cam	3	2	1	_____
Debbie	3	3	3	_____
Ed	2	2	2	_____
Vasily	1	3	4	_____
Ted	3	2	2	_____

RANGE

REVIEW

The **range** of a set of numbers is the largest value in the set minus the smallest value in the set. Note that the range is a single number, not many numbers.

For example, the hospital delivered six babies today. The weight in pounds of these newborns was 6, 9, 10, 8, 7, 5. Follow these steps to identify the range:

STEP 1: Locate the smallest number and the largest number.   5 and 10

STEP 2: Subtract the smallest number from the largest number. $10 - 5 = 5$

Answer: The range is 5.

Practice 24

Find the range in the following word problems.

1. The age of patients in the hospital fluctuates. Look at the data and calculate the range of patients' ages: 54, 94, 23, 46, 99, 100, 69, 18, 25, 75, 87, 58, 12.

2. The workforce at the Village Care Center is diverse in age. Look at the data and calculate the range of workers' ages: 18, 21, 24, 23, 45, 34, 16, 25, 31, 56, 64, 71, 49, 52, 59.

3. The breakfast meals served in the cafeteria vary in calories. Look at the data and calculate the range of calories in the meals: 120, 220, 280, 340, 440, 480, 90.

4. The public health nurse has a rural route to drive each week. What is the range that the daily miles, 7, 14, 23, 24, 16, 12, record?

5. The bandages sold in a local drugstore have a wide price range. Each bandage costs as follows: 50 cents, 35 cents, 78 cents, 89 cents, 99 cents, 12 cents, and 25 cents. What is the range in individual bandage costs?

Roman Numerals

In our daily lives, we use the **Arabic numerals** 0 to 9 and combinations of these digits to do most of our mathematical activities. In the health care field, **Roman numerals** are sometimes used along with Arabic numerals. Roman numerals are often found in prescriptions and in medical records and charts. Roman numerals consist of lower- and uppercase letters that represent numbers. For medical applications, Roman numerals are written in lowercase letters for the numbers 1 to 10. However, use uppercase letters when smaller numbers (0–9) are part of a number larger than 30 such as 60: LX not lx. Do not use commas in Roman numerals. Roman numerals are formed by combining the numbers.

1 = i or I	6 = vi or VI	$\frac{1}{2}$ = ss
2 = ii or II	7 = vii or VII	50 = L
3 = iii or III	8 = viii or VIII	100 = C
4 = iv or IV	9 = ix or IX	500 = D
5 = v or V	10 = x or X	1,000 = M

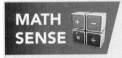 **MATH SENSE**   Use a mnemonic device to help remember the order of Roman numerals.

Note the pattern: 50–100–500–1,000

L = 50	Lovely
C = 100	Cats
D = 500	Don't
M = 1,000	Meow!

Roman numeral letters are arranged from the largest value to the smallest value. Each letter's value is added to the previous letter's value. Only powers of ten (I, X, C, M) can be repeated; however, these letters cannot be repeated more than three times in a row. Use the following basic Roman numeral concepts to accurately read and write Roman numerals.

CONVERTING ROMAN NUMERALS

Add Roman numerals of the same or decreasing value when they are placed next to each other. Read these from left to right.

EXAMPLES

vii = 5 + 2 = 7   xxi = 10 + 10 + 1 = 21

Practice 25

Write the numerals in Arabic or Roman numerals.

1. xiii _____

2. xv _____

3. xxxi _____

4. LV _____

5. xxvi _____

6. 3 _____

7. 12 _____

8. 120 _____

9. $1\frac{1}{2}$ _____

10. 11 _____

Subtract a numeral of decreasing or lesser value from the numeral to its right.

EXAMPLES

$$iv = 5 - 1 = 4 \qquad XC = 100 - 10 = 90$$

$$IM = 1,000 - 1 = 999 \qquad xix = 10 + 10 - 1 = 19$$

Practice 26

Write the numerals in Arabic or Roman numerals:

1. ixss _____

2. LXI _____

3. IX _____

4. LM _____

5. XCIX _____

6. 21 _____

7. 39 _____

8. $24\frac{1}{4}$ _____

9. 240 _____

10. 499 _____

When converting long Roman numerals to Arabic numerals, it is helpful to separate the Roman numerals into groups and work from both ends.

EXAMPLE

CDLXXIV → CD L XX IV

1. Start with the IV = 5 − 1 = 4   4

2. Next, X + X = 20   20

3. L = 50   50

4. C − D = 500 − 100 = 400   +400

5. Then add the elements.   474

Practice 27

Convert the following Roman numerals to Arabic numerals by working from both ends.

1. XXIV _____

2. XLI _____

3. DIV _____

4. MDCIXss _____

5. XXXIX _____

6. XLss _____

7. CDIV _____

8. MCML _____

9. DXCIIss _____

10. CMLXXIVss _____

This method of separating the elements and working from both ends also works well for converting from Arabic to Roman numerals.

◆

EXAMPLE

Convert 637 to Roman numerals

600	DC
30	XXX
7	VII

Then rewrite the Roman numeral from the largest number on the left to the smallest numbers on the right. → DCXXXVII

Practice 28

Convert the following Arabic numerals to Roman numerals by working from both ends.

1. $24\frac{1}{2}$_____

2. 75 _____

3. 14 _____

4. 125 _____

5. 1,000 _____

6. 789 _____

7. 450 _____

8. 76 _____

9. 17 _____

10. 1,294 _____

Practice 29

Convert between Roman numerals and Arabic numerals:

1. XCI _____

2. XXIVss _____

3. XVIII _____

4. 23 _____

5. 28 _____

6. 19 _____

7. 201 _____

8. CCLIVss _____

9. 66 _____

10. MVII _____

11. 45 _____

12. 13 _____

13. 362 _____

14. 16 _____

15. 99 _____

16. XXXIXss _____

17. LXXVIII _____

18. $209\frac{1}{2}$ _____

19. 2,515 _____

20. What should you do to convert a number with decimal 0.5 in it to a Roman numeral?

_____

◆◆◆◆ Time in Allied Health

Universal (military) time is used in many health care facilities. The Universal time system avoids confusion over A.M. and P.M. Universal time is based on the 24-hour clock, which begins at 0001, which is one minute after midnight.

Colons are not used between these numbers. Compare the two clocks below:

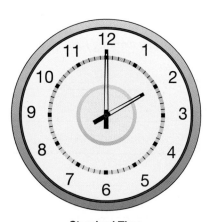

Standard Time
2:00 O'clock AM
2:00 O'clock PM

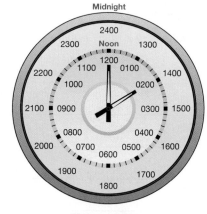

Universal Time
0200 AM
1400 PM

HOW TO CONVERT TO UNIVERSAL TIME

The hours have four digits:

1 A.M. or 1:00 A.M. = 0100
10 A.M. or 10:00 A.M. = 1000

Add 1200 to any time after noon.

2 P.M. or 2:00 P.M. = 1400
2 + 1200 = 1400 in Universal time
5:36 P.M. or 5:36 P.M. = 1736 in Universal time

Practice 30

Complete the chart.

Standard Time	Universal or Military Time
1:31 A.M.	1. _____
3:29 P.M.	2. _____
8:24 A.M.	3. _____
10:32 P.M.	4. _____
12:45 P.M.	5. _____
8:17 A.M.	6. _____
5:57 P.M.	7. _____
1:23 A.M.	8. _____
9:25 P.M.	9. _____
11:03 P.M.	10. _____

Practice 31

Complete the following.

Universal or Military Time	Standard Time
1408	1. _____
0013	2. _____
1001	3. _____
1452	4. _____
0037	5. _____
2400	6. _____
1524	7. _____
2006	8. _____
0912	9. _____
1630	10. _____

UNIT REVIEW

◆◆◆◆ Critical Thinking with Whole Numbers

Thinking in math requires taking time to look at the relationships among numbers and determining what the outcome is supposed to be.

Add the math symbols (+ − × ÷) to make each statement true.

1. 12 _____ 18 _____ 5 = 25

2. 75 _____ 2 _____ 3 = 50

3. 7 _____ 9 _____ 4 _____ 2 = 18

4. 42 _____ 3 _____ 6 _____ 5 = 125

5. 225 _____ 5 _____ 2 = 90

Use the numbers in the Number Set column to find the mean, mode, range, and median for each set of numbers.

Number Set	Mean	Mode	Range	Median
6. 10, 20, 20, 15, 5				
7. 60, 84, 98, 90, 98				
8. 96, 62, 97, 100, 96, 87, 85				
9. 15, 12, 11, 15, 13, 10, 15				
10. 75, 65, 34, 84, 230, 34				

List two instances when one would see Roman numerals

11. _____

12. _____

Consider the following statements. Circle true or false. Explain your answer.

13. True or False In addition and multiplication, the order of numbers in the problem has no bearing on the final answer.

_____

14. True or False The larger number in division is always what is divided into.

_____

15. True or False 225 is divisible by 3, 5, and 9.

_____

◆◆◆◆ Professional Expertise

- Whole numbers can be easily misread. Ensure proper formation of numbers that may be misread such as 1 and 7.
- Follow the number with the name of the unit involved such as 12 pounds or 34 kilograms.

WHOLE NUMBER POST-TEST

1. Complete this number statement. 724 + _____ + 48 = 1,621

2. An activity director in a long-term care facility is purchasing recreational supplies. Find the sum of the purchases: 3 Bingo games at $13 each, 10 puzzles at $9 each, 24 jars of paint at $3 each, and 2 rolls of paper for $31 each.

3. Using the information from problem 2 above, determine the mean (average) cost of these supplies. Round to the nearest dollar.

4. A medical coding student needs 432 hours of practical work experience to complete the college's course. If the student has completed 184 hours, how many hours remain to fulfill the requirement?

5. Three certified nursing assistants assist 16 rooms of patients on the Saturday morning shift. If each room has 3 patients, how many patients does each assistant care for if the patients are equally divided among the staff?

6. Uniform jackets are required at Valley Pharmacy. Each pharmacy technician is asked to purchase two jackets at $21 per jacket and one name badge for $8. What is the cost of these items for each pharmacy technician?

7. The medical clerk is asked to inventory the digital thermometers. In the six examination rooms, the clerk finds the following number of digital thermometers: 2, 4, 5, 2, 1, and 3. The total inventory is _____.

8. The dental assistants in a new office are setting up their free patient sample display. They order the following:

	Quantity	Unit	Item	Per Unit Cost (in dollars)	Total Cost
a.	1,500	each	toothbrush	1	_____
b.	100	each	floss (smooth)	2	_____
c.	75	each	floss (glide)	2	_____
d.	1,000	per 100	information booklet	10	_____
e.	25	each	poster	15	_____
f.				Subtotal	_____

9. After a mild heart attack, Mary spent 3 days in a coronary care unit. Her room bill was $2,898. What was her daily room rate?

10. White blood cell (WBC) count can indicate illness or health. The WBC count of patient B is checked. Before surgery, the WBC count of the patient was 12,674; post-surgery, he had a count of 6,894. What is the difference in patient B's count before and after surgery?

11. The cook has a variety of meals to prepare for Villa Center's residents. She averages 16 vegetarian meals every day of the week. Round the number of weekly meals to the nearest 10.

12. The newest staff member at the hospital is a surgery technologist. Her pay is approximately $14 an hour. If she is scheduled to work 36 hours a week, what is her weekly pay before deductions?

13. Read the number: 8$\underline{7}$5,420.

The place value of the underlined digit is _____.

14. Convert 10:37 P.M. to Universal time.

15. Write the Roman numeral xixss as an Arabic numeral.

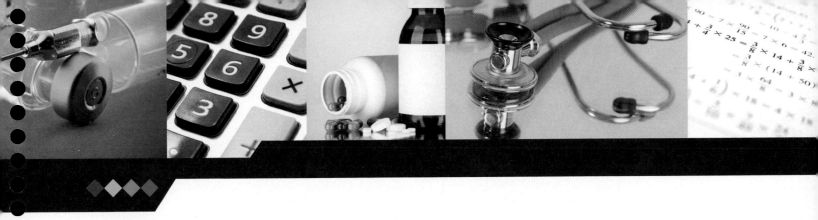

UNIT

2 Fractions

STUDENT LEARNING OUTCOMES

After completing the tasks in this unit, you will be able to:

2-1 Write part-to-whole relationships in fractional form

2-2 Use the terminology of fractions

2-3 Find common denominators

2-4 Create equivalent fractions

2-5 Order fractions

2-6 Reduce or simplify fractions

2-7 Use cancellation to reduce larger fractions

2-8 Add fractions with like and unlike denominators

2-9 Subtract fractions, including using borrowing, with like and unlike denominators

2-10 Multiply fractions and mixed numbers

2-11 Divide fractions and mixed numbers

2-12 Complete word problems that have fractions

2-13 Convert between Celsius and Fahrenheit degrees

2-14 Reduce/simplify and solve complex fraction problems

2-15 Complete measurement conversions with fractions

2-16 Read a ruler

PRE-TEST

1. This month has thirty days. Four days is what fractional part of this month?

2. $4\dfrac{1}{4} + 2\dfrac{3}{5} =$

3. $42 - 13\dfrac{1}{6} =$

4. $3\dfrac{1}{2} \times 2\dfrac{1}{5} =$

5. $3\dfrac{1}{3} \div 5 =$

31

6. $50\,°C =$ _____ $°F$

7. Order from the largest to the smallest: $\dfrac{7}{8}, \dfrac{1}{8}, \dfrac{3}{4}, \dfrac{15}{16}$

8. $\dfrac{\frac{1}{3}}{\frac{1}{4}} \times 7 =$

9. $\dfrac{\frac{1}{4}}{200} =$

10. The doctor orders $\dfrac{1}{2}$ tablet of medicine. There are 90 milligrams in a tablet. Is one-half tablet more or less than 50 milligrams of medication?

11. Reduce the fraction to the simplest form: $14\dfrac{22}{66}$

12. Change the mixed number to an improper fraction. $7\dfrac{5}{12}$

13. Look at the drug label below. What information from the label could be represented as a fraction?

erythromycin ethylsuccinate

100 mL
ORAL SUSPENSION
(when mixed)

Erythromycin activity
200 mg per 5 mL
when reconstituted

Rx only

100 mL | NDC 0074-6302-13

PL Pharmaceuticals 02-8472-2/R9

Practice Label

Before mixing, store below 86°F (30°C).

DIRECTIONS FOR MIXING: Add 53 mL water and shake vigorously. This makes 100 mL of suspension. For best taste mix at least 15 to 20 minutes before dosing. After mixing, refrigeration not required; store below 77° F (25° C).

Contains erythromycin ethylsuccinate equivalent to 4 g erythromycin. Child-resistant closure not required; exemption approved by U.S. Consumer Product Safety Commission.
When mixed as directed, each teaspoonful (5 mL) contains: Erythromycin ethylsuccinate equivalent to erythromycin ....200 mg in a fruit-flavored, aqucous vehicle.

DOSAGE MAY BE ADMINISTERED WITHOUT REGARD TO MEALS.

USUAL DOSE: Children: 30-50 mg/kg/day in divided doses. See enclosure for adult dose and full prescribing information.

May be taken before, after or with meals.

Shake well before using. Oversize bottle provides shake space. Keep tightly closed. **Refrigeration not required.**

Store below 77°F (25°C) and use within 35 days.

3 00746 30213 1
Lot   Exp.

14. In one month, Bella earned 3,250 dollars. That is $\dfrac{1}{12}$ of her annual income. What is her annual income?

15. Use cancellation to reduce each fraction to its lowest terms. Do not solve the problem.

$$\dfrac{4}{11} \times \dfrac{16}{48} \times \dfrac{44}{48}$$

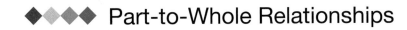

◆◆◆◆ Part-to-Whole Relationships

A **fraction** is a number that has two components: a part and a whole. A minute is 1 part of 60 minutes in a whole hour. This relationship of part to whole can be shown in a fraction:

$$\frac{1}{60} \quad \begin{array}{l} \leftarrow \text{numerator (the part)} \\ \leftarrow \text{denominator (the whole)} \end{array}$$

The 1 is called the **numerator**, and it represents the part of the whole. The 60 is the **denominator**, and it represents the whole or sum of the parts. Take another common part-to-whole relationship. Many people sleep an average of 8 hours a night. The relationship of sleeping hours to total hours in a day is 8 to 24, or $\frac{8}{24}$, or a reduced fraction of $\frac{1}{3}$.

Fractions are important to understand because you will come across them many times in health care occupations. Fractions appear in medication dosages, measurements, sizes of instruments, work assignments, and time units. For example, note the fraction in the following drug label:

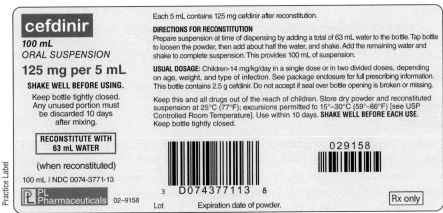

Reading fractions on drug labels is a workplace necessity. Notice the 125 mg per 5 mL on the label, which means that every 5 milliliters of the oral suspension has 125 milligrams of cefdinir. Sometimes this information appears in words: for example, 125 mg per 5 milliliter.

This translates to $\frac{125\,\text{mg}}{5\,\text{mL}}$ as a fraction.

Practice writing out the numerator (part)-to-denominator (whole) relationships:

EXAMPLE

$$\frac{1}{12} = \text{one part to twelve total parts}$$

Practice 1

Write the numerator-to-denominator relationships in the following problems.

1. $\frac{7}{8}$ = _____

2. $\frac{1}{6}$ = _____

3. $\dfrac{3}{5} =$ _____

4. $\dfrac{16}{21} =$ _____

Proper or **common fractions** are fractions with a numerator that is less than the denominator: $\dfrac{3}{7}, \dfrac{24}{47}, \dfrac{9}{11}$. The value of any proper or common fraction will be less than 1.

Mixed numbers are fractions that include both a whole number and a proper fraction: $3\dfrac{3}{4}, 12\dfrac{9}{11}, 101\dfrac{13}{22}$.

An **improper fraction** has a numerator equal to or larger than the denominator: $\dfrac{17}{12}, \dfrac{33}{24}, \dfrac{9}{9}$. Improper fractions are equal to 1 or larger. Improper fractions are used in the multiplication and division of fractions. Answers that appear as improper fractions need to be reduced so that the answer is a mixed number.

◆◆◆◆ Equivalent Fractions

REVIEW

Understanding **equivalent fractions** is important when making measurement decisions. Equivalent fractions represent the same relationship of part to whole, but there are more pieces or a variation of the parts involved. If you sliced a pizza into 8 pieces and then decided to cut each eighth in half, you would have sixteenths, not eighths. So the number of pieces in one pizza can change from $\dfrac{8}{8}$ to $\dfrac{16}{16}$, yet these fractions still represent one pizza, which means that the fractions involved are equal. The size of the pieces or parts is what varies.

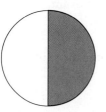

2 large pieces
$\dfrac{1}{2}$ is shaded

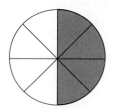

8 smaller pieces
$\dfrac{4}{8}$ are shaded

The shaded areas are the same size; the number of parts varies. Making fractions equal is easy using multiplication. Look at the fractions $\dfrac{1}{6}$ and $\dfrac{?}{18}$. The denominators are 6 and 18. Ask: 6 times what = 18? The answer is 3, so multiply the numerator by 3, and you will have formed an equivalent fraction. Thus, $\dfrac{1}{6} = \dfrac{3}{18}$.

The key to getting the correct answer is remembering that the number the denominator is multiplied by must also be used to multiply the numerator. If this method is difficult for you, then divide the smaller denominator into the larger one; your answer will then be multiplied by the first numerator to get the second numerator.

$$\frac{1}{6} = \frac{?}{18} \quad 6\overline{)18}, \quad \text{then } 3 \times 1 = 3$$

Another way to work this problem is:

$$\frac{1 \ (\times 3)}{6 \ (\times 3)} = \frac{3}{18}$$

Thus, $\frac{1}{6} = \frac{3}{18}$.

Practice 2

Use multiplication to solve for the missing numerators and denominators.

1. $\frac{1}{2} = \frac{?}{12}$

2. $\frac{1}{4} = \frac{?}{16}$

3. $\frac{1}{5} = \frac{?}{40}$

4. $\frac{2}{14} = \frac{?}{28}$

5. $\frac{5}{9} = \frac{?}{27}$

6. $\frac{1}{13} = \frac{?}{39}$

7. $\frac{4}{8} = \frac{?}{72}$

8. $\frac{1}{5} = \frac{?}{100}$

9. $\frac{7}{9} = \frac{42}{?}$

10. $\frac{1}{3} = \frac{8}{?}$

The skill of making equivalent fractions will be used in adding, subtracting, and comparing fractions.

◆◆◆◆ Reducing to Lowest or Simplest Terms

REVIEW

As in making fractions equivalent, reducing fractions to their lowest or simplest terms is another important fraction skill. Most tests and practical applications of fractions require that the answers be in the lowest terms. **Lowest terms** means that the fraction is the lowest proper fraction possible and can be reduced no further. For example, $\frac{4}{8}$ is not reduced to its lowest terms; however, $\frac{1}{2}$ is reduced to its lowest. After each calculation of addition, subtraction, multiplication, or division, you will need to reduce the answer to its lowest terms. Two methods will help you find the lowest terms.

MULTIPLICATION METHOD

To use the multiplication method, look at the numbers in the fraction. Find a number that divides into both the numerator and denominator evenly. Such numbers are called **factors** of the numbers. Write out the multiplication for the numerator and denominator. Cross out the two identical numbers in the multiplication problems. What is left will be the reduced fraction.

$$\frac{2}{16} = \frac{2 \times 1}{2 \times 8} \rightarrow \frac{\cancel{2} \times 1}{\cancel{2} \times 8}$$

So, $\frac{2}{16} = \frac{1}{8}$.

Depending on the multiple you choose, you may need to reduce the fraction more than once.

$$\frac{8}{24} = \frac{4 \times 2}{4 \times 6} = \frac{2}{6} \rightarrow \frac{1}{3}$$

In the example above, two sets of reduction occurred. Try to choose the largest multiple to avoid the need for excessive steps in reduction.

In the example below, the largest possible multiple is used, which reduces the simplification to one step.

$$\frac{8}{24} = \frac{8 \times 1}{8 \times 3} = \frac{1}{3}$$

Sometimes students only partially reduce a fraction, so try to find the largest possible factor of the numbers when you are reducing.

DIVISION METHOD

Look at the numbers in the numerator and the denominator. Choose a number that divides into both the numerator and the denominator. Next, divide the numerator and denominator by that number. Check to ensure that the resulting fraction is in its lowest form.

$$\frac{2}{16} = \frac{2 \div 2}{16 \div 2} = \frac{1}{8}$$

$$\frac{8}{24} = \frac{8 \div 4}{24 \div 4} = \frac{2}{6}$$

Then, $\frac{2}{6} \rightarrow \frac{\cancel{2} \times 1}{\cancel{2} \times 3}$.

The final reduced answer is $\frac{1}{3}$. This fraction is reduced to its lowest form.

How do you decide on the best method to use?

Choose your stronger skill—multiplication or division—and use that one to reduce fractions. You will make fewer errors if you select one method and use it consistently.

> **MATH SENSE**
>
> Choose the largest possible multiple to avoid having to repeat the steps in reduction.

Practice 3

Reduce the following fractions to the lowest terms.

1. $\frac{6}{24}$

2. $\frac{5}{20}$

3. $\frac{5}{10}$

4. $\frac{13}{39}$

5. $\dfrac{25}{100}$

8. $\dfrac{63}{90}$

6. $\dfrac{64}{72}$

9. $\dfrac{15}{45}$

7. $\dfrac{24}{48}$

10. $\dfrac{5}{255}$

When working with a mixed number, set aside the whole number. Handle the fraction portion of the number first, and then place it beside the whole number.

$$14\dfrac{3}{9} \rightarrow 14 \quad \text{and} \quad \dfrac{3}{9} \rightarrow \dfrac{3}{9} = \dfrac{1 \times 3}{3 \times 3} = \dfrac{1}{3} \rightarrow 14\dfrac{1}{3}$$

> **SET-UP HINT**
>
> Set aside the whole number, reduce the fraction, and then place the whole number next to the reduced fraction.

Practice 4

Reduce the following mixed numbers to the lowest terms.

1. $14\dfrac{5}{10}$

6. $5\dfrac{14}{64}$

2. $9\dfrac{15}{35}$

7. $2\dfrac{11}{99}$

3. $4\dfrac{11}{66}$

8. $10\dfrac{30}{80}$

4. $6\dfrac{18}{20}$

9. $6\dfrac{45}{90}$

5. $3\dfrac{3}{12}$

10. $4\dfrac{22}{30}$

Fractional parts or relationships are common in health care.

EXAMPLE

In a class of 30 people, 13 students are male and 17 are female. To write the relationship of the number of males to the total number of students, we place the part (13) over the whole (30), or the total number of students.

$$\dfrac{13}{30}$$

Write the fractional part that represents the relationship of the part to the whole. Then reduce all your answers to the lowest form.

1. Fifty of the 86 patients see the physical therapist each week.

2. The dietitian uses 35 six-ounce glasses and 50 eight-ounce glasses at breakfast. Represent in fraction form the relationship of six-ounce glasses to eight-ounce glasses used at breakfast.

3. Thirty out of the 120 patients at the short-term care facility are women. What is the fractional part of women to total patients?

4. Fourteen female babies and 16 male babies were born on Saturday. Express the number of female babies to male babies as a fraction.

5. About 500 medicine cups are used daily at a long-term care facility. The nurse claims that approximately 4,000 medicine cups are used a week. What is the day-to-week use rate of medicine cups?

◆◆◆◆ Improper Fractions

Working with improper fractions also requires reducing fractions. An **improper fraction** is a fraction that has a larger numerator than denominator.

$$\frac{16}{8} = \frac{8 \times 2}{8 \times 1} = \frac{2}{1} \to 2$$

If the numerator and the denominator do not have a common number by which they can be multiplied, simply divide the denominator into the numerator.

$$\frac{11}{8} \qquad 8\overline{)11}^{\,1\frac{3}{8}} \\ \underline{8} \\ 3$$

The remainder, 3, is a whole number. Place it on top of the divisor to form a fraction.

Improper fractions are either whole numbers or mixed numbers.

Improper fractions are used for dividing mixed numbers.

Practice 6

Reduce the following improper fractions.

1. $\dfrac{25}{3}$

6. $\dfrac{7}{3}$

2. $\dfrac{24}{5}$

7. $\dfrac{19}{8}$

3. $\dfrac{29}{5}$

8. $\dfrac{16}{2}$

4. $\dfrac{104}{7}$

9. $\dfrac{100}{100}$

5. $\dfrac{66}{7}$

10. $\dfrac{23}{18}$

◆◆◆◆ Adding Fractions with Like Denominators

REVIEW

Addition of fractions with the same denominator is straightforward. Follow the two steps below:

STEP 1: Line up the fractions vertically, add the numerators, and place the sum over the common, or like, denominator.

STEP 2: Reduce, if necessary. Check your work to ensure accuracy. Notice the first-column example does not require reducing, while the second example does.

$$\begin{array}{r} \dfrac{3}{6} \\[6pt] +\dfrac{2}{6} \\[6pt] \hline \dfrac{5}{6} \end{array} \qquad \begin{array}{r} \dfrac{4}{8} \\[6pt] +\dfrac{5}{8} \\[6pt] \hline \dfrac{9}{8} \end{array} \quad \text{Reduce by } 9 \div 8 = 1\dfrac{1}{8}$$

STEP 1: $\begin{array}{r} \dfrac{12}{15} \\[6pt] +\dfrac{18}{15} \\[6pt] \hline \dfrac{30}{15} \end{array}$

STEP 2: $\dfrac{30}{15} = \dfrac{\cancel{15} \times 2}{\cancel{15} \times 1} \qquad \dfrac{2}{1} = 2$

> **MATH SENSE**
>
> When reducing an answer, you find that the result is a whole number with a 1 for its denominator. In this case, use the numerator, a whole number, alone. Do not include the 1 since the answer is actually a whole number rather than a fraction.

If a whole number goes with the fractions, simply add it separately and place the fraction next to the whole number. The whole number will be affected only if the fraction answer is larger than 1—in that case, the whole number resulting from the fraction addition is added to the whole number answer.

EXAMPLE

$$14\frac{2}{8}$$
$$+7\frac{1}{8}$$
$$\overline{21\frac{3}{8}}$$

Add the fractions: $\dfrac{2}{8} + \dfrac{1}{8} = \dfrac{3}{8}$

Add the whole numbers: $14 + 7 = 21$

Write the answer. No reduction is necessary.

EXAMPLE

$$10\frac{2}{4}$$
$$+4\frac{3}{4}$$
$$\overline{14\frac{5}{4}}$$

Add the fractions: $\dfrac{2}{4} + \dfrac{3}{4} = \dfrac{5}{4}$

Add $10 + 4 = 14$, and then set this part of the answer aside as you handle the improper fraction.

$\dfrac{5}{4}$ must be reduced. It is an improper fraction.

Divide 5 by 4 $= 1\dfrac{1}{4}$. The whole number, 1, is added to 14 $(14 + 1 = 15)$, and the fraction $\dfrac{1}{4}$ is placed next to the whole number, giving the answer $15\dfrac{1}{4}$.

Practice 7

Add the following fractions. Reduce as necessary:

1. $\dfrac{3}{6} + \dfrac{2}{6}$

2. $\dfrac{3}{5} + \dfrac{4}{5}$

3. $\dfrac{7}{10} + \dfrac{6}{10}$

4. $\dfrac{1}{13} + \dfrac{4}{13}$

5. $\dfrac{3}{12} + \dfrac{4}{12}$

6. $\dfrac{2}{5} + \dfrac{3}{5}$

7. $\dfrac{3}{13} + \dfrac{4}{13}$

8. $13\dfrac{8}{12} + 2\dfrac{2}{12}$

9. $10\dfrac{1}{6} + 12\dfrac{4}{6}$

10. $11\dfrac{1}{4} + \dfrac{3}{4}$

11. $\dfrac{3}{5} + \dfrac{1}{5}$

12. $\dfrac{2}{7} + \dfrac{3}{7} + \dfrac{4}{7}$

13. $\dfrac{3}{8} + \dfrac{4}{8} + \dfrac{1}{8}$

14. $2\dfrac{1}{12} + 3\dfrac{5}{12} + 6\dfrac{4}{12}$

15. $101\dfrac{3}{4} + 33\dfrac{1}{4} + 5\dfrac{1}{4}$

◆◆◆◆ Finding the Common Denominator

Adding and subtracting fractions requires that the denominator be of the same number, also referred to as a *common denominator*. The lowest common denominator is the smallest number or multiple that both of the denominators of the fractions can go into.

Using multiplication, find the smallest number or multiple that the numbers can go into.

STEP 1:

$$\dfrac{2}{3} \quad \dfrac{}{3 \times 2} = \dfrac{?}{6}$$

$$+\dfrac{1}{6} \rightarrow \qquad \dfrac{1}{6}$$

In the above problem, 3 and 6 are the denominators. $3 \times 2 = 6$, so 6 is the common denominator.

SET-UP HINT 💡

Fewer errors occur if the setup is vertical. You can see the numbers and their relationships easier.

STEP 2: Once you have the common denominator in place, multiply the numerator by the same number with which you multiplied the denominator. The result will be equivalent fractions, so the number relationships remain the same.

$$\frac{2}{3} \qquad \begin{array}{l} 2 \times 2 = 4 \\ 3 \times 2 = 6 \end{array}$$

$$\begin{array}{r} +\frac{1}{6} \rightarrow \\ \hline \end{array} \qquad \begin{array}{r} +\frac{1}{6} \\ \hline \frac{5}{6} \end{array}$$

Practice 8

Find the common denominator in the following pairs of numbers. Set the problems up vertically and think about their multiples to find the common denominators.

1. $\frac{2}{4}$ and $\frac{1}{5}$

2. $\frac{3}{8}$ and $\frac{1}{16}$

3. $\frac{22}{44}$ and $\frac{1}{11}$

4. $\frac{1}{9}$ and $\frac{5}{45}$

5. $\frac{2}{5}$ and $\frac{3}{25}$

6. $\frac{3}{7}$ and $\frac{9}{49}$

7. $\frac{1}{200}$ and $\frac{5}{20}$

8. $\frac{4}{50}$ and $\frac{10}{150}$

9. $\frac{3}{9}$ and $\frac{4}{27}$

10. $\frac{1}{6}$ and $\frac{4}{18}$

Practice 9

Find the common denominator, and then add the following fractions with unlike denominators:

1. $\frac{3}{5} + \frac{1}{4}$

2. $\frac{1}{2} + \frac{4}{6}$

3. $\frac{4}{9} + \frac{2}{3}$

4. $\frac{7}{10} + \frac{3}{5}$

5. $\frac{11}{30} + \frac{2}{15}$

6. $\frac{5}{25} + \frac{1}{5}$

7. $\dfrac{4}{7} + \dfrac{1}{21}$

8. $\dfrac{2}{5} + \dfrac{1}{10} + \dfrac{3}{10}$

9. $\dfrac{3}{5} + \dfrac{1}{3} + \dfrac{2}{15}$

10. $\dfrac{2}{3} + \dfrac{1}{12} + \dfrac{2}{4}$

11. $\dfrac{1}{10} + \dfrac{1}{2} + \dfrac{4}{5}$

12. $12\dfrac{1}{6} + \dfrac{3}{4}$

13. $55\dfrac{1}{3} + 51\dfrac{5}{9}$

14. $5\dfrac{1}{2} + 2\dfrac{4}{5} + 5\dfrac{3}{10}$

15. $4\dfrac{3}{4} + 1\dfrac{1}{16} + 3\dfrac{2}{32}$

DIFFICULT COMMON DENOMINATORS

Sometimes one must consider a wider range of possible numbers for common denominators. For example, you may have a pair of fractions in which one of the denominators cannot be multiplied by a number to get the other denominator. In this case, it is often easiest to simply multiply the two denominators by each other. The result will be a common denominator.

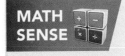

MATH SENSE

To find the more difficult common denominators, multiply the denominators by each other.

EXAMPLE

$$\dfrac{3}{13} \text{ and } \dfrac{1}{4}$$

What is the common denominator? If you multiply 13×4, your answer is 52. Use that number as the common denominator.

$$\dfrac{3}{13} \rightarrow 13 \times 4 = 52$$

$$\dfrac{1}{4} \rightarrow 4 \times 13 = 52$$

Then multiply each numerator by the same number that you multiplied its denominator by. Do this for each fraction, and the result will be a common denominator.

$$\dfrac{3}{13} \rightarrow \dfrac{3 \times 4 = 12}{13 \times 4 = 52}$$

$$\dfrac{1}{4} \rightarrow \dfrac{1 \times 13 = 13}{4 \times 13 = 52}$$

By finding the common denominator, you have also created equivalent fractions.

Practice 10

Find the common denominator for each of the following sets of fractions:

1. $\dfrac{3}{4}$ and $\dfrac{2}{5}$

2. $\dfrac{7}{8}$ and $\dfrac{1}{3}$

3. $\dfrac{24}{32}$ and $\dfrac{1}{6}$

4. $\dfrac{1}{7}$ and $\dfrac{4}{8}$

5. $\dfrac{3}{5}$ and $\dfrac{7}{9}$

6. $\dfrac{2}{26}$ and $\dfrac{1}{3}$

7. $\dfrac{3}{9}$ and $\dfrac{1}{4}$

8. $\dfrac{2}{5}$ and $\dfrac{6}{9}$

9. $\dfrac{3}{10}$ and $\dfrac{2}{3}$

10. $\dfrac{1}{9}$ and $\dfrac{7}{8}$

Practice 11

Find the common denominator, and then add the following mixed fractions:

1. $3\dfrac{2}{3} + 6\dfrac{1}{4}$

2. $10\dfrac{1}{2} + 13\dfrac{5}{22}$

3. $9\dfrac{1}{6} + 4\dfrac{3}{9}$

4. $11\dfrac{7}{8} + 2\dfrac{1}{7}$

5. $\dfrac{1}{2} + 4\dfrac{1}{7} + 2\dfrac{1}{14}$

6. $12\dfrac{3}{5} + 22\dfrac{1}{30}$

7. $10\dfrac{4}{5} + 8\dfrac{1}{6}$

8. $3\dfrac{4}{9} + 1\dfrac{2}{3} + 5\dfrac{2}{9}$

9. $11\dfrac{2}{5} + 7\dfrac{1}{2}$

10. $7\dfrac{11}{16} + 3\dfrac{4}{8} + \dfrac{1}{2}$

11. $2\frac{2}{9} + 6\frac{1}{3} + 8\frac{2}{27}$

12. $6\frac{2}{3} + 8\frac{4}{5} + 3\frac{6}{10}$

13. $6\frac{1}{4} + 13\frac{2}{3} + 19\frac{1}{2}$

14. $6\frac{7}{16} + \frac{3}{24} + 2\frac{1}{48}$

15. $\frac{3}{5} + \frac{6}{30} + 12\frac{2}{3}$

16. $8\frac{9}{11} + 3\frac{1}{33} + \frac{2}{66}$

17. $3\frac{5}{16} + \frac{5}{8} + \frac{2}{4}$

18. $\frac{5}{6} + 3\frac{3}{9} + 7\frac{2}{3}$

19. $4\frac{5}{6} + \frac{2}{5} + \frac{4}{15}$

20. $55\frac{4}{17} + 101\frac{3}{51}$

Practice 12

Solve the following word problems.

1. The certified nurse assistants weigh patients each month. Mrs. Smith weighed 120 pounds last month. Over the last two months, she gained $1\frac{1}{2}$ and $\frac{1}{4}$ pounds. What is Mrs. Smith's current weight?

2. The lab technician uses a cleaning solution daily. The technician used $4\frac{1}{2}$ ounces, $1\frac{1}{3}$ ounces, and 5 ounces of the cleaning solutions. What is the total amount of solution used?

3. A new baby grew $\frac{3}{4}$ of an inch in June and $\frac{7}{16}$ of an inch in July. How many total inches did the baby grow during these two months?

4. A sick child drinks $\frac{1}{2}$ cup of juice and an hour later $\frac{3}{4}$ cup of water. At dinner, the child drinks $1\frac{1}{4}$ cups more of water. What is the child's total fluid intake?

5. The nurse gives a patient $1\frac{1}{2}$ grains of medication followed by $2\frac{1}{3}$ grains. What is the total dosage the nurse has dispensed to the patient?

◆◆◆◆ Ordering Fractions

Different health care fields require the comparison of fractions. For example, you may need to compute sizes of medical items or pieces of equipment. It is useful to be able to determine the size relationships of instruments and place them in order for a surgeon before a surgery. This is accomplished by using the common denominator method.

Know these symbols: $<, =, >$

$$3 \text{ is less than } 4 \text{ is represented by } 3 < 4$$

$$7 \text{ is greater than } 5 \text{ is represented by } 7 > 5$$

$$\frac{2}{2} \text{ equals } 1 \text{ is represented by } \frac{2}{2} = 1$$

EXAMPLE

Which is larger, $\frac{1}{4}$ or $\frac{3}{8}$?

STEP 1: Convert the fractions to give each a common denominator.

$$\frac{1}{4} \rightarrow \frac{1 \times 2 = 2}{4 \times 2 = 8}$$

$$\frac{3}{8} \rightarrow \qquad \frac{3}{8}$$

STEP 2: Order by the numerators now that the fractions have the same denominator.

3 is larger than 2, so $\frac{3}{8} > \frac{2}{8}$ or $\frac{1}{4}$.

Practice 13

Order the following fractions from largest to smallest.

1. $\dfrac{1}{4}, \dfrac{2}{9}, \dfrac{4}{12}$

2. $\dfrac{9}{22}, \dfrac{5}{11}, \dfrac{8}{11}$

3. $\dfrac{6}{25}, \dfrac{20}{50}, \dfrac{33}{100}$

4. $\dfrac{7}{8}, \dfrac{2}{16}, \dfrac{3}{4}, \dfrac{1}{2}$

◆◆◆◆ Subtraction of Fractions

Subtraction of fractions follows the same basic principles as addition of fractions. The fractions must have common denominators before any subtraction can be done.

EXAMPLE

STEP 1: Make a common denominator if necessary.

$$\frac{7}{8} - \frac{5}{8} = \underline{\qquad} \text{ (8 is the common denominator.)}$$

STEP 2: Subtract the numerators and then reduce if necessary.

$$\frac{7}{8} - \frac{5}{8} = \frac{2}{8}, \text{ which is reduced to } \frac{1}{4}.$$

Practice 14

Find the common denominator, and then subtract the following fractions.

1. $\frac{3}{9} - \frac{2}{9}$

2. $\frac{5}{8} - \frac{2}{8}$

3. $\frac{3}{11} - \frac{1}{11}$

4. $\frac{22}{44} - \frac{11}{44}$

5. $10\frac{5}{12} - 8\frac{3}{12}$

6. $25\frac{3}{4} - 20\frac{1}{4}$

7. $101\frac{13}{24} - 56\frac{10}{24}$

8. $6\frac{6}{7} - \frac{3}{5}$

9. $\frac{15}{16} - \frac{7}{16}$

10. $20\frac{5}{6} - 12\frac{2}{6}$

11. $\frac{3}{4} - \frac{1}{2}$

12. $\frac{6}{8} - \frac{1}{4}$

13. $12\frac{1}{2} - \frac{3}{10}$

14. $20\frac{6}{14} - 2\frac{3}{7}$

15. $39\frac{11}{18} - 8\frac{3}{6}$

16. $25\frac{1}{3} - 20\frac{1}{8}$

17. $124\dfrac{11}{12} - \dfrac{5}{6}$

18. $18\dfrac{3}{4} - 12\dfrac{2}{3}$

19. $200\dfrac{9}{11} - 188\dfrac{2}{3}$

20. $500\dfrac{4}{5} - 150\dfrac{2}{9}$

BORROWING IN SUBTRACTION OF FRACTIONS

Two specific situations require that a number be borrowed in the subtraction of fractions:
(1) subtraction of a fraction from a whole number, and (2) after a common denominator is
established and the top fraction of the problem is less or smaller than the fraction that is
being subtracted from it.

Recall that the borrowing in whole numbers is accomplished as shown below. Set
the problem up vertically.

$$124 - 8 = \underline{\hspace{2cm}}$$

STEP 1: Borrow 1 from the tens column. Add it to the ones column.

STEP 2: Subtract.

$$\begin{array}{r} 1^1\,2^1\,4 \\ -8 \\ \hline 116 \end{array}$$

In fractions, the same borrowing concept is used; the format varies only slightly. The
difference is that the borrowed number must be put into a fractional form.

MATH SENSE

Any whole number over itself equals 1. So
$\dfrac{101}{101} = 1$, $\dfrac{3}{3} = 1$,
$\dfrac{12}{12} = 1$.

EXAMPLE

$$\begin{array}{r} 17\dfrac{3}{8} \\ -14\dfrac{4}{8} \\ \hline \end{array}$$

In the example above, the numerator 4 in the second fraction cannot be subtracted from
the first fraction's numerator 3. Thus, borrowing is required in the first fraction.

$$\begin{array}{r} 1^6\,7\dfrac{3}{8} + \dfrac{8}{8} \\ -14\dfrac{4}{8} \\ \hline \end{array}$$

STEP 1: Borrow 1 from the whole number. Convert the 1 into an improper fraction having
the same common denominator as the first fraction. Then add the two fractions.

STEP 2: Rewrite the problem so it incorporates the changes, and then subtract the
numerator only. Place it over the denominator. Reduce as necessary.

$$\begin{array}{r} 16\dfrac{11}{8} \\ -14\dfrac{4}{8} \\ \hline 2\dfrac{7}{8} \end{array}$$

> **SET-UP HINT**
>
> **BORROWING IN SUBTRACTION RULES**
> 1. Must have a common denominator.
> 2. To borrow from the whole number, make it a fractional part.
> 3. Add fractional parts.
> 4. Subtract; reduce if necessary.

Practice 15

Find the common denominator, and then solve the following subtraction problems using borrowing as needed.

1. $11 - \dfrac{5}{6}$

2. $9 - \dfrac{3}{5}$

3. $10 - \dfrac{2}{8}$

4. $13 - \dfrac{5}{9}$

5. $15 - \dfrac{7}{13}$

6. $30 - \dfrac{4}{11}$

7. $8\dfrac{2}{7} - 2\dfrac{3}{7}$

8. $14\dfrac{3}{12} - 10\dfrac{10}{12}$

9. $15\dfrac{1}{5} - 4\dfrac{4}{5}$

10. $9\dfrac{2}{4} - 5\dfrac{3}{4}$

Remember that when you are subtracting, the first rule is that you must have a common denominator. Once the common denominator is in place, borrow if necessary. Then subtract, placing the answer over the denominator; reduce as necessary.

Practice 16

Solve the following problems.

1. $14\dfrac{2}{5} - 6\dfrac{3}{4}$

2. $34\dfrac{1}{4} - 10\dfrac{4}{5}$

3. $36\dfrac{1}{6} - 16\dfrac{3}{5}$

4. $13\frac{3}{4} - 7\frac{7}{8}$

5. $16\frac{3}{11} - 10\frac{1}{2}$

6. $19\frac{1}{2} - 15\frac{7}{12}$

7. $112\frac{1}{2} - \frac{11}{15}$

8. $18\frac{3}{7} - 2\frac{7}{14}$

9. $45\frac{3}{8} - 13\frac{3}{4}$

10. $125\frac{2}{12} - 28\frac{5}{6}$

11. $29\frac{1}{4} - 12\frac{5}{12}$

12. $12\frac{1}{6} - 1\frac{4}{5}$

13. $90\frac{4}{9} - 13\frac{3}{4}$

14. $28\frac{1}{7} - 4\frac{6}{7}$

15. $13\frac{2}{20} - 6\frac{6}{10}$

16. $12\frac{1}{2} - 4\frac{7}{8}$

17. $14 - \frac{3}{7}$

18. $12\frac{1}{16} - 2\frac{5}{16}$

19. $20\frac{2}{3} - 10\frac{7}{9}$

20. $54\frac{1}{2} - 42\frac{3}{4}$

21. $22\frac{3}{5} - 17\frac{5}{6}$

22. $87 - 14\frac{2}{7}$

23. $225\frac{1}{4} - 34\frac{3}{8}$

24. $90\dfrac{1}{3} - 6\dfrac{3}{4}$

25. $45 - \dfrac{15}{16}$

Practice 17

Solve the following word problems.

1. A patient is on a low-sodium, low-fat diet. Three months ago the patient weighed $210\dfrac{1}{4}$ pounds. Now the patient weighs $198\dfrac{3}{4}$ pounds. How many pounds did the patient lose?

2. The school nurse encourages all students to drink at least 4 pints of water daily. Most students drink at least $1\dfrac{1}{2}$ pints. How much additional water should the students consume?

3. The pharmacy technician helps with annual inventory. If there were 125 boxes of computer labels at the beginning of the inventory period and $25\dfrac{3}{4}$ remain, how many boxes of labels were used throughout the year?

4. The dietitian had a 100 pound bag of unbleached flour at the beginning of the month. If she used $73\dfrac{1}{2}$ pounds of it, how much flour does she have left?

5. The recreation center is helping residents make placemats for the holidays. Each resident is given 45 inches of decorative edging per placemat. If each placemat uses $41\dfrac{1}{2}$ inches of decorative edging, how much edging is left over from each placemat?

◆◆◆◆ Multiplication of Fractions

REVIEW

To facilitate multiplication and division of fractions, set up the problems horizontally.

One of the simplest computations in fractions is multiplying a common fraction. No common denominator is needed.

EXAMPLE

STEP 1: Set up the problem horizontally and multiply the fraction straight across.

$$\dfrac{7}{8} \times \dfrac{1}{4} \begin{array}{c} \rightarrow \\ \rightarrow \end{array} = \dfrac{7}{32}$$

STEP 2: Reduce to the lowest terms, if necessary. $\dfrac{7}{32}$ does not need to be reduced.

Practice 18

Multiply the following fractions.

1. $\dfrac{3}{4} \times \dfrac{1}{12}$

6. $\dfrac{12}{48} \times \dfrac{1}{2}$

2. $\dfrac{1}{2} \times \dfrac{4}{5}$

7. $\dfrac{6}{9} \times \dfrac{2}{3}$

3. $\dfrac{7}{9} \times \dfrac{4}{5}$

8. $\dfrac{10}{100} \times \dfrac{2}{5}$

4. $\dfrac{2}{3} \times \dfrac{4}{6}$

9. $\dfrac{1}{3} \times \dfrac{13}{22}$

5. $\dfrac{1}{5} \times \dfrac{3}{7}$

10. $\dfrac{4}{5} \times \dfrac{1}{20}$

Review some number concepts in fractions that will help ensure accurate answers.

MATH SENSE

Any number over itself equals 1: $\dfrac{8}{8}$, $\dfrac{128}{128}$, and $\dfrac{14}{14}$ all equal 1.

Any numerator that has 1 as its denominator should be represented as a whole number:

$$\dfrac{4}{1} = 4, \dfrac{6}{1} = 6, \dfrac{51}{1} = 51, \text{ and } \dfrac{102}{1} = 102$$

MATH SENSE

Any whole number can become a fraction by placing a 1 as the denominator. $14 = \dfrac{14}{1}$.

MULTIPLYING A FRACTION BY A WHOLE NUMBER

To multiply a fraction by a whole number, follow these steps:

EXAMPLE

$$\dfrac{1}{6} \times 2 = \underline{\qquad}$$

STEP 1: Make the whole number into a fraction by placing a 1 as its denominator.

$$\dfrac{1}{6} \times \dfrac{2}{1}$$

STEP 2: Multiply straight across and then reduce if necessary.

$$\dfrac{1}{6} \times \dfrac{2}{1} = \dfrac{2}{6} \rightarrow \dfrac{1}{3}$$

Reduce to $\dfrac{1}{3}$.

Practice 19

Multiply the following fractions and whole numbers.

1. $\dfrac{1}{4} \times 6$

2. $3 \times \dfrac{2}{5}$

3. $\dfrac{7}{15} \times 35$

4. $24 \times \dfrac{2}{7}$

5. $7 \times \dfrac{8}{10}$

6. $16 \times \dfrac{1}{3}$

7. $\dfrac{5}{9} \times 21$

8. $\dfrac{5}{30} \times 200$

9. $\dfrac{1}{8} \times 32$

10. $\dfrac{11}{50} \times 20$

REDUCING BEFORE YOU MULTIPLY AS A TIMESAVER

When multiplying, you can expedite your work by reducing before you multiply. This is useful because it relies on the multiples of the numbers to reduce the numbers you are multiplying. This saves time at the end of the problem because you won't have to spend so much time reducing the answer.

Look at the numbers involved in $\dfrac{2}{5} \times \dfrac{3}{4}$. If a numerator number can go into a denominator number evenly, then canceling is possible.

$$\dfrac{\overset{1}{2}}{5} \times \dfrac{3}{\underset{2}{4}} \quad \text{The 2 goes into the 4 twice because } 2 \times 2 = 4.$$

Then multiply the changed numerals straight across.

$$\dfrac{1 \times 3}{5 \times 2} = \dfrac{3}{10}$$

The answer is $\dfrac{3}{10}$. If the problem was done without canceling, the answer after multiplication would be $\dfrac{6}{20}$, which needs to be reduced to $\dfrac{3}{10}$. Reducing first saves time by allowing you to work with smaller numbers. For more complicated problems, it may be easier to cancel by writing out the number involved.

EXAMPLE

STEP 1: Write out the multiples of each number to find numbers that each can go into evenly.

$$\begin{array}{cc} (10 \times 1) & (3 \times 1) \\[4pt] \dfrac{10}{15} \times & \dfrac{3}{100} \\[4pt] (3 \times 5) & (10 \times 10) \end{array}$$

(continued on next page)

STEP 2: Then, begin by crossing out the matching numbers, working from top to bottom.

$$(\cancel{10} \times 1) \qquad (\cancel{3} \times 1)$$
$$\frac{10}{5} \quad \times \quad \frac{3}{100}$$
$$(\cancel{3} \times 5) \qquad (\cancel{10} \times 10)$$

STEP 3: Then multiply the remaining numbers straight across.

$$(\cancel{10} \times 1) \quad (\cancel{3} \times 1) \qquad \rightarrow 1 \times 1 = \underline{1}$$
$$\frac{10}{15} \quad \times \quad \frac{3}{100} \qquad \qquad \qquad \left.\begin{array}{c}\end{array}\right\} \frac{1}{50}$$
$$(\cancel{3} \times 5) \quad (\cancel{10} \times 10) \qquad \rightarrow 5 \times 10 = 50$$

When there are more than two fractions, reducing fractions can occur anywhere within the fractions as long as the reducing is done in the top and bottom numbers. There can be multiple reductions of fractions as well.

EXAMPLE

$$\frac{11}{16} \times \frac{3}{12} \times \frac{8}{66} \rightarrow \quad \text{Set the problem up using the factors for each number.}$$

$$(11 \times 1) \quad (3 \times 1) \quad (2 \times 4)$$
$$\frac{11}{16} \quad \times \quad \frac{3}{12} \quad \times \quad \frac{8}{66}$$
$$(2 \times 8) \quad (4 \times 3) \quad (6 \times 11)$$

$$\left.\begin{array}{ccc}(\cancel{11} \times 1) & (3 \times 1) & (\cancel{2} \times \cancel{4}) \\ \dfrac{11}{16} \quad \times & \dfrac{3}{12} \quad \times & \dfrac{8}{66} \\ (\cancel{2} \times 8) & (\cancel{4} \times \cancel{3}) & (6 \times \cancel{11})\end{array}\right\} \quad \text{After reducing, multiple to get } \frac{1}{48}$$

Practice 20

Multiply the following fractions; remember to reduce before you multiply.

1. $\dfrac{4}{5} \times \dfrac{15}{7}$

2. $\dfrac{12}{20} \times \dfrac{4}{24}$

3. $\dfrac{3}{7} \times \dfrac{21}{36}$

4. $\dfrac{5}{6} \times \dfrac{3}{30}$

5. $\dfrac{11}{15} \times \dfrac{3}{44}$

6. $\dfrac{3}{7} \times \dfrac{7}{11}$

7. $\dfrac{14}{20} \times \dfrac{10}{28}$

8. $\dfrac{1}{3} \times \dfrac{3}{6} \times \dfrac{2}{4}$

9. $\dfrac{11}{16} \times \dfrac{4}{12} \times \dfrac{22}{44}$

10. $\dfrac{9}{10} \times \dfrac{1}{3} \times \dfrac{8}{13}$

11. $\dfrac{8}{14} \times \dfrac{25}{48} \times \dfrac{7}{50}$

12. $\dfrac{5}{12} \times \dfrac{33}{34} \times \dfrac{17}{20} \times \dfrac{60}{66}$

◆◆◆◆ Multiplication of Mixed Numbers

REVIEW

Mixed numbers are whole numbers with fractions. Multiplication involving mixed numbers requires that the mixed number be changed to an improper fraction.

EXAMPLE

Change $1\dfrac{3}{4}$ into an improper fraction.

STEP 1: Multiply the whole number times the denominator; then add the numerator.

$$1\dfrac{3}{4} \rightarrow\ 1 \times 4 + 3 = 7$$

STEP 2: Place the answer from step 1 over the denominator.

$$1\dfrac{3}{4} \rightarrow\ 1 \times 4 + 3 = 7\ \rightarrow\ \dfrac{7}{4}$$

$$\text{So } 1\dfrac{3}{4} = \dfrac{7}{4}$$

This improper fraction cannot be further reduced or changed. It may now be multiplied by another fraction.

Practice 21

Change these mixed numbers into improper fractions.

1. $8\frac{1}{4}$

6. $4\frac{3}{8}$

2. $5\frac{2}{3}$

7. $3\frac{5}{9}$

3. $17\frac{3}{5}$

8. $12\frac{1}{4}$

4. $24\frac{4}{7}$

9. $4\frac{5}{12}$

5. $2\frac{3}{12}$

10. $10\frac{1}{3}$

After converting mixed numbers to improper fractions, continue by following the same rules as for multiplying common fractions.

EXAMPLE

$$\frac{1}{3} \times 5\frac{1}{4}$$

STEP 1: Change the mixed number into an improper fraction.

$$5\frac{1}{4} \rightarrow 5 \times 4 = 20 + 1 = \frac{21}{4}$$

STEP 2: Reduce, if possible.

$$\frac{1}{3} \quad \times \quad \frac{21}{4}$$

(3×1) (3×7)

STEP 3: Multiply straight across.

$$1 \times 7 = 7$$
$$1 \times 4 = 4$$

STEP 4: Change the improper fraction to a mixed fraction.

$$\frac{7}{4} \rightarrow 7 \div 4 = 1\frac{3}{4}$$

EXAMPLE

$$3\frac{1}{4} \times 5\frac{2}{5}$$

STEP 1: Change to improper fractions.

$$3\frac{1}{4} \rightarrow 3 \times 4 = 12 + 1 = \frac{13}{4} \text{ and}$$

$$5\frac{2}{5} \rightarrow 5 \times 5 = 25 + 2 = \frac{27}{5}$$

STEP 2: Reduce, if possible.

$$\frac{13}{4} \times \frac{27}{5} \text{ — not possible}$$

STEP 3: Multiply straight across.

$$\frac{13}{4} \times \frac{27}{5} = \frac{351}{20}$$

STEP 4: Reduce—divide 351 by 20. Write it as a mixed fraction.

$$
\begin{array}{r}
17\frac{11}{20} \\
20\overline{)351} \\
20\downarrow \\
\hline
151 \\
140 \\
\hline
11
\end{array}
\qquad \text{Answer: } 17\frac{11}{20}
$$

Practice 22

Follow the steps you just learned to solve the following multiplication problems.

1. $2\frac{5}{12} \times \frac{1}{7}$

2. $4\frac{2}{3} \times \frac{4}{5}$

3. $\frac{3}{10} \times 1\frac{3}{4}$

4. $2\frac{1}{8} \times \frac{6}{11}$

5. $\frac{4}{9} \times 1\frac{2}{3}$

6. $3\frac{5}{7} \times 2\frac{5}{14}$

7. $17\frac{1}{4} \times 2\frac{1}{3}$

8. $1\frac{1}{4} \times 2\frac{1}{5}$

9. $2\frac{1}{5} \times 1\frac{3}{4}$

10. $3\frac{1}{6} \times 3\frac{1}{4}$

Practice 23

Use multiplication to solve the following word problems.

1. A bottle of medicine contains 30 doses. How many doses are in $2\frac{1}{3}$ bottles?

2. The nurse worked a total of $2\frac{1}{4}$ hours overtime. She is paid $32 an hour for overtime work. What are her overtime earnings?

3. One tablet contains 250 milligrams of pain medication. How many milligrams are in $3\frac{1}{2}$ tablets?

4. One cup holds 8 ounces of liquid. If a cup is $\frac{2}{3}$ full, how many ounces are in the cup?

5. The dietitian is working in a long-term care residence. Each day she prepares a high-protein drink for 25 residents. If each drink measures $\frac{3}{4}$ cup, how many total cups of the drink will she prepare a day?

◆◆◆◆ Division of Fractions

REVIEW

To divide fractions, two steps are required to compute the answer.

EXAMPLE

Solve:

$$\frac{1}{8} \div \frac{1}{4} = \underline{\hspace{1cm}}$$

STEP 1: Change the ÷ sign to a × sign.

$$\frac{1}{8} \div \frac{1}{4} \rightarrow \frac{1}{8} \times \frac{1}{4}$$

STEP 2: Invert the fraction to the right of the changed ÷ sign (now the × sign).

$$\frac{1}{8} \div \frac{1}{4} \rightarrow \frac{1}{8} \times \frac{4}{1}$$

This inversion causes the fraction to change from $\frac{1}{4}$ to $\frac{4}{1}$, which is called the reciprocal of $\frac{1}{4}$.

STEP 3: Follow the steps of multiplication of fractions: Reduce if possible; then multiply straight across and reduce as necessary.

$$\text{Reduce} \quad \frac{1}{8} \times \frac{\overset{(4 \times 1)}{4}}{\underset{(4 \times 2)}{1}} = \frac{1}{2}$$

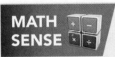 **MATH SENSE** The reciprocal of any fraction is its inverse:

$$\frac{2}{3} \rightarrow \frac{3}{2} \quad \frac{12}{35} \rightarrow \frac{35}{12} \quad \text{and} \quad \frac{9}{11} \rightarrow \frac{11}{9}$$

EXAMPLE

Solve:

$$\frac{4}{9} \div \frac{1}{3} = \underline{\hspace{2cm}}$$

STEP 1: Change the ÷ sign to a × sign.

$$\frac{4}{9} \times \frac{1}{3}$$

STEP 2: Invert the fraction after the changed ÷ sign (now the × sign).

$$\frac{4}{9} \times \frac{3}{1}$$

STEP 3: Multiply straight across.

$$\frac{4}{9} \times \frac{3}{1} = \frac{12}{9} \qquad \begin{array}{r} \text{Reduce} \\ 1\frac{3}{9} \\ 9{\overline{)12}} \\ \underline{-9} \\ 3 \end{array}$$

The answer is $1\frac{3}{9}$. Note that $\frac{3}{9}$ reduces to $\frac{1}{3}$, so the answer is $1\frac{1}{3}$.

Practice 24

Solve the following division problems.

1. $\dfrac{3}{7} \div \dfrac{3}{5}$

2. $\dfrac{5}{35} \div \dfrac{11}{21}$

3. $\dfrac{3}{12} \div \dfrac{6}{7}$

4. $\dfrac{7}{9} \div \dfrac{4}{5}$

5. $\dfrac{8}{9} \div \dfrac{1}{9}$

6. $33 \div \dfrac{11}{12}$

7. $\dfrac{1}{3} \div 15$

8. $6 \div \dfrac{1}{3}$

9. $\dfrac{7}{28} \div 30$

10. $8\dfrac{6}{10} \div 1\dfrac{4}{5}$

11. $4\dfrac{3}{8} \div 1\dfrac{2}{16}$

12. $7\dfrac{1}{2} \div 3\dfrac{1}{5}$

13. $12\dfrac{4}{8} \div 4\dfrac{1}{2}$

14. $12\dfrac{4}{10} \div 3\dfrac{1}{3}$

15. $5\dfrac{1}{2} \div 1\dfrac{1}{8}$

16. $3\dfrac{5}{8} \div 2\dfrac{1}{2}$

17. $2\dfrac{3}{14} \div 9\dfrac{2}{7}$

18. $1\dfrac{7}{9} \div \dfrac{8}{11}$

19. $10\frac{6}{7} \div 7\frac{1}{2}$

20. $1\frac{9}{12} \div \frac{1}{12}$

Practice 25

Use division to solve the following word problems.

1. A lab technician worked $45\frac{3}{4}$ hours in 5 days. He worked the same number of hours each day. How many hours a day did he work?

2. How many $\frac{1}{4}$ gram doses can be obtained from a $7\frac{1}{2}$ gram vial of medication?

3. The pharmacy technician's paycheck was for $1,123.85. If the technician worked $84\frac{1}{2}$ hours, what is the hourly rate of pay?

4. The nurse must give a patient 9 milligrams of a medication. If the tablets are 2 milligrams each, how many tablets are needed?

5. The pharmacy has 5 gram vials of medication. How many $\frac{1}{2}$ gram doses are available?

◆◆◆◆ Converting Temperatures Using Fraction Formulas

REVIEW

Fractions are very useful in converting between measurement systems. One example of this is converting between the Celsius and Fahrenheit temperatures. Fractions are more accurate than decimals because there is no change in the numbers as a result of rounding the decimals.

Follow these two setups:

To convert Celsius to Fahrenheit: $\left(°C \times \frac{9}{5}\right) + 32 = °F$

To convert Fahrenheit to Celsius: $\left(°F - 32\right) \times \frac{5}{9} = °C$

The decimal unit (Unit 3) will include the formula for handling temperature conversions using decimals.

Follow these steps to change a Fahrenheit temperature to a Celsius temperature:

EXAMPLE

$$5\,°C = \underline{\hspace{1.5cm}}\,°F$$

STEP 1: Solve within the parentheses first (per the order of operations), and then work left to right.

$$\left(°C \times \frac{9}{5}\right) + 32 = °F$$

$$°C \times \frac{9}{5} \rightarrow \quad 5 \times \frac{9}{5} = \frac{45}{5} \qquad 5\overline{)45} = 9 \quad \frac{9}{}$$
$$\underline{45}$$

STEP 2: Add 32 to the step 1 answer to get the °C.

$$9 + 32 = 41\,°F$$

Practice 26

Use the correct fraction conversion formula to convert the following Celsius temperatures to Fahrenheit.

1. $20\,°C = \underline{\hspace{1.5cm}}\,°F$

2. $35\,°C = \underline{\hspace{1.5cm}}\,°F$

3. $25\,°C = \underline{\hspace{1.5cm}}\,°F$

4. $60\,°C = \underline{\hspace{1.5cm}}\,°F$

5. $40\,°C = \underline{\hspace{1.5cm}}\,°F$

6. $45\,°C = \underline{\hspace{1.5cm}}\,°F$

7. $80\,°C = \underline{\hspace{1.5cm}}\,°F$

8. $15\,°C = \underline{\hspace{1.5cm}}\,°F$

Follow these steps to change a Fahrenheit temperature to a Celsius temperature:

EXAMPLE

$$122°F = \underline{\hspace{1.5cm}}\,°C$$

STEP 1: Solve within the parenthesis first. $(°F - 32) \times \frac{5}{9} = °C$

$$°F - 32 = \underline{\hspace{1.5cm}} \qquad \text{Subtract 32 from the Fahrenheit temperature.}$$
$$122°F$$
$$\underline{-32}$$
$$90$$

STEP 2: Multiply the step 1 answer by $\frac{5}{9}$ to get the °C.

$$90 \times \frac{5}{9} = \frac{450}{9} \text{ Divide 450 by 9.}$$

$$\begin{array}{r} 50 \\ 9\overline{)450} \\ 45\downarrow \\ \hline 00 \end{array}$$

So, 122°F is 50°C.

Practice 27

Use the correct fraction conversion formula to convert the following Fahrenheit temperatures to Celsius.

1. 104°F = _____°C

2. 32°F = _____°C

3. 50°F = _____°C

4. 113°F = _____°C

5. 59°F = _____°C

6. 131°F = _____°C

7. 86°F = _____°C

8. 122°F = _____°C

Some temperatures will require working with decimals. Additional practice will be provided in Unit 3: Decimals.

◆◆◆◆ Complex Fractions

REVIEW

Complex fractions are used to help nurses and pharmacy technicians compute exact dosages of medications. A complex fraction is a fraction within a fraction. Complex fractions may also more efficiently solve difficult problems. For example, some doctors and pharmacists continue to use grains as a measurement in their prescriptions even as the industry has converted to the use of milligrams and micrograms in dosages. A typical problem may be that a doctor prescribes $\frac{1}{8}$ grain, but the supply on hand is $\frac{1}{6}$ grain per milliliter. The setup would include a complex fraction. $\dfrac{\frac{1}{8}\text{ grain}}{\frac{1}{6}\text{ grain}} \times 1$ milliliter. A grain is a measure of weight. Occasionally, you may see metric units and grains appear in fraction form.

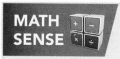

MATH SENSE

Whole numbers require you to place a 1 as a denominator prior to any division or multiplication of their digits.

EXAMPLE

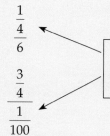

$$\dfrac{\frac{1}{4}}{6}$$

$$\dfrac{\frac{3}{4}}{\frac{1}{100}}$$

The fraction bars separating the fractional parts, numerator and denominator, should be viewed as division signs.

Complex fractions are solved by using the rules of division. These examples become:

$$\frac{1}{4} \div 6 \rightarrow \frac{1}{4} \div \frac{6}{1} \rightarrow \frac{1}{4} \times \frac{1}{6} = \frac{1}{24}$$

$$\frac{3}{4} \div \frac{1}{100} \rightarrow \frac{3}{4} \div \frac{1}{100} \rightarrow \frac{3}{4} \times \frac{100}{1} = \frac{300}{4} \quad \text{reduces to} \quad \frac{75}{1} = 75$$

Practice 28

Solve these complex fractions. Reduce to the lowest terms.

1. $\dfrac{\frac{3}{8}}{4}$

2. $\dfrac{\frac{1}{8}}{100}$

3. $\dfrac{\frac{1}{300}}{50}$

4. $\dfrac{40}{\frac{1}{25}}$

5. $\dfrac{\frac{1}{50}}{\frac{1}{60}}$

6. $\dfrac{\frac{3}{4}}{\frac{2}{3}}$

7. $\dfrac{\frac{1}{125}}{\frac{2}{200}}$

8. $\dfrac{\frac{1}{2}}{\frac{1}{4}}$

9. $\dfrac{\frac{1}{80}}{\frac{1}{75}}$

10. $\dfrac{\frac{1}{10}}{\frac{1}{100}}$

Dosage problems will also combine complex fractions with whole numbers and decimal numbers to compute the correct dosage. This work will be further covered in Unit 11: Dosage Calculations.

$$\frac{\dfrac{1}{300}}{\dfrac{1}{100}} \times 200$$

EXAMPLE

These types of problems appear to be more difficult than they actually are. Group the work into sections so that it is manageable, and you will be able to track your progress.

STEP 1: First solve the complex fraction by dividing it.

$$\frac{1}{300} \div \frac{1}{100} \rightarrow \frac{1}{300} \times \frac{100}{1} = \frac{100}{300} \rightarrow \text{Reduce to } \frac{1}{3}$$

STEP 2: Next, rewrite the entire problem.

$$\frac{1}{3} \times 200 \qquad \text{Then work this portion of the problem.}$$

$$\frac{1}{3} \times \frac{200}{1} = \frac{200}{3} \qquad \text{Reduce by dividing 200 by 3.}$$

The answer is $66\frac{2}{3}$. If the problem has a fraction in it, the answer may have a fraction in it. Do not convert this fraction to a decimal number.

Practice 29

Solve these problems.

1. $\dfrac{\dfrac{5}{8}}{\dfrac{1}{4}} \times 2$

2. $\dfrac{\dfrac{1}{200}}{\dfrac{1}{100}} \times 80$

3. $\dfrac{\dfrac{15}{500}}{\dfrac{1}{100}} \times 4$

4. $\dfrac{\dfrac{1}{125}}{\dfrac{1}{500}} \times 25$

5. $\dfrac{\dfrac{1}{3}}{\dfrac{1}{2}} \times 1\frac{1}{2}$

6. $\dfrac{\dfrac{1}{100}}{\dfrac{2}{25}} \times 10\frac{1}{4}$

MEASUREMENT IN FRACTIONS

Fractions are common in the measurement systems we use every day. For example, we use fractions in time such as $\frac{1}{2}$ hour, $7\frac{1}{2}$ minutes, and $4\frac{1}{2}$ hours. We also use fractions for our household measurements such as $1\frac{1}{2}$ cups, $\frac{1}{2}$ teaspoon, and 3 pints as well as in weights in pounds and ounces such as $34\frac{1}{2}$ ounces and $12\frac{1}{2}$ ounces. Using addition or multiplication, we can covert fractions between these units. For example, the doctor orders $1\frac{1}{2}$ quarts of medical preparation before a scheduled CT scan. The patient uses a cup to measure the liquid.

$$\text{Think: 1 quart has 4 cups} \qquad \frac{1 \text{ quart}}{4 \text{ cups}} = \frac{1\frac{1}{2} \text{ quart}}{X \text{ cups}}$$

Multiply $1\frac{1}{2}$ quarts times 4 cups to get the number of cups.

$$1\frac{1}{2} \times 4 = \frac{3}{2} \times \frac{4}{1} = \frac{12}{2} \qquad \text{Reduced, the final answer is 6 cups.}$$

It is very important to remember to add the unit of measure because doing so ensures that whoever reads the number knows which unit of measure was used.

Another way to complete these conversions is with a conversion chart.

To Convert From	To	Operation
Gallons	Quarts	Multiply by 4
Quarts	Cups	Multiply by 4
Tablespoons	Teaspoons	Multiply by 3
Cups	Pints	Divide by 2
Cups	Ounces	Multiply by 8
Pounds	Ounces	Multiply by 16
Feet	Inches	Multiply by 12
Yards	Feet	Multiply by 3
Yards	Inches	Multiply by 36

Learn some common measurement equivalencies. These often have fractional parts.

Practice 30

Make the following conversions:

COMMON MEASUREMENTS AND THEIR EQUIVALENTS	
1 yard = 3 feet	1 gallon = 4 quarts
1 foot = 12 inches	1 quart = 2 pints
1 tablespoon = 3 teaspoons	1 pint = 2 cups
1 pound = 16 ounces	1 cup = 8 ounces

1. $3\frac{1}{2}$ gallons = _____ quarts

2. $4\frac{1}{4}$ cups = _____ pints

3. $15\frac{1}{2}$ cups = _____ ounces

4. $5\frac{1}{2}$ tablespoons = _____ teaspoons

5. $8\frac{1}{3}$ feet = _____ inches

6. $14\frac{1}{2}$ yards = _____ feet

7. $7\frac{1}{3}$ cups = _____ ounces

8. $22\frac{3}{4}$ pounds = _____ ounces

9. $4\frac{1}{2}$ yards = _____ inches

10. $5\frac{1}{3}$ quarts = _____ cups

We also use this knowledge in common word problems in health care.

Practice 31

Solve the following word problems.

1. Dilly works in the accounting office at Health Valley Medical Center. She is trying to calculate the amount of time each week that each employee has allotted for lunch and break times. Each employee has $\frac{1}{4}$ hour for a morning break plus $\frac{1}{2}$ hour for lunch. If the employees each work 5 days a week and there are 27 employees, how much time does each employee spend each week at lunch and break? _____ How much time does the entire group of employees spend each week at lunch and break? _____

2. Ms. Smith was asked by her doctor to track her consumption of caffeinated beverages. She has consumed $12\frac{1}{2}$ ounces of cola, $9\frac{1}{3}$ ounces of coffee, and $12\frac{1}{4}$ ounces of black tea today. How much caffeinated beverage has she consumed today? _____

3. Kellie is on a strict diet in preparation for surgery. She has to monitor her weight daily for five days. She weighed $235\frac{1}{2}$ pounds on Monday. She lost $\frac{1}{8}$ pound on Monday. She gained $1\frac{1}{4}$ pounds on Tuesday, and on Wednesday she lost $1\frac{3}{4}$ pounds. Thursday, she lost $\frac{3}{4}$ of a pound, and on Friday she gained $1\frac{1}{2}$ pounds. How much did she weigh on the Friday after she weighed herself? _____

4. Sometimes medications are dispensed in ounces. We know that one cup contains 8 ounces. Mary took $\frac{1}{2}$ ounce of Maalox at breakfast, $\frac{1}{2}$ ounce of Maalox at lunch, and $\frac{3}{4}$ ounce at dinner. Is this more or less than one-fourth cup of medication? _____

5. A mail-order company likes to dispense orders in 120-day supplies. If Mary takes $\frac{1}{2}$ tablet three times a day, how many tablets would she need to fill the 120-day supply?_____

More details and practice on conversion will be given in Unit 6 and Unit 10.

UNIT REVIEW

◆◆◆◆ Critical Thinking with Fractions

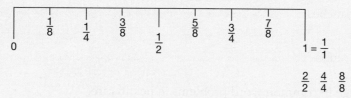

Read the following rulers and note the place on each where the arrow is located:

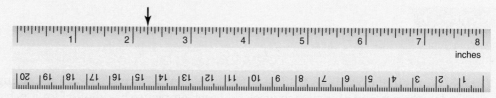

1. _____ inches

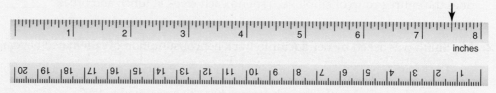

2. _____ inches

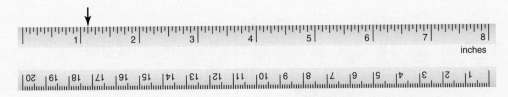

3. _____ inches

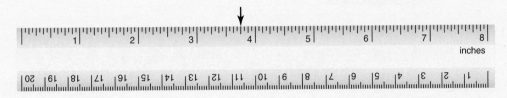

4. _____ inches

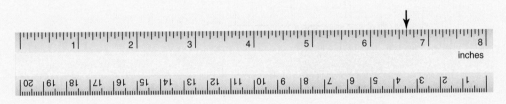

5. _____ inches

Solve the following problems using your fraction and whole number skills.

6. $1 \div m = \dfrac{7}{60}$

7. $\dfrac{2}{13} = 5 \div x$

8. $\dfrac{61}{x} = 5\dfrac{6}{11}$

9. $3\dfrac{8}{12} = \dfrac{z}{6}$

10. $\dfrac{15}{28} = \dfrac{6}{7}z$

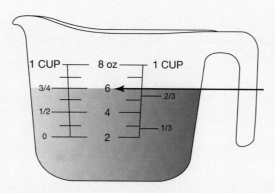

11. Look at the point of the arrow. This is what fractional part of a cup? _____

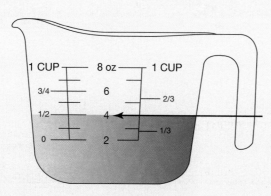

12. Look at the point of the arrow. This is what fractional part of a cup? _____

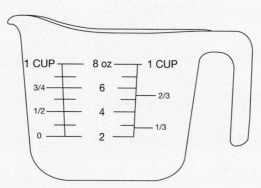

13. How many ounces is $\frac{2}{3}$ cup? _____

14. How many ounces is $\frac{1}{8}$ cup? _____

15. How many ounces is $2\frac{1}{4}$ cups? _____

◆◆◆◆ Professional Expertise

- All fractions should be written in reduced or simplified form.
- Include the unit of measure with each number when possible. In other words, it is $2\frac{1}{2}$ feet, not simply $2\frac{1}{2}$.
- When adding or subtracting fractions, set the problem up vertically to avoid making careless errors.
- Only addition and subtraction require a common denominator.
- Only subtraction has borrowing; first get a common denominator, then borrow.
- When multiplying or dividing fractions, set the problem up horizontally to expedite cancellation.
- When multiplying and dividing a whole number, start by setting the whole number as a fraction. The whole number is the numerator, and 1 is the denominator. Thus $3\frac{1}{2} \times 2$ becomes $3\frac{1}{2} \times \frac{2}{1}$. This keeps the numbers properly aligned.
- Household measures are always given in whole numbers and/or fractions.
- Write fractions with a horizontal fraction bar, $\frac{12}{13}$, not with a slanted fraction bar, $^{12}\!/_{13}$.

FRACTION POST-TEST

Reduce all answers to lowest terms.

1. A day has 24 hours. Six hours is what fractional part of the 24 hours?

2. Write two equivalent fractions for $\frac{1}{6}$.

3. Reduce $\frac{122}{11}$.

4. $8\frac{1}{6} + 3\frac{3}{4}$

5. $52 - 12\frac{1}{5}$

6. $14\frac{1}{2} \times 2\frac{1}{8}$

7. $5\frac{2}{6} \div 12$

8. $77°F = $ _____ °C

9. Order from smallest to largest: $\frac{3}{8}, \frac{1}{3}, \frac{1}{4}, \frac{2}{12}$

10. Solve: $\dfrac{\frac{1}{4}}{\frac{1}{8}} \times 25$

11. The doctor orders $\frac{1}{8}$ grain of a medicine. The nurse has $\frac{1}{6}$ grain on hand in the medicine cabinet. This is a comparison problem of what is ordered and what is available. Will the nurse give more or less of the dose on hand? _____

12. The physical therapist asks Mr. Smith to walk 20 minutes in one hour to improve his ambulation. What fractional part of an hour is Mr. Smith to exercise? _____

13. Among the fractions $\frac{1}{3}, \frac{1}{5}, \frac{5}{8}$, which one is equivalent to $\frac{15}{24}$?

14. On the dietitian's beverage tray are 16 filled six-ounce glasses. Four glasses contain prune juice and two glasses contain red wine. What fractional part of the glasses contains some beverage other than prune juice or red wine? Express the answer as a fraction. _____

15. Sally works in a nursery. Her job includes recording an accurate weight for each baby. One baby weighs $7\frac{1}{3}$ pounds, two babies weigh $6\frac{1}{2}$ pounds, and a fourth baby weighs $5\frac{7}{8}$ pounds. What is the current total weight of the babies? _____

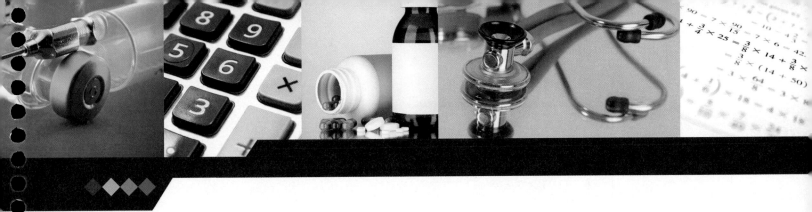

3 Decimals

STUDENT LEARNING OUTCOMES

After completing the tasks in this unit, you will be able to:

3-1 Read and write decimal numbers

3-2 Compare decimals

3-3 Read syringes in decimals

3-4 Add decimal numbers

3-5 Subtract decimal numbers

3-6 Multiply decimal numbers

3-7 Divide decimal numbers, including using zero as a place holder

3-8 Calculate decimal numbers in word problems

3-9 Use simplified multiplication and division

3-10 Convert scale units from decimals to fractions

3-11 Convert fractions to decimal numbers

3-12 Convert Celsius to Fahrenheit temperatures

3-13 Solve mixed fraction and decimal number problems

◆◆◆◆ Overview

Decimals are used every day in health care settings. Understanding the applications of decimals provides a strong foundation for measurement conversions, the metric system, medication dosages, and general charting work. Most medication orders and medical equipment such as syringes are written using the metric system, which relies on decimals.

PRE-TEST

1. Write the decimal 3.87 in words.

2. Round 32.575 to the nearest hundredth.

3. Which is smaller, 0.7850 or 0.7805?

4. $15.8 + 1.4 + 21 + 2.0 =$

5. $12 - 0.89 =$

6. $32.05 \times 7.2 =$

7. $749.7 \div 21 =$

8. $32.85 \times 10 =$

9. Convert 0.035 to a fraction.

10. $108\,°F =$ _____°C

11. $\dfrac{0.08}{0.04} \times 15.2 =$

12. Divide 4,298.9 by 1,000.

13. If 1 kilogram equals 2.2 pounds, what is the weight in pounds of a person who weighs 14.8 kilograms?

14. Convert 15 minutes of an hour into a decimal number.

15. The digital scale reads 146.5 pounds. Write that weight as a mixed fraction.

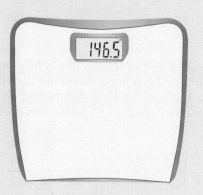

Decimals are also seen in drug labels, providing the details about the amount of a medication in metric units per tablet or capsule. These amounts may appear as a decimal number + milligram/tablet, as shown in the labels below. However, not all medications are listed in terms of decimal numbers.

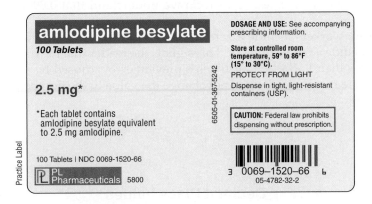

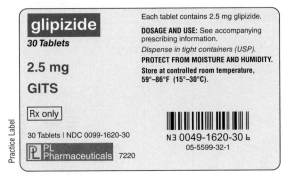

◆◆◆◆ Decimals

REVIEW

A **decimal** represents a part or fraction of a whole number. Decimal numbers are parts of 10s, 100s, 1,000s, and so on. In other words, decimals are multiples of ten. The decimal point (•) represents the boundary between whole numbers and decimal numbers.

Decimal Place Values

whole numbers					decimal numbers				
thousands	hundreds	tens	ones	and	tenths	hundredths	thousandths	ten-thousandths	hundred-thousandths
	1	0	4	•	9	9			

Consider $104.99. We understand this number to be one hundred four dollars and ninety-nine cents. The decimal point is the *and* if we write the number in words.

Any number to the left of the decimal point is always a whole number, and any number to the right of the decimal point is a decimal number. Without a whole number, a decimal number is always less than 1. So we understand that 0.89 and 0.123 are less than 1.

Health care workers include a zero to the left of the decimal point for any decimal that does not include a whole number. This signals the reader that the dose, measurement, or amount is less than 1. The zero also helps prevent errors caused by misreading a decimal number. Note that this zero does not change the value of the number.

EXAMPLE

Decimal Place Values

	whole numbers				**decimal numbers**				
thousands	hundreds	tens	ones	and	tenths	hundredths	thousandths	ten-thousandths	hundred-thousandths
		4	2	•	1	2	5		

Reading decimal numbers is simple if you follow these tips: Say the numbers from left to right as if they were whole numbers, and then add the decimal place value.

42.125 → read as forty-two and one hundred twenty-five thousandths.

MATH SENSE

Identify decimal numbers by looking for words that end in "th" or "ths."

Practice 1

Write the decimals in words.

1. 0.14 _____

2. 0.2 _____

3. 0.08 _____

4. 2.5 _____

5. 103.82 _____

6. 15.002 _____

7. 125.14 _____

8. 53.07 _____

9. 18.08 _____

10. 0.126 _____

Practice 2

Write the following words in decimal numbers:

1. three tenths _____

2. fourteen thousandths _____

3. six hundred and twelve thousandths _____

4. twenty hundredths _____

5. eight and five hundredths _____

   To double-check your work, make sure that the final or last number is placed in the place value spot of the words used to describe it. If it is hundredths, then the second decimal place must have a number in it.

EXAMPLE

fifty-six thousandths
0.056
↑ thousandths place

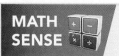

MATH SENSE

Care must be taken not to round too much or too often when calculating dosages. It is best to work a problem all the way to the end and then round the final answer. This avoids changing the actual figures that should be used to calculate an exact dosage.

◆◆◆◆ Rounding Decimals

REVIEW

Decimals are rounded in health care to create manageable numbers. We may have a difficult time visualizing a number such as 14.39757; however, we can easily understand the number 14.4 or 14.40. Rounding to a specific decimal place is accomplished in the same way that whole numbers are rounded. In general, health care workers round decimal numbers to the nearest tenth or the nearest hundredth.

EXAMPLE

Round 1.75 to the nearest tenth.

STEP 1: Underline the place to which you are rounding.

$$1.7\underline{5}$$

STEP 2: Circle one number to the right of the underlined number. If the circled number is 5 or greater, add 1 to the underlined number, and drop all the numbers to the right of the changed number.

$$1.7\text{⑤} \qquad \rightarrow 1.8$$

If the circled number is less than 5, do not change the underlined number, but drop all the numbers to the right of that number.

Sometimes a health care worker will round to the tenths place value and the whole number will be affected.

EXAMPLE

Round 4.97 to the nearest tenth.

STEP 1: $\qquad 4.\underline{9}7$

STEP 2: $4.9\boxed{7} \qquad 4.9\,(\text{Add 1 to 9}) = 5.0 \text{ or } 5$

Practice 3

Round to the nearest tenth:

1. 7.25 _____

2. 245.39 _____

3. 0.95 _____

4. 3.825 _____

5. 25.02 _____

6. 128.09 _____

7. 0.0943 _____

8. 349.37_____

9. 9.89 _____

10. 0.087 _____

Practice 4

Round to the nearest hundredth:

1. 18.358 _____

2. 0.899 _____

3. 4.290 _____

4. 0.0650 _____

5. 0.0074 _____

6. $2,104.556 _____

7. 35.708 _____

8. 9.56741 _____

9. 46.085 _____

10. 4.719 _____

When and which place value to round to is a frequently asked question. General guidelines for rounding will be provided in Unit 11: Dosage Calculations.

◆◆◆◆ Comparing Decimals

REVIEW

Comparing decimals is valuable in health care occupations because many different pieces of equipment are used that may be in metric measurements. Decimals are part of the metric system; thus understanding them is necessary to determine which instrument or measurement is larger or smaller. Comparing decimals is a skill that is also useful in sorting and ordering inventory items by size.

To compare decimals, you will rely on your eyes rather than on any specific math computation.

EXAMPLE

Which is larger: 0.081 or 0.28?

STEP 1: Line the decimals up like buttons on a shirt. This will help make the decimal numbers appear to have the same number of decimal places.

0.081
0.28

STEP 2: Add zeros to fill in the empty place values so that the decimals have the same number of places or digits.

0.081
0.280

STEP 3: Disregard the decimal point for a moment and read the numbers as they are written from left to right, including the added zero place value.

0.081 → eighty-one
0.280 → two hundred eighty

So, 0.28 is larger than 0.081.

Practice 5

Which decimal number is smaller?

1. 1.2 or 1.02 _____

2. 0.075 or 0.75 _____

3. 4.25 or 4.2505 _____

4. 0.4 or 0.04 _____

5. 0.0033 or 0.03 _____

Practice 6

Which decimal number is larger?

1. 0.0895 or 0.89 _____

2. 0.497 or 4.97 _____

3. 0.6 or 0.066 _____

4. 100.75 or 100.07 _____

5. 0.0679 or 0.675 _____

Practice 7

Using the same method, arrange the sets of numbers from largest to smallest:

1. 0.25, 2.5, 2.025, 0.025 _____

2. 0.01, 1.01, 10.01, 1.001 _____

3. 0.5, 5.15, 5.55, 5.05, 0.05 _____

4. 0.04, 0.004, 0.4, 0.044 _____

Syringes are often in decimal units. Syringes measure volume, and the unit of measure is milliliters. Read the syringes on the next page:

Practice 8

Write the measure on the line below each syringe:

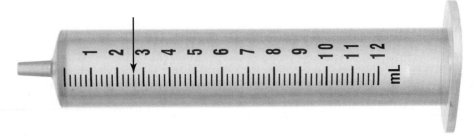

1. _____ milliliters

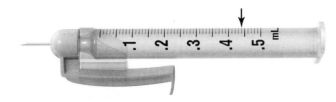

2. _____ milliliters

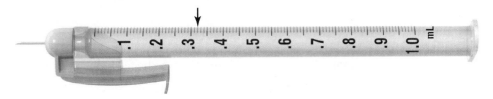

3. _____ milliliters

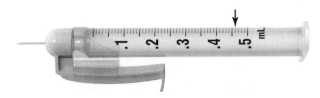

4. _____ milliliters

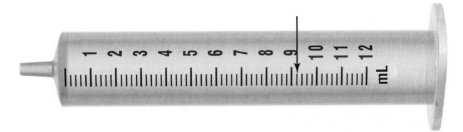

5. _____ milliliters

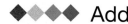 **Addition of Decimals**

To add decimals, first line up the decimal points, and then add. This might mean that a problem presented in a horizontal pattern needs to be rewritten in a vertical pattern.

A whole number always has a decimal point to the right side of the final number: 56 = 56.

$$2.32 + 0.14 = ? \rightarrow \quad \begin{array}{r} 2.32 \\ +0.14 \\ \hline 2.46 \end{array}$$

$$48 + 1.75 = \underline{\quad} \rightarrow \quad \begin{array}{r} 48.00 \\ +1.75 \\ \hline 49.75 \end{array} \quad \begin{array}{l} \leftarrow \text{Place a decimal point and fill} \\ \text{the empty spaces with zeros.} \end{array}$$

Lining up the decimals is the first step in ensuring the correct answer for the addition of decimals.

$$2.46 + 0.005 + 1.3 = \underline{\quad} \rightarrow \quad \begin{array}{r} 2.460 \\ 0.005 \\ +1.300 \\ \hline 3.765 \end{array} \quad \begin{array}{l} \text{Fill the empty spaces} \\ \text{with zeros.} \end{array}$$

STEP 1: Line up the decimals. The order of the numbers to be added is unimportant.

STEP 2: Add the numbers and bring the decimal point straight down.

Add the following decimals.

1. 0.8 + 15 + 3.5 = _____

2. 10.25 + 12 + 0.75 = _____

3. 0.15 + 32 + 0.15 = _____

4. 12.75 + 0.99 + 0.25 = _____

5. 0.0092 + 25.1 + 20 = _____

6. 0.849 + 1.6 + 56.3 = _____

7. 14.28 + 16.24 + 97 = _____

8. 0.75 + 23.87 + 124.07 = _____

9. 13.75 + 0.001 + 200.53 = _____

10. 35.01 + 76.02 + 0.0998 = _____

Practice 10

Solve the following word problems by adding the decimals.

1. A 25-year-old patient receives the following medication dosages daily: 1.5 milligrams, 2.25 milligrams, and 0.75 milligrams. What is his total dosage?

2. Two months ago, a child weighed 15.9 kilograms. Since then, the child has gained 0.9 and 1.5 kilograms. What is the child's current weight?

3. Patient Smith receives 4 tablets of medication dosages daily: One tablet is 225 milligrams, two tablets are 0.125 milligrams each, and one tablet is 0.75 milligrams. What is the patient's total daily dosage of medication in milligrams?

4. One tablet is labeled 124 milligrams and another is labeled 0.5 milligrams. What is the total dosage of these two tablets?

5. A child measured 122 centimeters at a semi-annual checkup with the doctor. What would be the child's height at the next office visit if the child grows by 2.54 centimeters?

◆◆◆◆ Subtraction of Decimals

REVIEW

To subtract decimals, follow two steps:

$$95.5 - 0.76 = \underline{\hspace{2cm}}$$

STEP 1: Set the problem up vertically. Put the larger number, or the number from which the second number is to be subtracted, above the second number, and then line up the decimals.

$$\begin{array}{r} 95.50 \\ -0.76 \end{array} \quad \leftarrow \text{Fill in the empty places with zeros.}$$

STEP 2: Subtract and then bring the decimal straight down.

$$\begin{array}{r} 9^4\,5.^{14}\,5^10 \\ -0.\ \ 7\ 6 \\ \hline 94.\ \ 7\ 4 \end{array}$$

Practice 11

Subtract the following decimals.

1. $6.4 - 4.52 = $ _____

2. $50.4 - 5.24 = $ _____

3. $25 - 0.754 =$ _____

4. $0.90 - 0.459 =$ _____

5. $5.8 - 0.250 =$ _____

6. $15 - 2.505 =$ _____

7. $0.2 - 0.025 =$ _____

8. $14.47 - 0.3108 =$ _____

9. $87.56 - 0.124 =$ _____

10. $0.07 - 0.007 =$ _____

Practice 12

Solve the following word problems by subtracting the decimals.

1. A patient started with a 1 liter bag of IV solution. When the doctor checked in on the patient, the bag contained 0.35 liters of solution. How much solution had been infused into the patient?

2. A bottle of medicine contains 30 milliliters. After withdrawing 2.25 milliliters for an injection, how many milliliters of medicine remain in the bottle?

3. A patient is to receive 4.25 milligrams of a drug daily. The patient has already received 2.75 milligrams. What is his remaining dosage in milligrams?

4. Patient B is on a low-fat diet. He weighed 89.9 kilograms last month. This month he weighs 88.45 kilograms. How many kilograms has he lost?

5. A patient had a temperature of 101.4°F. If after medication, the patient's temperature is 99.6°F, what is the decrease in temperature?

◆◆◆◆ Multiplication of Decimals

REVIEW

To multiply decimals, use the same process as in whole number multiplication, but do not line up the decimals. In decimal multiplication, the decimal places are counted, not aligned.

EXAMPLE

$$4.75 \times .4$$

STEP 1: Write the problem vertically.

$$\begin{array}{r} 4.75 \\ \times \quad .4 \\ \hline \end{array}$$

STEP 2: Multiply the numbers.

$$\begin{array}{r} 4.75 \\ \times \quad .4 \\ \hline 1900 \end{array}$$

STEP 3: Count the total number of decimal places in the two numbers multiplied together. Count these places from the right to the left. Then begin at the right of the answer and count over the same number of places and place the decimal point.

$$\begin{array}{r} 4.75 \\ \cup\cup \;\; 2 \text{ places} \\ 0.4 \\ \cup \;\; 1 \text{ place} \\ \hline 1.9\,0\,0 \\ \cup\cup\cup \end{array}$$

Place the decimal point three places from the right. The extra zeros are dropped unless they serve a particular purpose, such as place holders for money in dollar figures.

$$\begin{array}{ll} 17.750 & \rightarrow 17.75 \\ 205.12600 & \rightarrow 205.126 \\ \$12.00 & \rightarrow \$12.00 \end{array}$$

Practice 13

Set up the multiplication problems vertically and then solve them:

1. 12.5×3

2. 7.8×7

3. 25×1.6

4. 54×0.7

5. 10.2×12

6. 0.752×50

7. 6.74×0.12

8. 3.190×0.56

9. 0.278×1.7

10. 4.79×2.2

11. 0.07×0.03

12. 2.4×0.28

13. 5.175×29.2

14. $3,764 \times 13.75$

15. 9.708×0.17

16. 114.6×22.6

17. 190.8×0.04

18. 827.9×1.9

19. 574×12.095

20. 0.135×73.7

21. 53.9×24.9

22. 204.7×13.87

23. 0.347×28.95

24. 94.13×32.09

Practice 14

Use multiplication to solve the following word problems.

1. Village Center health care workers' earnings start at $10.52 an hour. If the employees work 40 hours per week, what is the minimum amount that each worker could earn in a week?

2. One mile has 1.6 kilometers. How many kilometers are in 35.5 miles?

3. Sheila earns $13.05 an hour. If she works 124 hours in August, what are her gross earnings for the month?

4. One kilogram equals 2.2 pounds. If patient A weighs 79.5 kilograms, what is his weight in pounds?

5. The recreation department is making placemats. The cost of materials for each placemat is $1.28. The activity director is estimating the cost of materials for 100 placemats. What is the estimated budget needed for this project?

◆◆◆◆ Division of Decimals

REVIEW

To divide decimals, one needs to place the decimal point first, and then divide the numbers. Once the decimal point is placed, it is not moved. Students have a tendency to want to move the decimal point once the division process is underway; the result is an error in decimal placement.

Follow the steps below to divide a number that has a decimal in the dividend:

STEP 1: Move the decimal point straight up to the same place in the quotient. Place the decimal point and then divide the numbers.

$$6\overline{)2.58}$$

STEP 2: Divide, adding a zero in front of all decimal numbers that do not include a whole number.

$$
\begin{array}{r}
0.43 \\
6\overline{)2.58} \\
\underline{24} \\
18 \\
\underline{18} \\
0
\end{array}
$$

Practice 15

Divide the following decimals to solve. Round to the nearest thousandth, if needed.

1. $6\overline{)44.35}$

2. $7\overline{)103.5}$

3. $4\overline{)0.649}$

4. $21\overline{)9.03}$

5. $12\overline{)1.44}$

6. $4\overline{)68.4}$

7. $32\overline{)1676.8}$

8. $17\overline{)51.17}$

9. $25\overline{)75.50}$

10. $34\overline{)2603.72}$

SET-UP HINT

Remember in division problem setup:

475 ÷ 4.5 =

→ *4.5)475

*The last number in the problem divides into the first number. You would read this as 475 divided by 4.5.

ZEROS AS PLACE HOLDERS IN DECIMAL DIVISION

Health care students may need some practice in dividing decimals that involve zeros in the quotient. This is one area where errors are commonly made. To avoid making these errors, recall that after you have brought a number down from the dividend, you must apply the divisor to that number. Place the decimal point and then divide the number. If the divisor does not go into the dividend, then you must place a zero in the quotient. Use a zero to hold a space.

EXAMPLE

$$
\begin{array}{r}
2.405 \\
14\overline{)33.67} \\
28\downarrow \\
\hline
56 \\
56\downarrow \\
\hline
07 \\
0\downarrow \\
\hline
70 \\
70 \\
\hline
0
\end{array}
$$

Because 14 cannot go into 7, place a zero in the quotient.

To divide a decimal number by a decimal number, change the divisor to a whole number by moving the decimal point to the right. Then move the decimal point in the dividend the same number of places. Use zeros as place holders if needed. Then place the decimal point and divide.

For example, $0.42\overline{)0.6216}$

STEP 1: Move the decimal $0.42\overline{)0.6216}$ Rewrite → $42\overline{)62.16}$

STEP 2: Divide $42\overline{)62.16}$

Practice 16

Use division to solve the following problems. Remember to use zeros as place holders.

1. 640 ÷ 0.4

2. 0.084 ÷ 12

3. 24.03 ÷ 0.03

4. 0.081 ÷ 9

5. 0.025 ÷ 6

6. 0.6250 ÷ 5

7. 183.96 ÷ 6

8. 6.030 ÷ 3

9. 0.18891 ÷ 0.9

10. 12.24 ÷ 4

Practice 17

Use division to solve the following problems. Remember to use zeros as place holders.

1. $0.5\overline{)3.02}$

2. $0.04\overline{)82.04}$

3. $2\overline{)10.008}$

4. $0.65\overline{)8.4825}$

5. $25\overline{)26}$

6. $0.7\overline{)78.75}$

7. $0.02\overline{)8.078}$

8. $0.3\overline{)4.608}$

◆◆◆◆ Simplified Multiplication and Division of Decimals

REVIEW

Using the shortcuts of **simplified multiplication and division** can save time when working with decimals. Simplified multiplication and division use units of ten to either multiply or divide. The reason they are simplified is that the decimal place is modified by moving the decimal right for multiplication and left for division. In health care fields, this shortcut is important to your work in metrics and in efficiently working longer problems.

This shortcut works only with multiples of ten: 10, 100, 1,000, etc. The process is straightforward. To multiply, move the decimal point to the right. To divide, move the decimal point to the left. The number of spaces you move the decimal point depends on which multiple you are working with. Look at the number of zeros included in the multiple, and then move the decimal in either direction depending on the operation. For both multiplication and division, be sure to use the correct number of spaces and number of zeros.

SIMPLIFIED MULTIPLICATION

To multiply by 10, locate the decimal point and move it to the right by one place.

To multiply by 100, locate the decimal point and move it to the right by two places.

To multiply by 1,000, locate the decimal point and move it to the right by three places.

Whole numbers have their decimal places on the far right of the last digit: 9 = 9., 75 = 75., 125 = 125.

EXAMPLE

$$4.5 \times 10 = 45 \qquad 4.5$$
$$4.5 = 45 \qquad \underline{\times\ 10}$$
$$\cup \qquad\qquad 45.0 \quad \text{(The zero is dropped.)}$$

Note that the answer is the same if the problem is worked the long way. Sometimes zeros must be added as place holders.

   In simplified multiplication locate the decimal point, count the zeros in the divisor, and move the decimal point the same number of places to the right.

EXAMPLE

Zeros must fill the spaces if needed.

$$34.7 \times 1000 = \underline{\qquad}$$
$$34.7\ 0\ 0 =$$
$$\cup\ \cup\cup \rightarrow 34{,}700$$

Practice 18

Use simplified multiplication to solve the following problems.

1. 75.3×10

2. 14.23×100

3. 228.05×10

4. $1{,}000 \times 74.28$

5. 0.09×100

6. 0.523×10

7. $45.07 \times 1{,}000$

8. 0.875×100

9. $0.476 \times 1{,}000$

10. 87×10

11. 1.345×10

12. $98.345 \times 1{,}000$

13. 1.009×10

14. 32.901×100

15. $23.850 \times 1{,}000$

SIMPLIFIED DIVISION

To divide by 10, locate the decimal point and move it to the left by one place.

To divide by 100, locate the decimal point and move it to the left by two places.

To divide by 1,000, locate the decimal point and move it to the left by three places.

In simplified division, locate the decimal point, count the zeros in the divisor, and move the decimal point the same number of places to the left.

EXAMPLE

$9.5 \div 10 =$ _____ $0.75 \div 100 =$ _____

9.5   0 0 0.75 → 0.0075   Zeros must be used to fill

∪ → 0.95   ∪∪   in places if needed.

Practice 19

Use simplified division to solve the following problems.

1. $48.5 \div 10 =$ _____

2. $3.08 \div 100 =$ _____

3. $250 \div 10 =$ _____

4. $4,349.02 \div 1,000 =$ _____

5. $0.035 \div 10 =$ _____

6. $175.2 \div 100 =$ _____

7. $25.4 \div 100 =$ _____

8. $3,234 \div 10 =$ _____

9. $32.50 \div 100 =$ _____

10. $0.09 \div 10 =$ _____

11. $10,010 \div 1,000 =$ _____

12. $9,765 \div 1,000 =$ _____

13. $3.076 \div 100 =$ _____

14. $429.6 \div 1,000 =$ _____

15. $10.275 \div 100 =$ _____

Practice 20

Use what you've learned about decimals to solve the following word problems.

1. A nursing student spends $379.50 for textbooks. If the student purchases six textbooks, what is the average cost of each book?

2. A patient's goal is to lose 24.6 pounds. The doctor wants the patient to lose these pounds slowly, over a twelve-month period. How many pounds should the patient attempt to lose each month?

3. Doctor Brown prescribed a medication dosage of 4.5 grams. How many 1.5 gram tablets need to be administered?

4. The dietitian serves a protein dish at three meals. If the total daily grams of protein are 33.39 grams, what is the average meal's grams of protein, assuming that the grams are equally divided among the three daily meals?

5. Bob made $131.20 in 5 hours. What is his hourly wage?

6. Larry is working in the storeroom moving boxes of medical supplies. Each box weighs 10.4 pounds. There are 24 boxes in a carton. How many pounds would a carton of medical supplies weigh?

7. Each sheet of film is 0.005 inches thick. How many sheets of film would create a stack of film that is 5 inches high?

8. The billing office is trying to figure out the amount of 0.75 hour overtime for a worker who is paid $32.48 for a regular hourly rate. The overtime rate is 1.5 of his regular hourly rate. How much is 0.75 of an hour at the overtime rate for this individual?

9. The cost of examination gloves has increased. The box of 100 is now $3.58. If a case contains 20 boxes, how much is the total cost before tax for a case of examination gloves?

10. Patient gowns are $29.95 a dozen. What is the cost per gown?

◆◆◆◆ Changing Decimals to Fractions

REVIEW

It is important to be able to convert between number systems so that you are comfortable with comparing sizes of items or quantities of supplies. Changing decimals to fractions requires the use of decimal places and placing the numbers in fractions that represent the very same numbers.

EXAMPLE

Convert 0.457 to a fraction.

STEP 1: To convert a decimal to a fraction, count the number of decimal places in the decimal number.

0.4̲5̲7̲   Three decimal places means thousandths in decimal numbers.

STEP 2: Write the number 457 as the numerator and 1,000 as the denominator.

$$\frac{457}{1,000}$$

STEP 3: Reduce if necessary. Here, $\frac{457}{1,000}$ cannot be reduced. The answer is $\frac{457}{1,000}$.

EXAMPLE

Convert 2.75 to a fraction.

STEP 1: Place 2 as the whole number. Your answer is going to be a mixed number because there is a whole number. Count the decimal places in .7̲5̲ = two places.

$$2 \underline{}$$

STEP 2: Write 75 as the numerator and 100 as the denominator.

$$2\frac{75}{100}$$

STEP 3: Reduce the fraction to $2\frac{3}{4}$ because

$$\frac{75}{100} = \frac{\cancel{25} \times 3}{\cancel{25} \times 4} \rightarrow \frac{3}{4}$$

The answer is $2\frac{3}{4}$.

Practice 21

Convert the decimals to fractions and reduce if necessary:

1. 0.08

2. 0.075

3. 14.2

4. 3.75

5. 125.05

6. 15.06

7. 9.25

8. 0.28

9. 9.3

10. 100.46

Convert scale weights to fractions.

11.
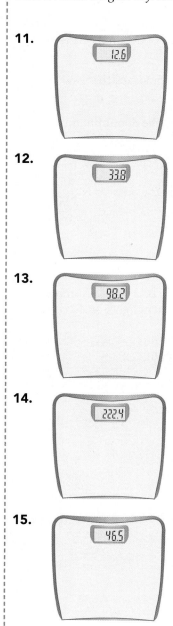

12.

13.

14.

15.

◆◆◆◆ Changing Fractions to Decimals

REVIEW

To change fractions to decimals, divide the denominator into the numerator. Critical to the success of this division is the placement of the decimal point. Once it is placed, do not move it.

EXAMPLE

Change $\frac{3}{4}$ to a decimal. Divide the denominator into the numerator. Place a decimal point after 3 and also in the quotient. Then add a zero after 3 and divide. Add zeros as needed to continue the division process.

$$
\begin{array}{r}
.75 \\
4\overline{)3.0} \\
28\downarrow \\
\hline
20 \\
20 \\
\hline
0
\end{array}
$$

EXAMPLE

Change $\frac{1}{3}$ to a decimal. Divide 3 into 1. Place the decimal point. Add zeros as needed to continue division. The division may not come out evenly but begin to repeat itself. After two places, make the remainder into a fraction by putting the remaining number over the divisor.

$$
\begin{array}{r}
.33\frac{1}{3} \\
3\overline{)1.0} \\
9\downarrow \\
\hline
10 \\
9 \\
\hline
1
\end{array}
$$

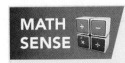

MATH SENSE

When the decimal answer is a number like 0.50, drop the final zero so that the answer is 0.5.

Practice 22

Change the following fractions to decimals.

1. $\frac{1}{2}$

2. $\frac{3}{5}$

3. $\frac{7}{8}$

4. $\frac{1}{6}$

5. $\frac{6}{25}$

6. $\frac{5}{12}$

7. $\frac{3}{15}$

8. $\dfrac{7}{10}$

9. $\dfrac{5}{6}$

10. $\dfrac{3}{18}$

◆◆◆◆ Temperature Conversions with Decimals

In some instances, you will need to make temperature conversions that include decimals. To perform these conversions, round the decimal numbers in temperatures to the nearest tenth place. The temperature conversion you reviewed in Unit 2: Fractions relied on fractions. The same fraction method can be converted into a decimal method. In deciding which method to use, select the method of fractions or decimals based on your stronger skill. Then consistently use that conversion formula.

DECIMAL CONVERSION FORMULA

To convert Celsius to Fahrenheit, (°C × 1.8) + 32 = °F

To convert Fahrenheit to Celsius, (°F − 32) ÷ 1.8 = °C

EXAMPLE

Convert from Celsius to Fahrenheit:

$$41°C = \underline{\hspace{1cm}} °F$$

STEP 1: Solve inside the parentheses first, and then work left to right. Multiply the Celsius temperature by 1.8. The number 1.8 is the decimal form of $\dfrac{9}{5}$.

$$
\begin{array}{r}
41 \\
\times\ 1.8 \\
\hline
328 \\
41\ \ \\
\hline
73.8
\end{array}
$$

STEP 2: Add 32 to the step 1 answer.

$$
\begin{array}{r}
73.8 \\
+32\ \ \\
\hline
105.8
\end{array}
$$

The answer is 105.8°F.

To convert from Fahrenheit to Celsius:

STEP 1: Subtract the 32 from the Fahrenheit temperature.

$$
\begin{array}{r}
107.6 \\
-32\ \ \\
\hline
75.6
\end{array}
$$

STEP 2: Divide the step 1 answer by 1.8.

$$\to 1.8\overline{)75.6} \to \qquad \begin{array}{r} 42. \\ 18\overline{)756.} \\ \underline{72} \\ 36 \\ \underline{36} \\ 0 \end{array}$$

The answer is 42°C.

Practice 23

Convert the following temperatures using the decimal conversion formula.

1. 12°C = _____°F

2. 42°C = _____°F

3. 69°C = _____°F

4. 101.5°C = _____°C

5. 46.6°F = _____°C

6. 40°F = _____°C

7. 100.4°F = _____°C

8. 69°C = _____°F

9. 12°C = _____°F

10. 105.8°F = _____°C

◆◆◆◆ ## Solving Mixed Fraction and Decimal Problems

REVIEW

Sometimes problems will include both fractions and decimals. The very same processes of solving the problems are still needed; however, the order of handling the parts of the problem may vary. Group the math computations inside the problem to best manage the separate operations.

SET-UP HINT

If the problem has a complex fraction multiplied by a decimal number, work the complex fraction first. Then complete the decimal multiplication.

EXAMPLE

$$\frac{\frac{1}{2}}{\frac{1}{5}} \times 2.2 =$$

STEP 1:
$$\frac{1}{2} \div \frac{1}{5} \rightarrow \frac{1}{2} \times \frac{5}{1} = \frac{5}{2}$$

Reduce to $2\frac{1}{2}$. Make the $\frac{1}{2}$ into 0.5 so that the multiplication is easy. Thus, the answer after first working the complex fraction is 2.5.

STEP 2: Then multiply 2.5 × 2.2.

$$
\begin{array}{r}
2.5 \\
\times\ 2.2 \\
\hline
50 \\
50 \\
\hline
5.50
\end{array}
$$

The answer to this mixed problem is 5.5.

SET-UP HINT

If the problem includes a decimal number, solve the decimals by first multiplying straight across, and then complete the process by dividing that answer by the denominator. This allows for the division of decimals only once, which saves time.

EXAMPLE

$$\frac{0.25}{0.5} \times 1.5$$

STEP 1: Multiply 0.25 × 1.5.

$$
\begin{array}{r}
0.25 \\
\times\ 1.5 \\
\hline
125 \\
25 \\
\hline
0.375
\end{array}
$$

STEP 2: Divide 0.375 by 0.5.

$$0.5\overline{)0.375}$$

$$
\begin{array}{r}
0.75 \\
0.5\overline{)0.375} \\
\underline{0.35} \\
0025 \\
\underline{0025} \\
0
\end{array}
$$

The answer is 0.75.

Practice 24

Solve the following mixed fraction and decimal problems.

1. $\dfrac{\frac{1}{200}}{\frac{1}{100}} \times 4.4$

5. $\dfrac{0.002}{0.125} \times 10.5$

2. $\dfrac{0.8}{0.64} \times 4.5$

6. $\dfrac{\frac{1}{12}}{\frac{1}{6}} \times 3.6$

3. $\dfrac{\frac{3}{4}}{\frac{1}{4}} \times 2.5$

7. $\dfrac{0.005}{0.01} \times 15.35$

4. $\dfrac{0.75}{0.15} \times 1.5$

8. $\dfrac{7\frac{1}{2}}{1\frac{1}{2}} \times 5.4$

UNIT REVIEW

◆◆◆◆ Critical Thinking Using Decimals

1. What is the largest number that can round up to 0.25?

2. Write pairs of decimal numbers to complete the chart below. Your answers will vary, as there are many ways to finish the chart:

Sums			Differences		
> than 1	= to 1	< than 1	> than 1	= to 1	< than 1

3. Estimate the product of 57.3 and 18.

4. What is the number of decimal places in the product of 8.46 and 0.4?

5. A graduated cylinder of 100 milliliters was on the table in the laboratory. The range of cylinders is 12 milliliters. What is the height of the shortest graduated cylinder in the lab?

6. Your heart pushes approximately 1.25 gallons of blood a minute through its chambers. How many gallons of blood are pushed through the heart in 8 hours?

7. Calculate how many tablets are needed to fill an order for 0.5 milligram of a medication with 0.25 milligram tablets. You will need _____ tablets.

8. Order from the smallest to the largest: $\frac{2}{3}, \frac{7}{8}, 0.5, \frac{2}{5}$.

9. A patient was given half of a 15 milligram tablet. This is equivalent to _____ milligrams.

10. 5.4 hours equals _____ hours and _____ minutes.

11–15.   Calculate the unit prices for the following items:

Item	Cost	Unit Price
Box of 100-count 1 milliliter syringes	$12.75	_____
Case of 1,000 latex-free size large gloves	$69.11	_____
Pack of 24 Silverlon adhesive strips	$14.25	_____
Pack of 200 4 × 4 sterile gauze sponges	$9.86	_____

◆◆◆◆ Professional Expertise

- Decimals look like periods, not commas.
- Use a zero as a place holder if there is no whole number given in a decimal number: 0.045, not .045.
- Align the decimals for addition and subtraction.

- Remember to move the decimal point in the divisor the same number of spaces in the number being divided into.
- Do not round more than needed because doing so might create an error. Round as close to the final step as possible.

DECIMAL POST-TEST

1. Write in words: 0.065

2. What is the sum of 1.7, 19, 0.25, and 0.8?

3. $29 - 0.075$

4. 75×1.8

5. $24.02 \div 0.2$

6. Round to the nearest hundredth: 978.735

7. Order these decimals from largest to smallest: 0.81, 0.080, 0.018, 8.018.

8. 10.009×100

9. A child receives 0.5 milligrams of a drug 4 times a day. How many milligrams is the child's daily dose?

10. A patient receives 2.25 grams of a medication daily. Tablets come in 0.75 gram dosages. How many tablets does the patient take daily?

11. Convert this decimal to a fraction: 0.125

12. Convert this fraction to a decimal: $\dfrac{13}{50}$

13. Convert this fraction to a decimal: $3\dfrac{5}{8}$

14. Convert 103° Fahrenheit to °Celsius.

15. Solve:

$$\dfrac{0.136}{0.2} \times 2.5$$

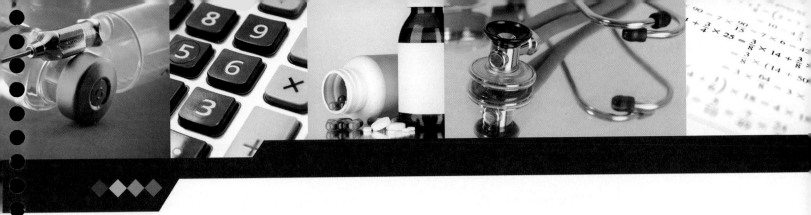

4 Ratio and Proportion

After completing the tasks in this unit, you will be able to:

4-1 Define ratio and proportion

4-2 Locate and decipher ratios in common health applications such as drug labels

4-3 Determine if two ratios are a proportion

4-4 Simplify ratios and complex ratios

4-5 Apply ratio definitions to express unit rates

4-6 Solve for x or an unknown in a proportion

4-7 Apply proportions to nutrition labels.

◆◆◆◆ Overview

Ratio is a way to show a relationship between two items. We are always counting and comparing items in our daily lives: hours at work versus hours away from work, number of yogurts we have eaten versus the number of yogurts still in the refrigerator, and so on. Ratios simply help us compare two items, objects, or amounts.

Proportion compares two equal ratios in a mathematical equation. We use proportion to either increase or decrease one part of the ratio in the equation so that the unit expressed or found is in the same relationship with the other part of the specific ratio and so that this ratio, when completed, shows the same relationship as the other ratio.

PRE-TEST

1. One kilogram equals 2.2 pounds. How many pounds equal 24.5 kilograms?

2. Solve for x. $48 : 64 = x : 124$.

3. One cup contains 8 ounces. How many full cups are in 138 ounces?

4. Solve for x. $\dfrac{1}{8} : 3 = \dfrac{1}{4} : x$

5. Solve for x. $x : 225 = 2 : 5$

6. Write the ratio that represents three registered nurses to twelve certified nursing assistants.

7. The patient's pulse is documented as 73 beats per minute. How many beats will be documented for five minutes if the rate remains the same?

8. Two tablespoons of peanut butter are used for each sandwich. One tablespoon has three teaspoons. If 49 sandwiches are made, how many teaspoons of peanut butter are needed to make these sandwiches?

9. Write the medication dosage for the amount on this label. Write it as a ratio. Include the unit of measures.

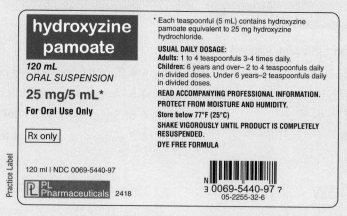

10. The tapioca recipe calls for $2\frac{1}{2}$ cups of milk to make six servings. How many cups of milk are needed for fifteen servings?

11. The dietitian ordered 4 ounces of chicken per patient for a dinner meal. The kitchen served 496 ounces of chicken this evening. How many patients received a 4 ounce portion of chicken?

12. The patient went to the laboratory to have blood drawn by a phlebotomist. Each tube of blood holds 2.5 milliliters of blood. Four tubes of blood were drawn. How many milliliters of blood were drawn?

13. On average, one registered nurse at Valley View uses 62 gloves a day to examine patients. In five days, how many gloves will that particular nurse use?

14. Solve for x. $\frac{4}{75} : 15 :: x : 20$

15. How many minutes are in 320 seconds? Your answer should be in minutes and seconds.

◆◆◆◆ Ratio

REVIEW

A ratio is used to show a relationship between two numbers or a comparison of two items. The numbers are separated by a colon (:) as in $x : y$. For example, 3 nurses and 4 medical assistants working a clinic shift can form a ratio. Ratios may be presented in three formats that provide the setup for solving proportions.

a. $3 : 4$ (3 nurses to 4 medical assistants)

b. $\dfrac{3}{4}$ (3 nurses to 4 medical assistants)

c. 3 is to 4 (3 nurses to 4 medical assistants)

The relationship can represent something as simple as the $1 : 3$ ratio commonly used to mix frozen juices. We use 1 can of frozen juice concentrate to 3 cans of water. Ratios are fractions that represent a part-to-whole relationship. Often when we work with ratios, we use the fraction format to reduce the ratio to its simplest form.

Ratios are always reduced to their lowest form. For example, 8 hours of sleep to 24 hours in a day would be expressed as

$$8 : 24 \rightarrow \frac{8}{24} \quad \frac{8 \times 1}{8 \times 3} = \frac{1}{3},$$ so the ratio is $1 : 3$.

SET-UP HINT

Writing your ratios in the proper order is important. Follow the order of each number of the ratio in the sentence or problem. It is a good idea to include the units. In that way, you can be sure that you have followed the same pattern in each ratio.

Practice 1

Write the following relationships as ratios using a colon. Reduce to lowest terms if necessary.

1. 6 days out of 7 days _____

2. twelve teeth out of thirty-two teeth _____

3. 8 students out of 15 students _____

4. 16 scalpels to 45 syringes _____

5. 7 inlays to 14 crowns _____

Simplifying ratios is an important skill. To simplify a ratio, divide the first number by the second.

For example, simplify the following ratio: $4\dfrac{1}{2} : 6$.

$$4\frac{1}{2} \div 6 \rightarrow \frac{9}{2} \div \frac{6}{1} \rightarrow \frac{9}{2} \times \frac{1}{6} = \frac{9}{12} \rightarrow \frac{3 \times 3}{3 \times 4} = \frac{3}{4} \quad \begin{array}{l} \text{which becomes } 3 : 4 \\ \text{as a simplified ratio} \end{array}$$

The answer is $3 : 4$.

As another example, simplify the following ratio: $11\frac{1}{4}$. Convert the mixed number into an improper fraction, and then reduce if necessary.

$$11\frac{1}{4} \rightarrow 11 \times 4 + 1 = 45 \rightarrow \frac{45}{4} = 45:4$$

The answer is $45:4$.

Practice 2

Simplify the following ratios. Write each answer as a ratio.

1. $24 : 3\frac{1}{4} = $ _____

2. $\frac{7}{8} : 14 = $ _____

3. $25 : \frac{5}{6} = $ _____

4. $\frac{1}{3} : 45 = $ _____

5. $0.8 : \frac{2}{5} = $ _____

6. $\frac{1}{2} : \frac{1}{8} = $ _____

7. $4\frac{1}{3} : 7 = $ _____

8. $0.875 : \frac{1}{4} = $ _____

9. $2\frac{1}{2} = $ _____

10. $\frac{2}{3} : 0.33 = $ _____

RATIOS IN HEALTH CARE

Drug labels are another place that ratios may be seen in health care. Careful reading of the drug label will help locate the dosage of medication per tablet or per amount of solution. Notice that each label uses a specific language indicating a ratio. These formats are milligrams/milliliters (mg/mL), micrograms/milligrams (mcg/mg), mg per tablet, milligrams in milliliters (mg in mL), etc. Careful reading will help identify what is in each tablet, each milliliter of medication, etc.

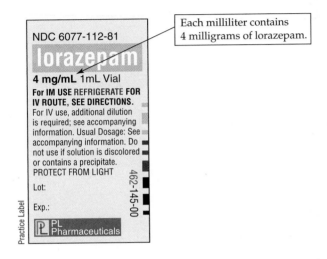

Each milliliter contains 4 milligrams of lorazepam.

Practice 3

Read the labels and write the ratio of the medication indicated in each label. Write the ratio in simplified form.

1. _____

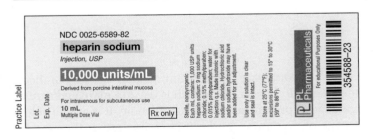

2. _____

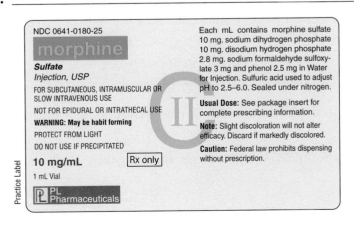

3. _____

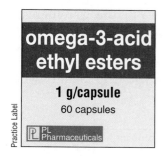

4. _____

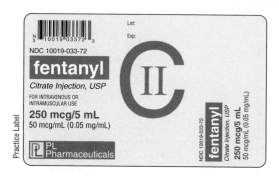

5. _____

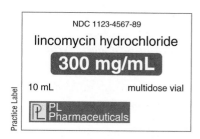

◆

Another example of ratio in health care comes from dealing with insurance coverage. There is something called a medical loss ratio, which is used in managed care to measure medical costs as a percentage of premium revenues or income. It is a type of loss ratio used to measure the percentage of premiums paid out in claims rather than expenses. A desirable ratio is 17 : 20 or 85% or less.

In addition, ratios can compare two items. For example, ratios are often used to find the unit rate, which is a rate having 1 as its denominator. Rate is a ratio of two measurements having different units.

$$\text{Example: } \frac{\$4.10\,(\text{a package of gauze strips})}{24\,(\text{individual number of strips})}$$

To get the unit rate, divide the bottom number (the denominator) into the top number (the numerator).

$$\$4.10 \div 24 = 0.170833 \text{ or } 17 \text{ cents per sheet of gauze}$$

17 cents : 1 sheet or 17 : 1

Practice 4

Express each as a unit rate.

1. $\dfrac{\$4{,}182 \text{ room bill for a hospital stay}}{3 \text{ days in the hospital}}$ _____

2. $\dfrac{120 \text{ pound goal to lose}}{52 \text{ weeks in a year}}$ _____

3. $\dfrac{24 \text{ ounces}}{3 \text{ cups}}$ _____

4. $\dfrac{14 \text{ cups of sugar}}{252 \text{ cookies}}$ _____

5. $\dfrac{14{,}235 \text{ patients}}{365 \text{ days}}$ _____

◆◆◆◆ Proportion

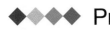 **REVIEW**

Proportions can be applied to almost every health care profession in one way or another. In addition to on-the-job applications, proportions provide a simple and quick method for solving many everyday math problems such as measurement conversions, recipe conversions for increasing or decreasing the amounts of ingredients, and map mileage.

Proportions are two or more equivalent ratios or fractions in which the terms of the first ratio/fraction have the same part-to-whole relationship as the second ratio/fraction.

EXAMPLE

If one box of gloves contains 100 gloves, then $4\frac{1}{2}$ boxes will contain how many gloves?

$$\frac{1 \text{ box}}{100 \text{ gloves}} = \frac{4\frac{1}{2} \text{ boxes}}{x \text{ number of gloves}}$$

Once you become well versed in the setup, you may drop the units. However, labeling the units is very helpful to ensure the proper setup.

$$\frac{3}{4} = \frac{15}{20} \text{ or } 3:4::15:20$$

Test the two ratios/fractions to see whether they are equivalent by multiplying diagonally (cross multiply).

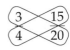 $4 \times 15 = 60$ and $3 \times 20 = 60$. This is a proportion.

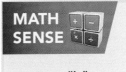 **SET-UP HINT**

Notice how the terms for each category (boxes and gloves) are across from each other. This is the proper setup: boxes across from boxes and gloves across from gloves.

MATH SENSE

: : means "is" or =

If the two numbers that are diagonal result in the same answer when they are multiplied, you are working with a proportion.

Proportions are powerful tools in health care. You can rely on them for solving a majority of your math conversions and problems.

Practice 5

Check to see if the following ratios are proportions:

Are these ratios proportions?

1. $5:2 = 4:1$ _____ Yes _____ No

2. $16:15 = 8:7$ _____ Yes _____ No

3. $40:30 = 4:3$ _____ Yes _____ No

4. $10:16 = 5:8$ _____ Yes _____ No

5. $100:1 = 50:2$ _____ Yes _____ No

◆◆◆◆ Solving for x

REVIEW

The ratio and proportion method is used to solve for x. Solving for x uses the known or given information to find what is not known or given. Since a proportion consists of two equal ratios, the relationship between the numerator and denominator of each fraction is the same for each ratio of the proportion. This is important to know when one must increase or decrease a solution or mixture because the ratio of ingredients must remain constant.

Solving for x is done in two steps.

STEP 1: Set the problems up like fractions. If units of measure such as inches and feet are given, place inches across from inches and feet across from feet. Then cross multiply (diagonally) the two numbers. Set the ratios up like fractions using a vertical line.

$$\frac{3}{4} = \frac{?}{16} \qquad 3 \times 16 = 48$$

STEP 2: Divide the answer from step 1 by the remaining number.

$$
\begin{array}{r}
12 \\
4\overline{)48} \\
\underline{4\downarrow} \\
8 \\
\underline{8} \\
\end{array}
$$

The quotient 12 is the answer to ? or x. This method is an easy way to find the answers for measurement conversions, dosage conversions, and math questions that provide part but not all of the information.

Practice 6

Solve for x or ?

1. $12 : 45 = x : 15$ _____

2. $x : 6 = 15 : 60$ _____

3. $25 : 45 = 75 : x$ _____

4. $7 : x = 21 : 24$ _____

5. $3 : 9 = ? : 81$ _____

6. $13 : 39 = 1 : ?$ _____

7. $2 : 11 = ? : 77$ _____

8. $x : 125 = 5 : 25$ _____

9. $2 : 26 = 4 : ?$ _____

10. $1 : x = 5 : 200$ _____

Using ratios is often the simplest method of solving other health care math problems, such as dosage calculations and measurement problems.

EXAMPLE

Zoe weighs 35 pounds. Her doctor prescribed a drug that relates milligrams of medication to kilograms of body weight. The pharmacy technician will need to convert pounds to kilograms. By using the ratio of 1 kilogram to 2.2 pounds, the answer is quickly computed.

$$\underset{\text{2.2 pounds}}{\overset{\text{1 kilogram}}{\underbrace{}}} \overset{known}{} = \underset{\text{35 pounds}}{\overset{\text{? kilograms}}{\underbrace{}}} \overset{unknown}{}$$

STEP 1: Multiply the numbers diagonally.

$$1 \times 35 = 35$$

STEP 2: Divide 35 by 2.2. The answer is 15.9 kilograms.

So 35 pounds equals 15.9 kilograms.

Converting between kilograms and pounds is a common procedure in health care.

Practice 7

Set up and solve these conversions using ratio and proportions. Round to the nearest tenth if necessary. Use the conversion 1 kilogram = 2.2 pounds.

1. Convert 16.4 kilograms to pounds. _____

2. Convert 125.8 kilograms to pounds. _____

3. Convert 35 kilograms to pounds. _____

4. Convert 75 kilograms to pounds. _____

5. Convert 83.5 kilograms to pounds. _____

6. Convert 16 pounds to kilograms. _____

7. Convert $25\frac{1}{2}$ pounds to kilograms. _____

8. Convert 108 pounds to kilograms. _____

9. Convert 215.6 pounds to kilograms. _____

10. Convert 165 pounds to kilograms. _____

EXAMPLE

How many pounds are in 24 ounces?

Set the problem up by placing what you know on the left side of the equation and what you do not know on the right side. If you set up all your problems with the known on the left and the unknown on the right, there will be less information for your brain to process because the pattern will be familiar to you.

$$\underset{\text{16 ounces}}{\frac{\overset{known}{\text{1 pound}}}{}} \qquad \underset{\text{24 ounces}}{\frac{\overset{unknown}{\text{? pounds}}}{}}$$

STEP 1: $1 \times 24 = 24$

STEP 2: $24 \div 16 = 1.5$

The answer is $1\frac{1}{2}$ pounds or 1.5 pounds.

The answer in a ratio may have a decimal or a fraction in it.

EXAMPLE

Bob is 176 centimeters (cm) tall. How tall is he in inches? Round the answer to the nearest tenth.

$$\underset{\text{2.54 cm}}{\frac{\overset{known}{\text{1 inch}}}{}} \qquad \underset{\text{176 cm}}{\frac{\overset{unknown}{\text{? inches}}}{}}$$

STEP 1: $1 \times 176 = 176$

STEP 2: $176 \div 2.54 = 69.29$

$$
\begin{array}{r}
69.29 \\
254\overline{)17600} \\
1524\downarrow \\
\overline{2360} \\
2286\downarrow \\
\overline{740} \\
508\downarrow \\
\overline{2320} \\
2286 \\
\overline{34}
\end{array}
$$

So, after the division: $176 \div 2.54 = 69.29$. Rounded to the nearest tenth, the answer is 69.3 inches.

Notice that the units in the metric system are often rounded to the nearest tenth. This is why the division problem above adds a decimal and zeros: to work out the dividend to the hundredths place so that the final answer is rounded to the tenth.

APPROXIMATE EQUIVALENTS

1 inch	= 2.54 centimeters	1 cup	= 8 ounces
1 foot	= 12 inches	1 pint	= 480 milliliters*
1 yard	= 3 feet	1 quart	= 32 ounces
1 pound	= 16 ounces	1 quart	= 960 milliliters*
1 kilogram	= 2.2 pounds	1 pint	= 2 cups
1 tablespoon	= 3 teaspoons	1 fluid ounce	= 30 milliliters
1 quart	= 2 pints	1 teaspoon	= 5 milliliters
1 gallon	= 4 quarts	1 fluid ounce	= 2 tablespoons

*Certain fields use rounded measures; for example, instead of 480 mL and 960 mL, they use 500 mL and 1,000 mL. Check with your instructor.

Notice that the conversions are set up so that the unit (1) elements are all on the left and that these will be placed on the top of the known part of the ratio and proportion equation. This simplifies the learning process, expedites learning, and helps recall of these conversions.

Practice 8

Using this ratio and proportion setup, solve the following conversions.

$$\frac{known}{\rule{1.5cm}{0.4pt}} = \frac{unknown}{\rule{1.5cm}{0.4pt}}$$

Set up these conversions using ratios and proportions.

1. 23 feet = _____ yards → $\dfrac{1 \text{ yd}}{3 \text{ ft}} = \dfrac{?}{23 \text{ ft}}$

2. 18 quarts = _____ gallons

3. 3 quarts = _____ pints

4. $2\dfrac{1}{4}$ pints = _____ cups

5. 3 tablespoons = _____ teaspoons

6. $2\dfrac{1}{2}$ quarts = _____ milliliters

7. $\dfrac{1}{2}$ cup = _____ ounces

8. 1 injection at \$29.50 = 3 injections at _____

9. $3\dfrac{1}{2}$ pounds = _____ ounces

10. 3 medicine cups = _____ milliliters
(One medicine cup equals 1 fluid ounce.)

11. 12.5 mL = _____ teaspoons

12. 5 fluid ounces = _____ tablespoons

13. _____ tablespoons = 15 teaspoons

14. 64 ounces = _____ cups

15. 750 milliliters = _____ pints

16. 48 inches = _____ feet

17. 5 pounds = _____ ounces

18. _____ quarts = 5000 milliliters

19. _____ kilograms = 11 pounds

20. 15 cups = _____ ounces

More practice with conversions of measurements between systems and with multiple steps in conversions will be given in Unit 6: Combined Applications.

◆◆◆◆ Word Problems Using Proportions

REVIEW

When solving word problems involving proportions, follow these three basic steps:

STEP 1: Set the problem up so that the same type of elements are directly across from one another.

EXAMPLE

If 12 eggs cost \$1.49, how much do 18 eggs cost?

$$\frac{\text{Eggs}}{\text{Cost}} = \frac{\text{Eggs}}{\text{Cost}} \rightarrow \frac{12 \text{ eggs}}{\$1.49} = \frac{18 \text{ eggs}}{\$?}$$

STEP 2: Multiply the diagonal numbers.
$$\$1.49 \times 18 = 26.82$$

STEP 3: Divide the answer from step 2 by the remaining number in the problem.
$$26.82 \div 12 = \$2.235 \text{ or } \$2.24$$

So, 18 eggs cost \$2.24.

EXAMPLE

How many milligrams of medication would a nurse administer to a 95-pound child if the prescribed dose was 30 milligrams for every 10 pounds?

STEP 1:

$$\frac{30 \text{ milligrams}}{10 \text{ pounds}} = \frac{x \text{ milligrams}}{95 \text{ pounds}}$$

STEP 2: $30 \times 95 = 2{,}850$

STEP 3: $2850 \div 10 = 285$ milligrams

So, the child would receive 285 milligrams of the medication.

EXAMPLE

The lab mixes a 12% solution for the physician. A 12% solution has a 3 : 25 ratio. This ratio includes 3 grams of powder in 25 milliliters of solution. How many grams of powder will be added to 65 milliliters of solution?

STEP 1:

$$\frac{3 \text{ grams}}{25 \text{ milliliters}} = \frac{x \text{ grams}}{65 \text{ milliliters}}$$

STEP 2: $3 \times 65 = 195$

STEP 3: $195 \div 25 = 7.8$ grams

So, 7.8 grams of powder will be used to mix 65 milliliters of the 3 : 25 solution.

Practice 9

Solve the following word problems.

1. A caplet contains 325 milligrams of medication. How many caplets contain 975 milligrams of medication?

2. If a dose of 100 milligrams is contained in 4 milliliters, how many milliliters are in 40 milligrams?

3. If 35 grams of a pure drug are contained in 150 milliliters, how many grams are contained in 75 milliliters?

4. Three tablets of ulcer medication contain 375 milligrams of medication. How many milligrams are in twelve tablets?

5. If 1 kilogram equals 2.2 pounds, how many kilograms are in 61.6 pounds?

◆◆◆◆ Solving for x in More Complex Problems Using Proportion

REVIEW

Decimals and fractions may appear in your proportion problems. Although the numbers may be visually distracting, the *very* same principles apply when solving these proportions.

EXAMPLE

$$0.25 \text{ mg} : 0.8 \text{ mL} = 0.125 \text{ mg} : x \text{ mL}$$

STEP 1: Place mg across from mg and mL across from mL. Place the known information on the left side of the equation and the unknown information on the right side.

$$\frac{\overset{known}{0.25 \text{ mg}}}{0.8 \text{ mL}} \quad \frac{\overset{unknown}{0.125 \text{ mg}}}{x \text{ mL}}$$

Cross multiply $0.8 \times 0.125 \text{ mg} = 0.1$.

STEP 2: $0.1 \div 0.25 = 0.4 \text{ mL}$

EXAMPLE

$$\frac{1}{8} : \frac{1}{2} :: 1 : x$$

STEP 1: Set up and cross multiply. Multiply $\frac{1}{2} \times 1 = \frac{1}{2}$.

$$\frac{\frac{1}{8}}{\frac{1}{2}} = \frac{1}{x}$$

STEP 2: Divide $\frac{1}{2}$ by $\frac{1}{8}$.

$$\frac{1}{2} \div \frac{1}{8} \rightarrow \frac{1}{2} \times \frac{8}{1} = \frac{8}{2}, \quad \text{which is reduced to 4.}$$

Sometimes you will find that medical dosages have both fractions and decimals. Analyze the situation and convert the numbers to the same system format. As a general rule, fractions are always more accurate for calculating than decimals because some decimal numbers have repeating digits, which create variable answers.

EXAMPLE

$$\frac{1}{16} : 1.6 :: \frac{1}{8} : x$$

STEP 1: Convert 1.6 into a fraction. So $1.6 = 1\frac{6}{10}$. Then multiply $1\frac{6}{10} \times \frac{1}{8} = \frac{2}{10}$

$$\frac{\frac{1}{16}}{1\frac{6}{10}} = \frac{\frac{1}{8}}{x} \qquad 1\frac{6}{10} \times \frac{1}{8} = \frac{16}{10} \times \frac{1}{8} = \frac{16}{80} \text{ or } \frac{2}{10}$$

STEP 2: Divide $\frac{2}{10}$ by $\frac{1}{16}$.

$$\frac{2}{10} \div \frac{1}{16} \rightarrow \frac{2}{10} \times \frac{16}{1} = \frac{32}{10} \quad \text{Reduced to } 3\frac{2}{10} \rightarrow 3\frac{1}{5}.$$

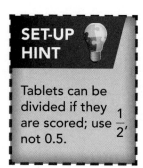

SET-UP HINT

Tablets can be divided if they are scored; use $\frac{1}{2}$, not 0.5.

Practice 10

Include a unit of measure in your answer. Round any partial unit to the nearest tenth.

1. 2.5 mg : 2 mL = 4.5 mg : x mL _____

2. 12 mg : 2.5 mL = 4 mg : x mL _____

3. 7.5 mg : 5 mL = 24 mg : x mL _____

4. 0.2 mg : 1 tab = 6 mg : x tabs _____

5. $\frac{1}{4}$ grains : 15 mg = ? grains : 60 mg _____

6. x mg : $\frac{1}{2}$ tab = 6 mg : 4 tabs _____

7. $\frac{1}{100}$ grains : 2 mL = $\frac{1}{150}$ grains : x mL _____

8. 600 mg : 1 cap = x mg : 2 caps _____

9. 1,000 units : 1 mL = 2,400 units : x mL _____

10. 1 tab : 0.1 mg = x tabs : 0.15 mg _____

11. A drug comes in 100 milligram tablets. If the doctor orders 150 milligrams daily, how many tablets should the patient receive daily?

12. A medical chart states that the patient weighs 78.4 kilograms. What is the patient's weight in pounds? Round to the nearest tenth.

Nutritional Application of Proportions

REVIEW

Carbohydrates, fats, and proteins provide fuel factors for our bodies. These factors are easily applied by using proportions to solve for the unknown.

> **SET-UP HINT**
>
> Carbohydrates → 4 calories per 1 gram
> Fats   → 9 calories per 1 gram
> Proteins   → 4 calories per 1 gram

EXAMPLE

400 carbohydrate calories = _____ grams

$$\underset{\text{known}}{\frac{1\ \text{gram}}{4\ \text{calories}}} = \underset{\text{unknown}}{\frac{?\ \text{grams}}{400\ \text{calories}}}$$

STEP 1: Multiply diagonally.

$$1 \times 400 = 400$$

STEP 2: Divide answer from step 1 (400) by the remaining number in the equation (4).

$$\begin{array}{r} 100 \\ 4\overline{)400} \\ \underline{4} \\ 00 \end{array}$$

So 400 carbohydrate calories are available in 100 grams of carbohydrates.

Practice 11

Use proportion to solve the following problems:

1. 81 calories of fat = _____ grams

2. 120 calories of protein = _____ grams

3. 36 calories of carbohydrate = _____ grams

4. 145 calories of carbohydrate = _____ grams

5. _____ calories are in 12 grams of protein.

6. _____ calories are in 99 grams of fat.

7. _____ calories are in 328 grams of carbohydrate.

8. _____ calories are in 2,450 grams of protein.

◆

Proportion is also useful in solving measurement problems that involve amounts of sodium, calories, fat, and protein in food or an amount in a drug dosage. The proportion will use the information in a scenario to solve for the unknown quantities of a specific amount.

EXAMPLE

If one glass of milk contains 280 milligrams of calcium, how much calcium is in $1\frac{1}{2}$ glasses of milk?

$$\frac{1 \text{ glass}}{280 \text{ milligrams}} = \frac{1\frac{1}{2} \text{ glasses}}{? \text{ milligrams}}$$

$$280 \times 1\frac{1}{2} = 420 \text{ mg of calcium}$$

Practice 12

Solve these nutritional problems using ratio and proportion.

1. One-half cup of baked beans contains 430 milligrams of sodium. How many milligrams of sodium are there in $\frac{3}{4}$ cup of baked beans?

2. Baked beans contain 33 grams of carbohydrates in a $\frac{1}{2}$ cup serving. How many milligrams of carbohydrates are in three $\frac{1}{2}$ cup servings?

3. A $\frac{1}{2}$ cup serving of fruit cocktail contains 55 milligrams of potassium. How many milligrams of potassium are in 2 cups of fruit cocktail?

4. If $\frac{1}{2}$ cup of fruit cocktail contains 13 grams of sugar, then $1\frac{1}{4}$ cup of fruit cocktail contains how many grams of sugar?

5. Old-fashioned oatmeal contains 27 grams of carbohydrates per $\frac{1}{2}$ cup of dry oats. How many grams of carbohydrates are available in $2\frac{1}{4}$ cups of the dry oats?

◆

◆◆◆◆ Practice with Food Labels

Knowing how to read food labels is important because patients often need to limit their salt, sugar, and fat intake to help ensure good health. Proportion is useful in figuring out the amounts of these ingredients when portioning—increasing or decreasing portions.

Practice 13

Carefully read the label and then use its information to solve each question.

Albert's Tomato Soup

Nutrition facts	Amount/serving %DV*	Amount/serving %DV*
Serving size ½ cup (120 mL) Condensed soup Servings about 2.5 Calories 90 Fat calories 0	Total fat 0 g 0%	Total carbohydrates 20 g 7%
	Saturated fat 0 g 0%	Fiber 1 g 4%
	Cholesterol 0 mg 0%	Sugars 15 g
	Sodium 710 mg 30%	Protein 2 g
	Vitamin A 12% · Vitamin C 12% · Calcium 0% · Iron 0%	

*Percent daily values (%DV) are based on a 2,000 calorie diet.

1. If $\frac{1}{2}$ cup of soup equals 120 milliliters, then how many milliliters (mL) are in $3\frac{1}{2}$ cups of soup?

2. If a can has 2.5 servings, how many cans are needed to serve 10 people?

3. One serving contains 90 calories; how many calories are in $4\frac{1}{2}$ servings?

4. One gram of fiber constitutes 4% of a daily dietary value. How many grams of fiber would be present in 25% of the daily value?

5. How many grams of carbohydrates are present if the portion meets 15% of the daily value of carbohydrates? Round to the nearest tenth.

Use the information from the label to complete these proportions.

Big Al's Organic Sweet and Juicy Dried Plums

Nutrition facts Serving size 1½ oz (40 g in about 5 dried plums) Servings per container about 30		Amount per serving Calories 100 Calories from fat 0	
	%DV*		%DV*
Total fat 0 g	0%	Potassium 290 mg	8%
Saturated fat 0 g	0%	Total carbohydrates 24 g	8%
Cholesterol 0 mg	0%	Dietary fiber 3 g	11%
Sodium 5 mg	0%	Soluble fiber 1 g	
Vitamin A 10% (100% as beta carotene)		Insoluble fiber 1 g	
Vitamin C 0%	.	Sugars 12 g	
Calcium 2%		Protein 1 g	
Iron 2%		**Big Al's Organic Sweet and Juicy Dried Plums/Prunes**	

*Percent daily values (%DV) are based on a 2,000 calorie diet. Your daily values may be higher or lower depending on your calorie needs.

6. How many total grams (g) of weight are present in 34 prunes?

7. If 100 calories are consumed with 5 prunes, how many calories are consumed with 12 prunes?

8. If 5 prunes have 290 milligrams (mg) of potassium and that accounts for 8% of percent daily value, how many prunes are needed to equal 15% of the percent daily value? Round to the nearest whole number.

9. If 5 prunes provide 10% of the Vitamin A needed daily, what percent of the daily percent of Vitamin A is present in 20 prunes?

10. If a serving size is $1\frac{1}{2}$ ounces (oz), how many ounces are five servings?

Use the information from the label to complete these proportions.

Jade's Soy Milk

Nutrition facts	Amount/serving %DV*		Amount/serving %DV*	
Serving size 1 cup (240 mL)	Total fat 4 g	6%	Total Carbohydrates 4 g	1%
Servings about 8 per 1.89 L	Saturated fat 0.5 g	3%	Fiber 1 g	4%
Calories 80	Trans fat 0 g		Cholesterol 0 mg	0%
Fat calories 35	Polyunsaturated fat 2.5 g		Sugars 12 g	
	Monounsaturated fat 1 g		Protein 7 g	
	Sodium 85 mg 4%		Potassium 300 mg	8%
	Vitamin A 10% · Vitamin C 0% · Calcium 30% · Iron 6%			
	Vitamin D 10% · Folate 6% · Magnesium 10% · Selenium 8%			

*Percent daily values (%DV) are based on a 2,000 calorie diet.

11. If 1 cup of soup contains 4 grams (g) total fat, then how many grams of total fat are in $2\frac{3}{4}$ cups of Jade's Soy Milk?

12. If a cup of soy milk contains 85 milligrams of sodium, and an individual consumes $2\frac{2}{3}$ cups of soy milk per day, what is the sodium intake from soy milk? Round to the nearest whole number.

13. If one serving of Jade's Soy Milk provides 1% of the amount of daily carbohydrates needed, how many milliliters make 5% of the daily carbohydrate intake?

14. One serving contains 80 calories; how many calories are in $3\frac{1}{4}$ servings?

15. If 1 cup of Jade's Soy Milk provides 1 gram of fiber and 4% of the recommended daily fiber intake, how many cups of this soy milk are needed to make up 25% of the dietary fiber?

UNIT REVIEW

◆◆◆◆ Critical Thinking With Ratio and Proportion

1. Use ratio and proportion to find x. $\dfrac{\frac{1}{8}}{\frac{3}{4}} = \dfrac{12}{x}$

2. The physician ordered Valium 3.5 milligrams intramuscularly every six hours as needed for anxiety. The pharmacist has Valium in his pharmacy in the following supply: 10 milligrams per 2 milliliters. How many milliliters will the patient receive in each dose for this drug order?

3. Using the information from problem 2, what would be a full dosage of medication, in milliliters, given on schedule for one day?

4. The average human heart beats 4,320 times every sixty minutes. Express this as a unit rate.

5. Write 450 calories in three servings as a unit rate.

6. Mixing infant formula is an important task. For every 2 ounces of instant infant formula, Mary needs 6 ounces of tepid, sterilized water. If the can of instant infant formula contains 8 ounces, how many ounces of sterilized water are needed?

7. At Valley View Center, there are three part-time employees for every two full-time employees. If there are 48 full-time employees, how many part-time employees are there?

8. The exercise pool at Care Vista has a pump that can drain 5,500 gallons of treated water from the pool in 90 minutes. How many gallons can it drain in two and a half hours? Round to the nearest whole number.

9. Greek yogurt has 140 calories in six ounces. What is the unit rate of calories in each ounce? Round to the nearest whole number.

10. There are 14 grams of protein in a 6 ounce container of Greek yogurt. What is the per-unit rate of grams of protein per ounce? Round to the nearest whole number.

11. In 12.5 hours, the patient had an even distribution of 750 milligrams of medication via intravenous solution. How many milligrams of medication did the patient receive per hour?

12. Write the following ratio as a decimal: 1 : 25

13. The dental assistant is to mix the modeling mix for a dental model. She has learned that she should use 50 milliliters of water for 100 milligrams of the modeling mix. How many milligrams of modeling mix are used with 75 milliliters of water?

14. The lab technician is working on a special research project. She can prepare 45 pipettes every hour for the project. If she works consistently at this rate, how many pipettes will she have ready in 45 minutes? Round to the nearest whole number.

15. A disinfectant solution has 10 grams of disinfectant powder to 100 milliliters of hot water. Keeping the ratio at 1 : 10, how many grams of disinfectant powder are used for 330 milliliters of hot water?

◆◆◆◆ Professional Expertise

- Always reduce ratios to their simplest form.
- Similar units in ratios should be across from each other when setting up two fractions as a proportion.
- Read the problem carefully to find out if you are solving for a ratio, a unit rate, or a proportion.

RATIO AND PROPORTION POST-TEST

Show all your work.

1. Write a definition for proportion. Provide one health profession application or example.

2. $30 : 120 = \ ? : 12$

3. 1 glass contains 8 ounces. How many full glasses are in 78 ounces?

4. $\dfrac{1}{2} : 4 = \dfrac{1}{3} : x$

5. $x : 625 = 1 : 5$

6. If 10 milligrams are contained in 2 milliliters, how many milligrams are contained in 28 milliliters?

7. A tablet contains 30 milligrams of medication. How many tablets will be needed to provide Ms, Smith with 240 milligrams of medication?

8. 100 micrograms of a drug are contained in 2 milliliters. How many milliliters are contained in 15 micrograms?

9. $\dfrac{1}{100} : 6 = \ ? : 8$

10. $0.04 : 0.5 = 0.12 : ?$

11. How many minutes are in 130 seconds? Your answer will have both minutes and seconds. Show your setup.

12. Four out of every six dental patients request fluoride treatment after their dental cleaning treatments. If 120 patients have dental cleanings this week, how many will choose to have fluoride treatments as well?

13. If the doctor's office uses 128 disposal thermometer covers each day, how many covers will be used in a five-day workweek?

14. Solve: $\dfrac{1}{125} : 3 : : \underline{\hspace{1cm}} : 12$

15. If the doctor ordered six ounces of cranberry juice four times a day for four days, how many total ounces would be served to the patient?

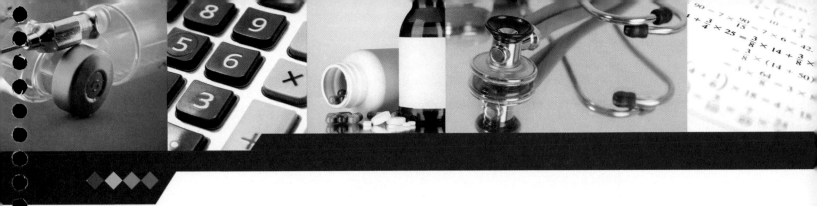

5   Percents

STUDENT LEARNING OUTCOMES

After completing the tasks in this unit, you will be able to:

5-1 Convert between percent and decimal numbers

5-2 Set up percent problems using the percent formula

5-3 Use proportion to solve percent problems

5-4 Calculate percent change

5-5 Solve single trade discount problems

5-6 Calculate percent strength problems

PRE-TEST

1. Write $35\frac{1}{4}\%$ as a decimal.

2. What is 32% of 140?

3. Write $\frac{1}{8}$ as a percent.

4. 120 is what percent of 440? Round to the nearest tenth if needed.

5. 75 is 15% of what number?

6. Express 35 : 50 as a percent.

7. The number of patients increased from 110 to 121. This is a _____% increase.

8. The wheelchair is priced at $475.00. How much would this wheelchair cost with a 15% discount? Do not worry about tax.

9. Convert $1\frac{1}{4}$ into a percentage.

10. Convert 2 into a percentage.

11. Convert $3\frac{2}{3}$% into a ratio.

12. The nurse at Vista Hills Center makes 38 dollars an hour. She will get a dollar and 15 cent raise per hour in June. This is a _____% raise. Round to the nearest whole number if needed.

13. There is a new cohort of nursing students at the university. There are 36 students, of whom 16 are male. What percentage is female? Round to the nearest whole percent if necessary.

14. Last year 40% of patients admitted to the hospital had had heart attacks. There were 2,200 patients admitted last year. How many patients had had heart attacks?

15. Write $\frac{1}{6}$ as a mixed or complex percent.

◆◆◆◆ Overview

Percents are another example of a part-to-whole relationship in math. **Percents** are parts of one hundred and are represented by the % sign. Percents can be written as fractions: 35 parts of 100 or $\frac{35}{100}$.

In our daily work in health care, we see percentages on medication labels and containers.

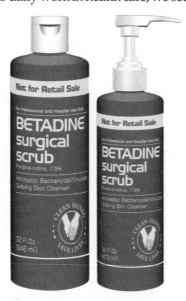

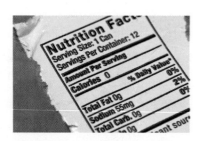

Knowledge of percents in health care will help you understand the percent strength of solutions for patient medications, interest on loans and taxes, and discounts and mark-ups in pharmacies and retail stores. In addition, medical insurance and accounts receivable departments use percentages regularly to determine what portion of an invoice is covered as well as to calculate preferred provider versus out-of-program provider rates and coverage. In general, though, general health care professionals see percent applications less frequently than fractions and decimals.

◆◆◆◆ Percent-to-Decimal Conversion

 REVIEW

To convert a percent to a decimal, shift the decimal point two places to the *left*. The process of doing this quick division replaces having to divide the number by 100. This is the same method of simplified division shown in Unit 3: Decimals.

EXAMPLE

$$75\% \rightarrow 7\ 5.\% \rightarrow 0.75$$

If a percent has a fractional part, the decimal occurs between the whole number and the fractional part.

EXAMPLE

$$33\frac{1}{3}\% \rightarrow 33.\frac{1}{3}\% \rightarrow 0.33\frac{1}{3}$$

Practice 1

Convert from percents to decimals.

1. 65%

2. 52%

3. $75\frac{1}{2}\%$

4. 28%

5. $44\frac{1}{2}\%$

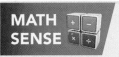

MATH SENSE

A whole number has its decimal to the far right of the final digit or number.

125% = 125.%
76% = 76.%

◆◆◆◆ Decimal-to-Percent Conversion

REVIEW

To convert a decimal to a percent, shift the decimal point two places to the *right*. This is the simplified multiplication method practiced in Unit 3: Decimals.

If a number has a decimal in it and you are converting from a decimal to a percent, use the existing decimal point as the starting point for the conversion. It is possible to have percents greater than 100.

SET-UP HINT

Begin counting from wherever the decimal is placed.

$$0.023 \rightarrow 02.3\% \quad 2.56 \rightarrow 256\%$$

Handle a mixed fraction by placing the decimal point between the whole number and the fraction, and then convert the fraction to a whole number by dividing the numerator by the denominator. Then move the decimal two places to the right and add a % sign.

$$14\frac{3}{4} \rightarrow 14.\frac{3}{4} \rightarrow 14.75 \rightarrow 1475\%$$

EXAMPLES

$$0.25 \rightarrow 0.25\% = 25\%$$

$$13 \rightarrow 13. \rightarrow 13.00 = 1300\%$$

Practice 2

Convert from decimals to percents.

1. 0.375

2. 5.64

3. 9.2

4. 10.8

5. 0.076

Practice 3

Convert to decimals or percents as directed.

1. 82.5% to a decimal

2. 0.07% to a decimal

3. 41% to a decimal

4. 6.35 to a percent

5. 0.078 to a percent

6. $9\frac{3}{4}$ to a percent

7. $1.25\frac{1}{4}$ to a percent

8. $78\frac{1}{9}\%$ to a decimal

9. 1.5% to a decimal

10. $0.67\frac{1}{4}$ to a percent

◆◆◆◆ Using Proportion to Solve Percent Problems

REVIEW

Proportions are also very useful in solving percent problems. To accomplish this, use the formula:

$$\frac{\%}{100} = \frac{\text{is (part)}}{\text{of (whole or total)}}$$

_____%	_____(is)
100	_____(of)

The box method for this formula will help you keep your numbers in the correct place. Notice that 100 is always in the bottom left corner, and that the % is always above it. The right-hand side has the part (the "is") over the whole (the "of").

$$\frac{\%}{100} = \frac{\text{is (the part)}}{\text{whole (the total)}}$$

To solve any percent problem, take the information from the problem and put it into the formula. There are three possible places that the information can go.

$$\frac{?}{100} = \frac{?}{?}$$

The 100 never changes because it indicates that every percent is part of 100. It is important to set up the problem correctly. The following questions ask for different information. Therefore, the setup of the problems will be different.

Problem	Setup
What is 25% of 75?	$\frac{25}{100} = \frac{?}{75}$
What % of 75 is 18.75?	$\frac{?}{100} = \frac{18.75}{75}$
18.75 is 25% of what?	$\frac{25}{100} = \frac{18.75}{?}$

Note that the ? is in a different place each time. When the problem is worked, each of the above answers will be different.

Practice 4

Set up the problems, but do not solve them.

1. What is 75% of 200?

_____%	_____(is)
100	_____(of)

2. 10 is what % of 125?

_____%	_____(is)
100	_____(of)

3. Find 8.5% of 224.

_____%	_____(is)
100	_____(of)

4. 40 percent of what number is 350?

_____%	_____(is)
100	_____(of)

5. 18 is what percent of 150?

_____%	_____(is)
100	_____(of)

6. What is $1\frac{1}{2}$% of 400?

_____%	_____(is)
100	_____(of)

7. 75 of 90 is what percent?

_____%	_____(is)
100	_____(of)

8. Out of 200, 140 is what percent?

_____%	_____(is)
100	_____(of)

9. 50% of what number is 75?

_____%	_____(is)
100	_____(of)

10. $8\frac{1}{3}$% of 144 is what?

_____%	_____(is)
100	_____(of)

PERCENT PROBLEMS IN HEALTH CARE

To solve percent problems in health care, one needs to be aware that the problem may include whole numbers, fractions, and decimals. The skills used in percents draw on the foundation you have in these areas of math computation. It is important to remember and apply the fraction concepts learned when dealing with fractions in percents because a fraction is more accurate and exact than a decimal number that has a repeating final digit.

To solve percent problems, use the proportion method studied in Unit 4: Ratio and Proportion.

EXAMPLE

Fifteen is what percent of 300?

$$\frac{x\%}{100} = \frac{15}{300}$$

STEP 1: Cross multiply the two numbers.

$$(100 \times 15 = 1,500)$$

STEP 2: Divide the step 1 answer by the remaining number—the number diagonal from the x or ?

$$1,500 \div 300 = 5$$

The answer is 5%. So we know that 15 is 5% of 300.

Practice 5

Use proportion to solve the following problems.

1. 35% of 120 is _____.

2. 12 is what percent of 44?

3. 50 is what percent of 248?

4. 60% of 120 is what?

5. What is 35% of 16.8?

6. Find 9% of 3,090.

7. 45 is what percent of 200?

8. 74 is what percent of 74?

9. What is 44% of 40?

10. 121 is what percent of 220?

COMPLEX PERCENT PROBLEMS

More complex percents include fractions, and the most efficient way of handling these percents is as complex fractions. By setting up the problem in proportion format, the work is put into manageable steps. A common error that students make is to multiply the first two numbers and consider their work done; however, there is always a final division step that must be performed.

EXAMPLE

What is $8\frac{1}{3}$% of 150?

$$\frac{8\frac{1}{3}}{100} = \frac{x}{150}$$

STEP 1: Multiply $8\frac{1}{3}$% and 150. Deal with the fraction; do not change it to a decimal because if you do, your answer will not be as exact. Convert the mixed fraction into an improper fraction. Multiply the whole number by the denominator and add the numerator. Place this number over the denominator. Then multiply this improper fraction by the number 150.

$$8\frac{1}{3} = \frac{25}{3} \times 150 = \frac{3,750}{3} = 1,250$$

STEP 2: Divide the step 1 answer of 1,250 by 100. Use simplified division, which moves the decimal 2 places to the left to divide by 100.

$$1,250 : 1,\underset{\cup\cup}{2\ 5\ 0} = 12.5 \text{ or } 12\frac{1}{2} \quad 0.5 \text{ equals } \frac{1}{2}.$$

Practice 6

Solve the following problems.

1. What is $5\frac{1}{3}\%$ of 125? Round to the nearest hundredth.

2. $12\frac{1}{2}\%$ of 400 is what?

3. $33\frac{2}{3}\%$ of 90 is what?

4. $35\frac{1}{4}\%$ is what part of 150? Round to the nearest hundredth.

5. $12\frac{1}{2}\%$ of 125 is what? Round to the nearest hundredth.

6. 50 is $83\frac{1}{3}\%$ of what number?

7. 160 is $12\frac{1}{2}\%$ of what number?

8. 45 is $15\frac{1}{3}\%$ of what number? Round to the nearest hundredth.

9. 200 is $37\frac{1}{2}\%$ of what number? Round to the nearest hundredth.

10. $87\frac{1}{2}\%$ of 120 is what?

Three other applications of percents are important for the health care student: percent change, the percent strength of a solution, and the single trade discount.

◆◆◆◆ Percent Change

Change is ever present in our lives. A percent change can represent an increase or a decrease. We calculate percent change for fees, medical doses, weight, income, and so on. You may use a simple formula to help determine percent change.

$$\frac{\text{Amount of change}}{\text{Original number}} = \text{Fraction of change}$$

STEP 1: Set up the fraction of change.

STEP 2: Use proportion to set up a percent conversion. Remember that percent means out of one hundred.

EXAMPLE

The twelve-year-old boy was told by his doctor to lose weight. He weighed 180 pounds. He needed to weigh 120 pounds. He went on a supervised diet and exercise plan. He lost 60 pounds in one year. What is the percent of change of the amount of weight he lost?

$$\frac{60\ (\textit{change in weight})}{180\ (\textit{original weight})} = \frac{x}{100}$$

STEP 1: $60 \times 100 = 6,000$

STEP 2: $6,000 \div 180 = 33\frac{1}{3}\%$

So, the 60 pounds he lost represent a $33\frac{1}{3}\%$ weight loss.

EXAMPLE

Mary ate 5 servings of fruits and vegetables a day. Her physician encouraged her to eat 9 servings of fruits and vegetables each day. This represents a _____ % change.

$$\frac{4\ (\textit{amount of change})}{5\ (\textit{original amount})} = \frac{x}{100}$$

STEP 1: $4 \times 100 = 400$

STEP 2: $400 \div 5 = 80\%$

So, the 4 servings of fruits and vegetables that she will add represent an 80% change.

Practice 7

Solve the following percent change problems.

1. Bella reduced her monthly workdays from 20 to 16. What is the percentage of change in the number of her monthly days of work?

2. The premature baby needed to gain weight before being released from the hospital. She weighed 3 pounds 6 ounces. She needed to weigh 5 pounds 8 ounces. What is the percent of change? Round to the nearest whole number.

3. The cost of pain medication increased from 17 cents to 21 cents per tablet. This is a
_____ % increase. Round to the nearest tenth.

4. The infant drinks 2 ounces of formula every four hours. The doctor wants the infant
to increase his intake to 4 ounces every four hours. What percent increase is this?

5. The insurance company reviewed a dental procedure claim of $624.00. If the patient
had used the preferred provider, the bill would have been reduced to $249.60. This
represents a _____% reduction in expense.

◆◆◆◆ Percent Strength of Solutions

REVIEW

The strength of solutions is an important application of percents. A **solution** is a liquid
that has had medication, minerals, or other products dissolved in it. Percent strength
refers to how much of a substance has been dissolved in a specific amount of liquid.

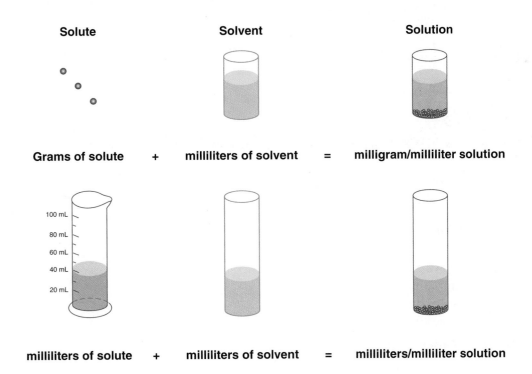

Solute	Solvent	Solution
Grams of solute +	**milliliters of solvent** =	**milligram/milliliter solution**
milliliters of solute +	**milliliters of solvent** =	**milliliters/milliliter solution**

Solution refers to a two-part substance: a **solute**, which is the drug, mineral, or
product, and a **solvent** or liquid, which can consist of a variety of mediums depending on
the medical application. **Solutes** will be either a dry drug measured in grams or a liquid
measured in milliliters. The total volume of the liquid is always in milliliters.

Key to percent strength is your knowledge of part-to-whole relationships: A percent
is x parts to 100 total parts.

EXAMPLE

A 15% drug solution has 15 parts of drug to 100 parts of solution. There are thus 15 grams of drug to 100 milliliters of solution.

$$15\% \text{ is } \frac{15}{100} = \text{Reduced, that is } \frac{15 = 5 \times 3}{100 = 5 \times 20} = \frac{3}{20}$$

As a ratio, this would be shown in the reduced form of 3 : 20.

Sometimes the solution will be given as a ratio rather than a percent. To express the solution strength as a percent, set up the problem as a proportion with 100 mL of the total solution. Recall that percent is always part of 100.

EXAMPLE

Write $2\frac{1}{4}\%$ as a ratio of pure drug to solution.

STEP 1: $\dfrac{2\frac{1}{4}}{100}$

STEP 2: $\dfrac{\frac{9}{4}}{100}$ which means $\dfrac{9}{4} \div \dfrac{100}{1}$

$\dfrac{9}{4} \times \dfrac{1}{100} = \dfrac{9}{400}$ or 9 : 400

So the final ratio is 9 grams to 400 milliliters of solution.

Practice 8

Percent strength: What is the ratio of pure drug to solution? Simplify, if necessary.

1. 8% solution _____

2. 0.9% solution _____

3. $5\frac{1}{2}\%$ solution _____

4. 7.5% solution _____

5. 5% solution _____

USING PROPORTION TO CONVERT SOLUTIONS

Knowledge of proportion is useful in converting to smaller or larger amounts of solution. In health care, professionals may not always require 100 mL of a solution. It is important to maintain the correct ratio of pure drug to solution to ensure that the patient is getting the medication or solution the doctor intended. Note that the ratio of pure drug remains consistent no matter how much solution is to be prepared.

EXAMPLE

Percent strength 8% means that there are 8 g of drug to 100 mL of solution. If the doctor orders 25 mL of an 8% strength solution, then a proportion may be used to ensure that the ratio of pure drug to solution represents 8%.

$$\underset{\text{100 mL solution}}{\overset{\text{8 g of drug}}{\overbrace{}}}^{\textit{known}} = \underset{\text{25 mL solution}}{\overset{\text{? g of drug}}{\overbrace{}}}^{\textit{unknown}}$$

STEP 1: $8 \times 25 = 200$

STEP 2: $200 \div 100 = 2$

So, to make 25 mL of an 8% solution using this ratio of pure drug to solution, 2 g of pure drug to 25 mL of solution are required. This keeps the percent strength of the medication consistent with the doctor's order for an 8% strength solution. Note that the amount of mixed solution changes, not the percent strength itself.

EXAMPLE

Ten grams of a drug are mixed in 25 mL of solution. What is the percent strength of this medication?

To convert this ratio into a percent, write it as a proportion. Then solve for x, which will become the percent.

$$\underset{\text{25 mL}}{\overset{\text{10 g}}{\overbrace{}}}^{\textit{known}} = \underset{\text{100 mL}}{\overset{x \text{ g}}{\overbrace{}}}^{\textit{unknown}}$$

Follow proportion steps to solve. Cross multiply $10 \times 100 = 1000$. Divide 1000 by $25 = 40$, so the answer is 40% strength.

Practice 9

Solve the following.

1. The doctor has ordered a 15% saline solution to be prepared. How many grams of pure drug will be needed to make each of these amounts of solution at the 15% strength?

   a. 25 mL of solution

   b. 35 mL of solution

   c. 65 mL of solution

   d. 125 mL of solution

2. Nine milliliters of pure drug are in 100 mL of solution.

   a. What is the percent strength of the solution?

   b. How many milliliters of drug are in 75 mL of that solution?

3. Fifteen grams of pure drug are in 50 mL.

   a. What is the percent strength of the solution?

   b. How many grams of pure drug are in 200 mL of the solution?

Practice 10

Solve the following.

1. A $7\frac{1}{2}$% strength solution has been prepared.

   a. How many grams of medication are in the $7\frac{1}{2}$% strength solution?

   b. How many milliliters of solution are in this $7\frac{1}{2}$% strength solution?

   c. Express this solution as a simplified ratio.

   d. How much pure drug is needed to create 35.5 mL of this solution? Round to the nearest tenth. Your answer will be in grams.

   e. How much pure drug is needed to create 80 mL of this solution? Your answer will be in grams.

   f. If you have 60 mL of solution, how many grams of pure drug will you need in order to keep the $7\frac{1}{2}$%? Round to the nearest tenth. Your answer will be in grams.

2. A 0.09% strength solution has been prepared.

   a. How many grams of medication are in the 0.09% strength solution?

   b. How many milliliters of solution are in this 0.09% strength solution?

   c. Express this solution as a simplified ratio.

   d. How much pure drug is needed to create 54 mL of this solution? Round to the nearest hundredth. Your answer will be in grams.

   e. How much pure drug is needed to create 24 mL of this solution? Round to the nearest hundredth. Your answer will be in grams.

   f. If you have 50 mL of solution, how many grams of pure drug will you need in order to keep the 0.09% solution? Round to the nearest hundredth. Your answer will be in grams.

3. A 78% strength solution has been prepared.

   a. How many grams of medication are in the 78% strength solution?

   b. How many milliliters of solution are in this 78% strength solution?

   c. Express this solution as a simplified ratio.

d. How much pure drug is needed to create 65.5 mL of this solution? Round to the nearest tenth. Your answer will be in grams.

e. How much pure drug is needed to create 90 mL of this solution? Round to the nearest tenth. Your answer will be in grams.

f. If you have 450 mL of solution, how many grams of pure drug will you need in order to keep the 78%? Your answer will be in grams.

◆◆◆◆ # Single Trade Discount

Single trade discounts are useful to individuals who handle products or inventory that must be marked up. The single trade discount provides the net price of items when a single discount has been given. Some health care organizations that use certain name brands receive these discounts from manufacturers of the products they use or sell most often.

EXAMPLE

What is the net price of a surgical instrument listed at $189.90 with a trade discount of 40%?

STEP 1: The percentage is first made into a decimal by moving the decimal point two places to the left. Then multiply the list price by the trade discount.

$$
\begin{array}{r}
\$189.90 \\
\times \quad .40 \\
\hline
00000 \\
75960 \\
\hline
\$75.96
\end{array}
$$

STEP 2: Subtract the amount of the discount (the answer from step 1) from the list price to get the net price.

$$
\begin{array}{r}
\$189.90 \\
-75.96 \\
\hline
\$113.94
\end{array}
$$

The net price of this instrument is $113.94.

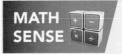

MATH SENSE

You may need to round your decimal number to the nearest cent.

Practice 11

Find the net price by using the single trade discount method. If necessary, round to the nearest penny. Show your work.

	List Price	Trade Discount	Amount of Discount	Net Price
1.	$17.30	15%	_____	_____
2.	$75.89	20%	_____	_____
3.	$45.90	12.5%	_____	_____
4.	$455.86	30%	_____	_____
5.	$352.90	25%	_____	_____
6.	$72.35	10%	_____	_____
7.	$250.40	45%	_____	_____
8.	$862.75	35%	_____	_____
9.	$158.00	40%	_____	_____
10.	$73.85	10%	_____	_____

UNIT REVIEW

◆◆◆◆ Critical Thinking in Percent

1. Express 24 : 36 as a reduced fraction; then convert the fraction into a percent. Show your work.

2. The child weighed 148 pounds before his pediatrician put him on a strict diet. After six weeks, he weighed 133 pounds. What was the percent of change? Round it to the nearest whole percent.

3. Change $2\frac{2}{3}$ into a complex percent.

4. Tom spent $485.00, 28% of his income, on medication last month. What was Tom's income last month?

5. If the regular price of a blood pressure cuff is $34.09 and you can save 12% with a coupon, what is the new price? Do not include sales tax.

6. The Hillside Health Club has 450 members. In December, 298 members came to a health club event. What percent of the club membership attended the event? Round to the nearest whole number.

7. Using the information from problem 6 above, what percentage of the members did not attend the event?

8. One family pays $640.00 a month for health insurance. The cost of their health insurance will rise by 25% in January. What will they pay each month at the new premium?

9. In a survey, 5,000 women were asked if they take a calcium supplement. Forty-five percent of these women reported that they do take a calcium supplement. How many women take calcium supplements?

10. Vinh has trouble remembering to take her daily vitamins. Last month she marked her calendar on each day after she took her vitamins. She discovered that 18 out 30 days, she took her vitamins. This is _____% of the days in the month.

11. Light mayonnaise has a ratio of 5 grams of fat in 50 calories per tablespoon. What is the percentage of fat per tablespoon?

12. If wheat bread has 80 calories per slice and 4 grams of protein per slice, what percentage of calories come from protein?

13. Sam weighs 225 pounds. He was told by his cardiologist that he should weigh 180 pounds. To the nearest percent, what percent of his current weight should he lose?

14. A child needs to increase her weight by 18%. She currently weighs 64 pounds. What will her new weight be once she has gained 18% of her current weight? Round to the nearest tenth.

15. Express $1\frac{1}{2} : 4$ as a percent.

◆◆◆◆ Professional Expertise

- Always check to make sure that the % sign is added when needed.
- Make sure the ratio of percent strength is in its reduced form.
- Add the units of measure mg/mL or mL/mL.

PERCENT POST-TEST

1. Write the definition of a percent. Provide one example.

2. Convert the following into percents:

   a. $66\frac{2}{3}$

   b. $\frac{5}{6}$

3. 75% of 325 is what number?

4. 8 is what % of 40?

5. 28 is 14% of what number?

6. What does $5\frac{1}{2}\%$ solution mean?

7. The doctor has ordered 25 mL of 9% saline solution. How much pure drug is needed to make this order?

8. The list price for a case of medicine is $129.50. Your pharmacy will receive a 12% trade discount.

   a. What is the amount of the discount? _____

   b. What is the net cost of a case of medicine? _____

9. What percent is 3 tablets of a prescription written for 36 tablets?

10. If a pharmacy gave a 15% discount on walkers, what would be the discount for a total bill of $326.00 for a six-month rental?

11. If a ratio of 3 : 25 is given for a solution, what percent strength is this solution?

12. What is $\frac{1}{2}$% of 500?

13. Express 8 : 125 as a percent.

14. What is $\frac{3}{4}$%?

15. 35 is 0.05% of what?

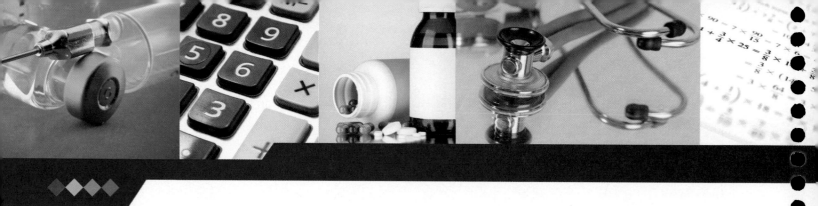

UNIT

6 Combined Applications

STUDENT LEARNING OUTCOMES

After completing the tasks in this unit, you will be able to:

6-1 Convert among fractions, decimal numbers, ratios, and percents

6-2 Learn the relationships among fractions, decimal numbers, ratios, and percents

6-3 Use ratio to convert between units of measure

◆◆◆◆ Overview

Health care workers rely on a variety of math systems to achieve their daily tasks. Knowing different ways to convert efficiently among math systems will benefit you on the job as your expertise grows and your level of responsibility increases. It is thus important to have the ability to convert among fractions, decimals, ratios, and percents. Previous units reviewed each of these skills separately; this unit brings them together to help you develop some strategies for performing these conversions in the most efficient way.

PRE-TEST

1. Convert $\frac{3}{18}$ to a decimal. Round to the nearest hundredth.

2. Covert $1\frac{1}{4}\%$ to a ratio.

3. Write 1.05 as a fraction.

4. Convert $2\frac{5}{6}$ to a ratio.

5. Convert $23\frac{3}{4}$ to a decimal.

6. Convert 16 : 300 to a percent. Round to the nearest tenth.

7. Convert 12.325 to a percent.

8. $7\frac{1}{4}$ cups = _____ ounces

9. $13\frac{1}{2}$ tablespoons = _____ fluid ounces

10. $2\frac{1}{4}$ feet = _____ centimeters

11. 5.5 hours = _____ minutes

12. $11\frac{1}{4}$ quarts = _____ cups

13. If a teaspoon has approximately 60 drops, how many drops are in $8\frac{1}{2}$ teaspoons?

14. $9\frac{1}{2}\% \times 0.67$ is what? Round to the nearest hundredth.

15. Simplify $\dfrac{-\frac{1}{2}\%}{5}$.

Every day, we convert between systems. Oftentimes we do this automatically.

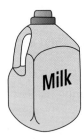
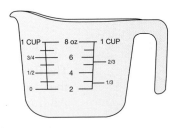

1 gallon = 16 cups

Conversions among Fractions, Decimals, Ratios, and Percents

REVIEW

In health care situations, we often have to convert among systems. Sometimes we need to convert fractions to decimals. For example, a person's weight might be recorded as $14\frac{1}{4}$ pounds, and we need to convert that to a decimal, which is 14.25. Another example is seen in insurance, when a patient's portion of a bill is 20% of $1,200.00. We need to explain that 20% actually means that the patient must pay $240.00 of the bill. Thus, we have used the percent formula to move from percentage to dollars. People understand dollars and cents; percentages of a bill are more difficult to comprehend. A third example is that of a patient who must have a 4-to-1 mix of medication and a substance such as juice or applesauce. The ratio will be converted to another measure such as teaspoons. Knowing how to convert measurements can expedite your math-processing time on the job.

Review the basics of conversion:

Conversion	Method/Formula
Fraction to decimal	Divide the denominator into the numerator.

$$\frac{3}{4} = \begin{array}{r} 0.75 \\ 4\overline{)3.0} \\ \underline{28\downarrow} \\ 20 \\ \underline{20} \\ 0 \end{array}$$

Decimal to fraction	Count the decimal places; place the number over 1 with enough zeros to match the same number of decimal places.

$$0.0\underline{2}\ (2\ \text{places}) \rightarrow \frac{2}{10\ \underline{0}}\ (2\ \text{zeros})$$

Reduce to $\frac{1}{50}$.

Proper fraction to ratio, ratio to proper fraction	Ratios are shown with : instead of /. Fractions and ratios are interchangeable by simply changing the symbol.

$$\frac{1}{8} \rightarrow 1:8 \text{ and } 4:31 \rightarrow \frac{4}{31}$$

The first ratio number is always the numerator, and the second ratio number is always the denominator. All fractions and ratios must be in lowest terms.

Mixed number to ratio, ratio to mixed number	If the fraction is a mixed number, the mixed number must first be made into an improper fraction before setting up the ratio.

$$1\frac{3}{4} \rightarrow 1 \times 4 + 3 = \frac{7}{4} \rightarrow 7:4$$

If a ratio is an improper fraction when a conversion needs to be made, change the fraction to a mixed number.

$$\frac{11}{4} \rightarrow 11 \div 4 = 2\frac{3}{4}$$

Decimal to percent

Move the decimal point two places to the right. Add the percent sign.

$$0.25 \rightarrow 25\% \quad 1.456 \rightarrow 145.6\%$$

Percent to decimal

Move the decimal point two places to the left. Add zeros if needed as placeholders.

$$90\% \rightarrow 0.9 \text{ and } 5\% \rightarrow 0.05$$

$$57\frac{1}{2}\% \rightarrow 0.57\frac{1}{2} \text{ or } 0.575$$

Fraction to percent

Convert the fraction to a decimal, and then to a percent.

Decimal to ratio

Convert the decimal to a fraction, and then change the percent sign to a colon.

CONVERTING TO FRACTIONS, DECIMALS, RATIOS, AND PERCENTS

Convert the following numbers as needed to fractions, decimals, ratios, and percents. Using the review sheet of conversion methods, try to compute only one math problem per line by carefully selecting the order of the conversions to be done. By carefully selecting this order, you will minimize extra work.

EXAMPLE

Fraction	Decimal	Ratio	Percent
_____	0.05	_____	_____

Figuring out the order takes a little practice. When 0.05 is changed to a percent first, no math calculation needs to be done: Simply move the decimal.

Fraction	Decimal	Ratio	Percent
_____	0.05	_____	5%

Next convert the decimal to a fraction. Count the number of decimal places and then place the 5 over a 1 with the same number of zeros as decimal places. Reduce the fraction to lowest terms.

Fraction	Decimal	Ratio	Percent
$\frac{5}{100} \rightarrow \frac{1}{20}$	0.05	_____	5%

Take the reduced fraction and write it in ratio form.

Fraction	Decimal	Ratio	Percent
$\frac{5}{100} \rightarrow \frac{1}{20}$	0.05	1 : 20	5%

EXAMPLE

Fraction	Decimal	Ratio	Percent
$7\frac{3}{5}$	_____	_____	_____

This mixed number must be made into an improper fraction before it can become a ratio.

$$\left(7 \times 5 + 3 = 38 \rightarrow \frac{38}{5}\right)$$

Change the sign from / to : to make the ratio.

Fraction	Decimal	Ratio	Percent
$7\frac{3}{5}$	_____	38 : 5	_____

Next change to a decimal. Handle the whole number 7 separately. Place it on the line as a whole number, and then divide the denominator into the numerator.

$$3 \div 5 = 0.6$$

Add this to the whole number to make the decimal 7.6.

Fraction	Decimal	Ratio	Percent
$7\frac{3}{5}$	7.6	38 : 5	_____

Finally, move the decimal point in the decimal number two places to the right. Add the percent sign.

Fraction	Decimal	Ratio	Percent
$7\frac{3}{5}$	7.6	38 : 5	760%

SET-UP HINT

Suggested Order of Operations

If starting with percent, move from → decimal → fraction → ratio.
If starting with ratio, move from → fraction → decimal → percent.
If starting with fraction, move from → ratio → decimal → percent.
If starting with decimal, move from → percent → fraction → ratio.

$$\frac{1}{2} \rightarrow 0.5 \rightarrow 50\%$$

$$\frac{1}{4} \rightarrow 0.25 \rightarrow 25\%$$

$$\frac{3}{4} \rightarrow 0.75 \rightarrow 75\%$$

$$\frac{1}{3} \rightarrow 0.33\frac{1}{3} \rightarrow 33\frac{1}{3}\%$$

$$\frac{2}{3} \rightarrow 0.66\frac{2}{3} \rightarrow 66\frac{2}{3}\%$$

Practice 1

Provide the following measures. Reduce to lowest terms as necessary. Round to the nearest hundredth if necessary.

	Fraction	Decimal	Ratio	Percent
1.	$\frac{5}{8}$	_____	_____	_____
2.	_____	_____	$3:25$	_____
3.	_____	_____	_____	25%
4.	_____	0.375	_____	_____
5.	_____	_____	$1:250$	_____
6.	$\frac{7}{8}$	_____	_____	_____
7.	_____	0.06	_____	_____
8.	_____	_____	_____	12.5%
9.	$\frac{1}{10}$	_____	_____	_____
10.	_____	_____	_____	$33\frac{1}{3}\%$
11.	_____	1.36	_____	_____
12.	$12\frac{1}{2}$	_____	_____	_____
13.	_____	_____	$2:5$	_____
14.	_____	$0.66\frac{2}{3}$	_____	_____
15.	_____	_____	$16:25$	_____
16.	_____	0.004	_____	_____
17.	$\frac{5}{6}$	_____	_____	_____
18.	_____	_____	_____	$7\frac{1}{4}\%$
19.	_____	0.01	_____	_____
20.	_____	_____	$7:3$	_____

◆◆◆◆ Using Combined Applications in Measurement Conversion

In health care, a solid working knowledge of weights and measures is essential. You will use three systems of measure in your work: household or standard measurement, metric measurement, covered in this unit, and apothecary measurement, covered in Unit 11: Dosage Calculations. For example, you may need to convert from a teaspoon to milliliters to calculate a dose. Critical to your success in measurement conversion is your ability to remember a few key conversions and the proportion method for solving conversions. Metric-to-metric conversions use a different conversion method, which is also covered in Unit 8.

HOUSEHOLD OR STANDARD MEASUREMENT

Household or **standard measurements** are used by all of us in our daily activities, and these are common measurements in health care as well. Household measures tend to be less accurate than either metric or apothecary measures because of their nature and our methods of using them. This means that household measures are used for the less critical measurements in health care, such as mixing a solution for a client's foot soak: 3 tablespoons of Epsom salt to 1 quart of water. Most households use the measures of teaspoon, tablespoon, cup, pint, quart, and so on.

MATH SENSE	To measure:	Units of Measure
	Height	Feet, inches, meters, centimeters
	Weight	Pounds, ounces, kilograms, grams
	Liquid volume	Gallons, quarts, pints, cups, tablespoons, teaspoons
	Medication dosages	Tablespoons, teaspoons, tablets, ounces, capsules, caplets

Abbreviations of units of measure are also used, and some abbreviations include the following:

Drop = gtt

Teaspoon = t (tsp)

Tablespoon = T (tbsp)

Cup = c

Write the word for each abbreviation.

1. ft = _____

2. yd = _____

3. oz = _____

4. T = _____

5. lb = _____

6. t = _____

7. qt = _____

8. pt = _____

9. gtt = _____

10. gal = _____

◆◆◆◆ Standard Units of Measure

REVIEW

The basics of standard measure conversion were covered in Unit 4: Ratio and Proportion. To refresh yourself on the application of proportion to measurement conversions, complete the review exercises.

TIME	
1 minute	= 60 seconds
1 day	= 24 hours
1 week	= 7 days
1 year	= 12 months

WEIGHT	
1 kilogram	= 2.2 pounds
1 pound	= 16 ounces

LINEAR MEASURE	
1 foot	= 12 inches
1 yard	= 3 feet
1 meter	= 39.4 inches
1 inch	= 2.5 or 2.54 centimeters

LIQUID MEASURE	
1 tablespoon	= 3 teaspoons
1 cup	= 8 ounces
1 pint	= 2 cups
1 quart	= 2 pints
1 gallon	= 4 quarts

APPROXIMATE EQUIVALENTS	
1 grain*	= 60 milligrams
1 teaspoon	= 5 milliliters
1 tablespoon	= 3 teaspoons
1 fluid dram*	= 4 milliliters
1 fluid ounce	= 8 fluid drams*
1 fluid ounce	= 2 tablespoons
1 fluid ounce	= 30 milliliters
1 cup	= 240 or 250 milliliters**
	= 8 fluid ounces
1 pint	= 480 or 500 milliliters**
	= 2 cups or 16 fluid ounces
1 quart	= 32 fluid ounces
	= 1 liter or 1000 milliliters
1 teaspoon	= 5 milliliters
1 kilogram	= 2.2 pounds
1 fluid ounce	= 2 tablespoons

*These units are from the **apothecary system**, a historical system of mass units that was used by physicians and apothecaries to express medical units. These units are being replaced by common metric measures so that the units used in medication dosages are more uniform. So instead of using grains for morphine, the labeling is now in milligrams. Using the metric system helps ensure accurate doses because the metric units of measure are in common units. These units, grain and dram, are included here because some professionals still use them occasionally.

**If 1 cup is 8 ounces, then the exact conversion to milliliters is 240 milliliters. In the past, this measure was rounded to 250 for uniform conversions and easy divisibility. Therefore, 1 cup equaled 250 milliliters and 1 pint equaled 500 milliliters. However, the *exact* conversion rate is 1 cup is 240 milliliters and 1 pint is 480 milliliters.

Using the ratio and proportion knowledge from Unit 4, let's look at some examples of measurement conversions in health care.

EXAMPLE

Convert 45 kilograms to pounds.

STEP 1: Set up the proportion. Locate the conversion 1 kilogram = 2.2 pounds and set it up as a ratio. This is what you know from the conversion chart. Then add the amount that you are converting to the unknown measure. Note that you need to place like units across from each other: Kilograms are across from kilograms, and pounds are across from pounds.

$$\frac{1 \, \text{kilogram}}{2.2 \, \text{pounds}} = \frac{45 \, \text{kilograms}}{? \, \text{pounds}}$$

STEP 2: Multiply the diagonal numbers.

$$\frac{1 \, \text{kilogram}}{2.2 \, \text{pounds}} = \frac{45 \, \text{kilograms}}{? \, \text{pounds}}$$ So that means 2.2 × 45 = 99.

STEP 3: Divide by the remaining number. Any number divided by 1 is itself. So the final answer is 45 kilograms equals 99 pounds.

EXAMPLE

$$4\frac{1}{2} \, \text{cups} = \underline{\hspace{1.5cm}} \, \text{ounces}$$

STEP 1: Set up as a proportion using the information from the problem and the conversion table.

$$\frac{1 \, \text{cup}}{8 \, \text{ounces}} = \frac{4\frac{1}{2} \, \text{cups}}{? \, \text{ounces}}$$

STEP 2: Multiply $8 \times 4\frac{1}{2}$. This is one example where knowing the conversions can expedite your work. Think: $4\frac{1}{2}$ is 4.5. So, 8 × 4.5 = 36.

STEP 3: Divide by 1, which leaves the final answer as 36 ounces.

Practice 3

Using the ratio and proportion setup from Unit 4, solve for the unknowns in these measurement conversions. Use the provided tables to assist you in proportion conversions.

1. 1550 milliliters = _____ pints. Round to the nearest pint.

2. 27 kilograms = _____ pounds

3. 13.8 inches = _____ centimeters. Round to the nearest hundredth.

4. _____ milliliters = 8 teaspoons

5. _____ ounces = 90 milliliters

6. 38.1 centimeters = _____ inches

7. _____ ounces = $1\frac{1}{2}$ pints

8. _____ quarts = 15 liters

9. _____ teaspoons = 12.5 milliliters

10. _____ milliliters = 15 teaspoons

MORE COMBINED APPLICATIONS

Sometimes measurement conversions require more than one conversion to get to the answer.

EXAMPLE

Two conversions are required to convert from ounces to teaspoons.

STEP 1: Convert the ounces to milliliters:

$$\overset{known}{\frac{1 \text{ ounce}}{30 \text{ milliliters}}} = \overset{unknown}{\frac{\text{ounces}}{? \text{ milliliters}}} \rightarrow 240 \text{ milliliters}$$

STEP 2: Convert milliliters to teaspoons.

$$\overset{known}{\frac{1 \text{ teaspoon}}{5 \text{ milliliters}}} = \overset{unknown}{\frac{? \text{ teaspoons}}{240 \text{ milliters}}} \rightarrow 48 \text{ teaspoons}$$

These problems cannot be solved by making a straight conversion from what is known to what is unknown. A path must be developed so that you can establish how to get the answer. Think about what conversions most closely match the problem itself, and then set up the problem.

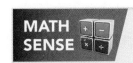

MATH SENSE

Do not rush through the two-step conversions. These require some forethought about how to get from what is known to what is unknown.

Plastic medicine cups are used in the health care industry to measure liquid dosages. A medicine cup is typically marked off in milliliters. Often, one medicine cup is 1 fluid ounce, which is 30 mL.

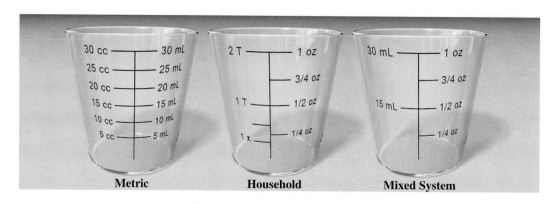

Metric   Household   Mixed System

Practice 4

Answer the following.

1. medicine cup = _____ tablespoons

2. 5 teaspoons = _____ drops

3. $2\frac{1}{4}$ pints = _____ ounces

4. $\frac{1}{2}$ cup = _____ teaspoons

5. 1 pint = _____ tablespoons

6. 15 tablespoons = _____ milliliters

7. 68000 grams = _____ pounds

8. 28 inches = _____ millimeters

9. _____ ounces = 24 teaspoons

10. $1\frac{1}{2}$ ounces = _____ teaspoons

11. 12 tablespoons = _____ fluid ounces

12. 9 teaspoons = _____ tablespoons

13. 14 fluid ounces = _____ pounds

14. 12 teaspoons = _____ milliliters

15. $10\frac{1}{2}$ pounds = _____ ounces

16. $4\frac{1}{4}$ pints = _____ cups

17. 5 cups = _____ fluid ounces

18. 72 inches = _____ feet

19. $12\frac{1}{4}$ ounces = _____ teaspoons

20. 30 drops = _____ teaspoons

Sometimes math problems require multiple setups. To solve these types of problems, group the work into the most logical format.

EXAMPLE

$$\frac{25\%}{\frac{1}{4}}$$

STEP 1: Look at the problem and decide what to do to make the units similar. Convert 25% into a fraction.

$$\rightarrow \frac{25}{100}$$

STEP 2: Review the problem to see what operation should be completed.

$$\frac{\frac{25}{100}}{\frac{1}{4}}$$

This problem is a complex fraction. Divide the denominator of $\frac{1}{4}$ into the numerator of $\frac{25}{100}$.

$$\frac{25}{100} \div \frac{1}{4} \rightarrow \frac{25}{100} \times \frac{4}{1} = \frac{100}{100} = 1$$

Practice 5

Answer the following.

1. Simplify: $\dfrac{75\%}{\frac{1}{4}}$

2. $\dfrac{1:150}{1:300} \times 2$

3. $12\frac{1}{2}\% \times \dfrac{\frac{1}{2}}{\frac{3}{4}}$

4. $\dfrac{\frac{1}{2}\%}{4} \times 1000$

5. $5\% \times \dfrac{1:2}{3:4}$

Practice 6

Converting among Systems Worksheet

Provide the following measures. Reduce to lowest terms as necessary.

	Fraction	Decimal	Ratio	Percent
1.	$\frac{1}{8}$	_____	_____	_____
2.	_____	_____	1 : 20	_____
3.	_____	_____	_____	65%
4.	$\frac{1}{17}$	_____	_____	_____
5.	_____	_____	2 : 5	_____
6.	$\frac{5}{6}$	_____	_____	_____
7.	_____	0.08	_____	_____
8.	_____	_____	_____	10.25%
9.	$\frac{3}{5}$	_____	_____	_____
10.	_____	_____	1 : 200	_____
11.	_____	1.625	_____	_____
12.	$\frac{1}{8}$	_____	_____	_____
13.	_____	_____	11 : 50	_____
14.	_____	0.15	_____	_____
15.	_____	_____	3 : 25	_____
16.	_____	0.008	_____	_____
17.	$\frac{1}{6}$	_____	_____	_____
18.	_____	_____	_____	$15\frac{1}{4}\%$
19.	_____	0.04	_____	_____
20.	_____	_____	9 : 10,000	_____

UNIT REVIEW

◆◆◆◆ Critical Thinking with Combined Applications

1. The kitchen helper at a long-term care facility was instructed by the dietitian to create a recipe that has a ratio of $\frac{1}{2}$ cup butter to 1 cup of sugar. Is this relationship a ratio, a proportion, or a fraction? Explain.

2. The blood bank kept on hand a ratio of 4 : 9 of Type O to Type B blood. What is 4 : 9 as a percentage? Round to the nearest whole number.

3. Write $16\frac{1}{3}\%$ as a simplified fraction.

4. For her client's 80th birthday gathering, a home health aide is making punch that has a 2 : 3 ratio of lemon spritzer to pineapple juice. If there are 9 cups of pineapple juice, how many cups of lemon spritzer are used?

5. Write $14\frac{2}{9}\%$ as a ratio.

6. Write $\frac{1}{400}$ as a decimal rounded to the nearest thousandth.

7. Write $\frac{1}{200}$ as a percent.

8. $16\,\text{patients} = \frac{1}{4}$ the number of people in the hospital wing. What fractional part of the wing would 24 patients make?

9. If a solution is a 0.5% concentration, how would this be written as a ratio?

10. Write $\frac{2}{7}$ as a percent rounded to the nearest hundredth.

11. Write $\dfrac{1}{6}$ as a complex percent.

12. The hospital has a ratio of 8 nursing assistants to 1 nurse. Today, there are 6 nurses working. How many nursing assistants are working today?

13. Write 8.3% as a decimal.

14. Does 25% of 84 equal 84 : 4?

15. Does $72 : 6 = 12\dfrac{1}{2}\%$ of 72?

◆◆◆◆ Professional Expertise

- Use your knowledge of each math system to work your complex problems step-by-step.
- Reduce the fractions.
- Round as directed.
- Include the units of measurement in your setup and also in your answer.
- Don't forget to add or drop the % sign depending on the problem.

COMBINED APPLICATIONS POST-TEST

Show all your work.

1. Convert $\dfrac{5}{25}$ to a decimal.

2. Convert $\dfrac{1}{4}\%$ to a ratio.

3. Convert 4.05 to a fraction.

4. Convert $4\dfrac{1}{8}$ to a ratio.

5. Convert $27\frac{1}{4}$ to a decimal.

6. Convert 12 : 200 to a percent.

7. Convert 14.25% to a ratio.

8. $3\frac{1}{4}$ cups = _____ ounces

9. 12 fluid ounces = _____ tablespoons

10. $3\frac{1}{2}$ feet = _____ centimeters. Use the conversion 1 in. = 2.54 cm. Round to the nearest tenth.

11. 18 hours = _____ minutes

12. 1 gallon = _____ cups

13. If a teaspoon has approximately 60 drops, how many drops are in $2\frac{1}{3}$ tablespoons?

14. Round 12% × 0.67 to the nearest hundredth.

15. Simplify: $\dfrac{15\%}{\frac{1}{2}}$

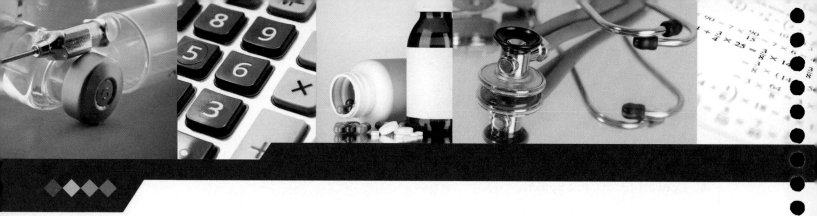

STUDENT LEARNING OUTCOMES

After completing the tasks in this unit, you will be able to:

7-1 Define basic terms in algebra: integer, number statement, expression, and coefficient

7-2 Learn the relationships between positive and negative numbers

7-3 Solve problems that include absolute value

7-4 Complete the integer operations of addition, subtraction, multiplication, and division

7-5 Calculate the square root

7-6 Use the order of operations to solve problems

7-7 Write expressions for word problems

7-8 Solve equations

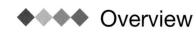 Overview

Algebra is the study, understanding, and use of symbolic reasoning, mathematical properties, processes, and calculations to problem solve for a variety of unknown situations. This unit lays the foundation for algebraic concepts. In health care, the use of algebra is seen in the use of formulas to solve problems. One such formula is the conversion between temperature systems. If you do not follow the order of operations, for example, when you are calculating with the temperature formula (see Units 2 and 3), you will not reach the correct solution. In addition, dimensional analysis (Appendix D) is an algebraic formula used to convert among measurement systems.

PRE-TEST

1. $-14 + 24 =$

2. $-25 - 12 =$

3. $3 + (2 \times 20) - 15 \div 3 =$

4. $15 - 50 \div 5 + 13 =$

5. $5^3 + 7^0 =$

6. $6^2 \times 2^3 =$

7. $\sqrt{144} =$

8. $\sqrt{64} \times 2 =$

9. $|-13| =$

10. $20 - 4 \times 3 + 12 \div 2 =$

11. The coefficient of $4xf$ is _____.

12. Write the expression: the product of some number x and 12.

13. $5 \times 5 \times 5 \times 5 \times 5$ can also be written as _____.

14. Maria made $250.00 more than her sister. Their incomes combined equal $57,000.00. How much did Maria earn?

15. $\dfrac{t}{-6} = 36; t =$ _____

◆◆◆◆ Integers

REVIEW

We use **integers** to solve many everyday math problems. The integers consist of the positive whole numbers (1, 2, 3, 4, 5, . . .), their negatives (−1, −2, −3, −4, −5, . . .), and the number zero. Zero is neither positive nor negative; it is neutral. Integers form a countable infinite set.

The **number line** is a line labeled with the integers in increasing order from left to right. The number line extends in both directions:

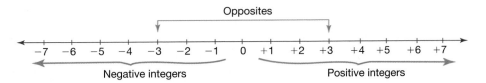

The (−) sign is used to indicate a negative number, and the (+) sign is used to indicate a positive number.

Remember that any integer on the right is always greater than the integer on the left.

We can use the + and − signs to illustrate numbers for information. For example, if the hospital adds three more staff, that can be illustrated as +3. Use the chart to help decide if the number is negative or positive.

MATH SENSE	Terms That Indicate a Negative Integer	Terms That Indicate a Positive Integer
	decrease	increase
	less	more
	loss	profit
	fewer	more

Practice 1

Write the integer for each of the following situations.

1. 18 more nurses _____

2. a 1 degree increase in temperature _____

3. a profit of four thousand dollars _____

4. a twelve pound loss in weight _____

5. 14 beats a minute less _____

Write the opposite of each integer:

6. −16 = _____

7. 12 = _____

8. +5 = _____

9. −100 = _____

10. +17 = _____

Practice 2

Provide two examples when positive or negative integers might be used to represent a health care situation.

1. _____

2. _____

We can use the symbols of $<$, $>$, and $=$ to represent the number relationships.

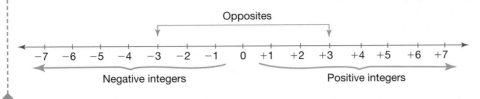

Opposites

Negative integers   Positive integers

For example,

$-8 > -12$ (Remember that the negative numbers increase
$-4 < 2$ in value closer to zero.)
$12 > -6$
$-3 = -3$

Practice 3

Compare the following using $<$, $>$, or $=$.

1. $+6$ _____ -6

2. -4 _____ -2

3. $+12$ _____ -16

4. -8 _____ -8

5. -24 _____ $+24$

ABSOLUTE VALUE

The **absolute value** of an integer indicates its distance from zero on the number line. The absolute value of a number such as 3 is shown as $|3|$. The straight bars indicate the distance of the number from zero. This is why absolute value is never negative; absolute value asks only, "How far?", whether the number is in a positive or a negative direction on the number line. This means that $|3| = 3$ because 3 is three units to the right of zero; also, $|-3| = 3$ because -3 is three units to the left of zero. So whether it is $|3|$ or $|-3|$, the distance from zero in both cases is 3.

For example,

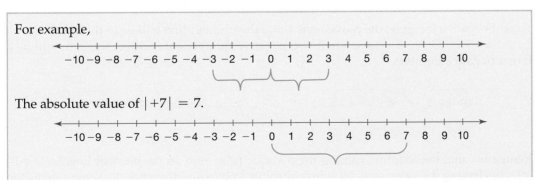

The absolute value of $|+7| = 7$.

(continued to next page)

The absolute value of $|-5| = 5$.

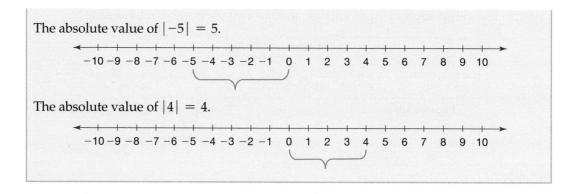

The absolute value of $|4| = 4$.

Practice 4

Write the absolute value of the following.

1. $|+12|$ = _____

2. $|-14|$ = _____

3. $|6|$ = _____

4. $|21|$ = _____

5. $|-476|$ = _____

INTEGER OPERATIONS

Integer operations use the basic mathematical functions addition, subtraction, multiplication, and division to solve math problems.

ADDING INTEGERS WITH LIKE SIGNS

Adding positive integers is just like adding whole numbers. For example, $2 + 7 = 9$ is the same as $+2 + +7 = +9$. Thus, the numbers move right on the number line.

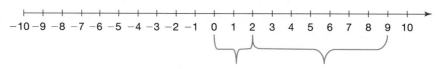

To add negative integers, the movement along the number line will be to the left of 0.

So $-4 + -3 = -7$. Thus, when two negative numbers are added, the sum will be a larger negative number.

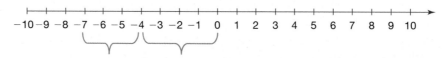

Remember that the absolute value is the distance from zero on the number line. So to add integers having the same sign, add their absolute values and then use the same sign as the numbers you are adding.

EXAMPLES

$5 + 4 = $ _____	$-7 + 0 = $ _____	$-7 + -5 = $ _____
The absolute values are $\lvert5\rvert + \lvert4\rvert = 9$	The absolute values are $\lvert7\rvert + \lvert0\rvert = 7$	The absolute values are $\lvert7\rvert + \lvert5\rvert = 12$
These are positive numbers being added.	Adding zero to any number does not change the number.	Add the sign of the numbers being added.
	Add the negative sign.	
$5 + 4 = 9$	$-7 + 0 = -7$	$-7 + -5 = -12$

Practice 5

Solve the following.

1. $4 + 17 = $ _____

2. $-9 + -27 = $ _____

3. $-8 + -4 = $ _____

4. $23 + 12 = $ _____

5. $-12 + -54 = $ _____

6. $(-5) + -18 = $ _____

7. $3 + 6 + 12 = $ _____

8. $(-9) + (-5) + (-12) = $ _____

9. $(-17) + (-2) + (-3) = $ _____

10. $(2) + 0 + (14) = $ _____

ADDING INTEGERS WITH UNLIKE SIGNS

The number line is very helpful when adding numbers with different signs. The number line below shows the sum of $-5 + 8$.

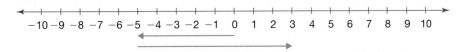

The integer -5 plus 8 equals 3. Note that the positive 8 is larger than the negative 5, so the answer will be $+3$ or 3.

Remember that the absolute value is the distance from zero on the number line. So to add integers having different signs, subtract their absolute values and then use the sign of the larger number.

EXAMPLES

$-7 + 6 =$ _____

$+9 + (-4) =$ _____

$(-8) + (-5) + 7 =$ _____

Subtract the absolute values.
$|7| - |6| = 1$

The -7 is larger than the 6.

The answer will be negative.

Subtract the absolute values.
$|9| - |4| = 5$

The $+9$ is larger than -4.

The answer will be positive.

Combine the integers with the same signs.
$(-8) + (-5) = -13$

Subtract the absolute values. $|13| - |7| = 6$

The -13 is larger than the 7. The answer will be negative.

$-7 + 6 = -1$

$+9 + (-4) = 5$

$(-8) + (-5) + 7 = -6$

Practice 6

Solve the following.

1. $25 + (-7) =$ _____

2. $-9 + 18 =$ _____

3. $13 + -8 =$ _____

4. $-7 + 13 =$ _____

5. $8 + (-12) + 10 =$ _____

6. $-3 + 4 + (-7) =$ _____

7. $6 + (-5) + (-11) =$ _____

8. $-28 + 45 + (+12) =$ _____

9. $98 + (-12) + (-2) =$ _____

10. $-7 + (0) + (-2) =$ _____

SUBTRACTING INTEGERS

Each integer has an opposite. For example, $+5$ has an opposite integer, -5. This concept of opposites is used in the subtraction of integers. To subtract an integer, add its opposite. Addition and subtraction are inverse or opposite operations.

Another way to understand how to subtract integers is to follow a three-step setup. Look at the math problem: $+5 - (-9) =$ _____

STEP 1: Change the math function sign from $-$ to $+$. $+5 + (-9) =$ _____

STEP 2: Change the number sign after the function sign. $+5 + (+9) =$ _____

STEP 3: Add to find the solution. $+5 - (-9) = 14$

If this seems confusing, count the spaces on the number line to discover the absolute value of each integer from 0.

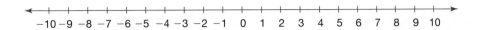

$$-10\ -9\ -8\ -7\ -6\ -5\ -4\ -3\ -2\ -1\ \ 0\ \ 1\ \ 2\ \ 3\ \ 4\ \ 5\ \ 6\ \ 7\ \ 8\ \ 9\ \ 10$$

EXAMPLES

$8 - (-3) = $ _____	$-9 - 4 = $ _____	$-12 - (-5) = $ _____
Change the minus sign to add	Change the minus sign to add	Change the minus sign to add
$8 + (-3) = $ _____	$-9 + 4 = $ _____	$-12 + (-5) = $ _____
Change to the opposite sign of (-3), which is $(+3)$.	Change to the opposite sign of (4), which is (-4).	Change to the opposite sign of (-5), which is $(+5)$.
Add	Add	Add
$8 + (+3) = 11$	$-9 + -4 = -13$	$-12 + (+5) = -7$

Practice 7

Solve the following.

1. $10 - (-7) = $ _____

2. $-9 - 7 = $ _____

3. $-12 - (-6) = $ _____

4. $-7 - (+13) = $ _____

5. $8 - (-12) = $ _____

6. $-3 - (-4) = $ _____

7. $6 - (-5) - (-11) = $ _____

8. $-18 - (-25) - (+12) = $ _____

9. $-12 - 12 = $ _____

10. $-7 - (0) - (-1) = $ _____

MULTIPLICATION OF INTEGERS

The multiplication of integers can be presented in a variety of ways. In whole numbers, we saw multiplication problems that looked like this: $2 \times 4 = 8$.

In integers, multiplication presents itself in a variety of formats. The multiplication sign $\times$ is not used because it can easily be confused with the variable x. A **variable** is an unknown number.

The important part of the multiplication of integers concerns determining if the product of the factors is positive or negative. Follow these rules:

SET-UP HINT	Problem	Workspace	Explanation of Sign
	+2(+3) or 2(3)	$2 \times 3 = 6$	The product of two positive factors is positive.
	−7(−6)	$7(6) = 42$	The product of two negative factors is positive.
	−5(+6)	$-5(6) = -30$	The product of a negative factor and a positive factor is negative.

EXAMPLES

$+7(12) =$ _____
$7 \cdot 12 =$ _____

$-8(-3) =$ _____
$8 \cdot 3 =$ _____

$-3(125) =$ _____
$3 \cdot 125 =$ _____

Two positive factors means the product will be positive.

Two negative factors means the product will be positive.

One positive factor times one negative factor means the product will be negative.

$7 \cdot 12 = +84$ or 84

$-8(-3) = +24$ or 24

$-3(125) = -375$

Practice 8

Multiply the following integers.

1. $-9(6) =$ _____

2. $7(3) =$ _____

3. $-8 \cdot 14 =$ _____

4. $5(-15) =$ _____

5. $-5(23) \cdot 2 =$ _____

6. $2(-9)(-3) =$ _____

7. $-5(-2)(-4) =$ _____

8. $9(2)\left(\dfrac{1}{2}\right) =$ _____

9. $3(2)(-4) =$ _____

10. $-1(2)(-4) =$ _____

DIVISION OF INTEGERS

The division symbol is usually not used in algebra. Instead, a fraction bar is used to show division.

$$\frac{28}{(7)} \quad \text{or} \quad \frac{128}{-4}$$

Problem	Workspace	Explanation of Sign
$+108 \div +3 = $ _____	$+108 \div +3 = +36 \text{ or } 36$	The product of two positive factors is positive.
$\dfrac{-51}{-3} = $ _____	$\dfrac{-51}{-3} = +17 \text{ or } 17$	The product of two negative factors is positive.
$\dfrac{-63}{3} = $ _____	$\dfrac{-63}{3} = -21$	The product of a negative factor and a positive factor is negative.

EXAMPLES

$$\frac{+150}{(+3)} = \underline{\quad\quad}$$
$$+150 \div (+3) = \underline{\quad\quad}$$

If the signs of both the divisor and the dividend are positive, then the quotient will be positive.

$$\frac{+150}{(+3)} = +50 \text{ or } 50$$

$$\frac{-18}{(-3)} = \underline{\quad\quad}$$
$$-18 \div (-3) = \underline{\quad\quad}$$

If the signs of both the divisor and the dividend are negative, then the quotient will be positive.

$$\frac{-18}{(-3)} = +6 \text{ or } 6$$

$$\frac{125}{-5} = \underline{\quad\quad}$$
$$125 \div (-5) = \underline{\quad\quad}$$

If the sign of the divisor or the dividend is negative and the other is positive, the quotient will be negative.

$$\frac{125}{-5} = -25$$

Practice 9

Divide the following integers.

1. $\dfrac{+300}{25} = $ _____

2. $\dfrac{63}{-9} = $ _____

3. $\dfrac{+164}{-2} = $ _____

4. $\dfrac{-14}{-2} = $ _____

5. $\dfrac{-90}{15} = $ _____

6. $\dfrac{-300}{-4} = $ _____

7. $\dfrac{12.6}{-3} = $ _____

8. $\dfrac{-1,000}{-5} = $ _____

9. $\dfrac{-24}{4} = $ _____

10. $\dfrac{180}{-10} = $ _____

EXPONENTIAL NOTATION

Exponential notation is a useful means for writing a product of many factors. The base is the number being multiplied, and the exponent is the number of times that the base is multiplied.

For example, $3 \cdot 3 \cdot 3 \cdot 3 \cdot 3$ becomes 3^5. The number 3 is the base and 5 is the exponent. The exponent tells us how many times the base is used as a factor. This number, 3^5, is read 3 to the fifth power.

So this example has three forms.

Exponential form (exponential notation)	3^5
Factor form (repeated multiplication)	$3 \cdot 3 \cdot 3 \cdot 3 \cdot 3$
Standard form	243

Some simple rules make using exponents easy.

RULE 1: Any number raised to the first power is always equal to itself. $7^1 = 7$

Any number without an exponent always has an understood exponent of 1.

RULE 2: If a number is raised to the second power, we say it is *squared*. 5^2 is read as 5 squared.

RULE 3: If a number is raised to the third power, we say it is *cubed*. 4^3 is read as 4 cubed.

RULE 4: Any number (except 0) raised to the zero power is equal to 1.

$9^0 = 1$ and $121^0 = 1$. However, note that $0^4 = 0 \times 0 \times 0 \times 0 = 0$

Practice 10

Complete the chart.

	Exponential Notation	Factor Form/Repeated Multiplication	Standard Form
1.	5^3	_____	_____
2.	_____	$10 \cdot 10 \cdot 10 \cdot 10$	_____
3.	_____	_____	16
4.	_____	$2 \cdot 2 \cdot 2 \cdot 2 \cdot 2 \cdot 2$	_____
5.	7^2	_____	_____
6.	_____	_____	144
7.	5^0	_____	_____
8.	_____	$15 \cdot 15$	_____
9.	_____	_____	1
10.	_____	$10 \cdot 10$	_____

SQUARE ROOTS

The **square root** sign is $\sqrt{}$. To find the square root of a number x, one finds the factor that, when multiplied by itself one time, equals the number x inside the square root sign. For example, $\sqrt{100}$: $10 \times 10 = 100$ or 10^2. Thus, the square root of $\sqrt{100}$ is 10. This is called a **perfect square** because the factors are whole numbers, and are the same whole number.

Practice 11

Determine the square root for each.

1. $\sqrt{16}$ _____

2. $\sqrt{36}$ _____

3. $\sqrt{81}$ _____

4. $\sqrt{225}$ _____

5. $\sqrt{121}$ _____

6. $\sqrt{49}$ _____

7. $\sqrt{196}$ _____

8. $\sqrt{256}$ _____

9. $\sqrt{289}$ _____

10. $\sqrt{64}$ _____

ORDER OF OPERATIONS

Mathematicians have developed a standard order of operations for calculations that have more than one arithmetic operation. Following the order of operations allows for only one correct answer for each problem.

STEP 1: Perform any calculations involving parentheses, fraction bars, exponents, and square roots.

STEP 2: Perform all multiplications and divisions, working from left to right.

STEP 3: Perform all additions and subtractions, working from left to right.

MATH SENSE
Some instructors use the mnemonic device "Please excuse my Dear Aunt Sally" (PEMDAS) to help students remember the correct order.

P: Parentheses and fraction bars
E: Exponents and roots
M: { Multiplication
D: { Division
A: { Addition
S: { Subtraction

In the following example, we can see why the order of operations is helpful.

$$5 + 7 \times 8 = \underline{\hspace{2cm}}$$

Following the order of operations (PEMDAS),

STEP 1: $7 \times 8 = 56$

STEP 2: $56 + 5 = 61$

If the order of operations is not followed, the answer would incorrectly come out to $5 + 7 = 12$ and $12 \times 8 = 96$. Thus, it is important to have a rule to ensure that a set pattern for calculating each operation is followed.

Practice 12

Solve the following operations.

1. $(4 \times 5) \times 12 = $ _____

2. $8 + 9 - (3 \times 6) = $ _____

3. $(15 \times 3) - 8 \div 2 = $ _____

4. $4 \times (12 - 8) + 3 = $ _____

5. $(500 - 250) \div 25 + 1 = $ _____

6. $(24 \div 3) \times 2 + 12 = $ _____

7. $10 - 6 \times (14 \div 2) = $ _____

8. $\dfrac{(124 \div 4)}{1} = $ _____

9. $\dfrac{(15 \times 3)}{(5 \times 1)} = $ _____

10. $352 - (34 - 2) + 2 \times 14 = $ _____

◆

ALGEBRAIC EXPRESSIONS

A **variable** is a letter or symbol that represents an unknown number. Letters such as p, t, x, or y are used to represent variables. For example, we can use s to represent the number of students when calculating the cost of educating a class of nurses for a year. A variable can be used in addition, subtraction, multiplication, and/or division problems. Some variables have **coefficients** like the -8 in $-8s$, where the coefficient, or number, -8 is multiplied by the unknown number s. If a variable appears by itself as s, or xy, it is understood to have a coefficient of 1 because $s = 1s$ and $xy = 1xy$.

EXPRESSIONS

An **expression** is a mathematical statement that may use numbers and/or variables. An **algebraic expression** is an expression that contains one or more variables.

The following are examples of expressions:

EXAMPLES

$$9 + z$$
$$xy$$
$$9(3 - r)$$
$$20 + (9 - x)$$

An expression is also used to build a mathematical statement from words, as in a word problem.

An LPN spends $240.00 on books and a dental assistant spends y on books. Write an expression for their combined amounts of dollars spent on books. The combined amount of an LPN's spending and a dental assistant's spending is $240.00 + y$.

Practice 13

For each problem, identify the variable and the coefficient.

Expression	Variable	Coefficient
1. $12a^3$	_____	_____
2. $25bcd$	_____	_____
3. $1.5x$	_____	_____
4. $7z^2$	_____	_____
5. $12ab^2c$	_____	_____
6. $22xy$	_____	_____
7. $2bc^3$	_____	_____
8. $-xyz$	_____	_____
9. $-7bc$	_____	_____
10. abc	_____	_____

To evaluate an expression for some number means that we replace or substitute the number for the variable in the expression and then simplify the expression.

Some common algebraic expressions are:

some number n increased by 2.7 $\rightarrow n + 2.7$

9 less than some number $x \rightarrow x - 9$

the sum of two numbers a and $b \rightarrow a + b$

some number q multiplied by 5 $\rightarrow 5q$

the product of x and $-9 \rightarrow -9x$

4 times the sum of three numbers x, y, and $z \rightarrow 4(x + y + z)$

The sum of two numbers y and z divided by $-8 \rightarrow \dfrac{y + z}{-8}$

Note: The variable is always written after the numeral.

Practice 14

Write the algebraic expression for each mathematical statement.

Word Phrase	**Algebraic Expression**
1. some number p decreased by 4.5	_____
2. some number c multiplied by 7	_____
3. the sum of two numbers a and b	_____
4. some number x divided by 5	_____
5. the sum of two numbers a and b divided by 6	_____
6. five times the sum of two numbers x and y	_____
7. the quotient of some number r and 3	_____
8. six less than some number x	_____
9. the sum of two numbers m and n multiplied by 2	_____
10. the sum of some number x and 24	_____

Practice 15

Let's practice moving from numbers to word expressions so that we can verbalize what we understand the number expressions to mean.

Write an algebraic expression in words for each number statement. For example,

$z(4) - 6$ would become z multiplied by 4 minus 6.

1. $a + b - z$ _____

2. $w(y + 2)$ _____

3. $\dfrac{x}{y} - 15$ _____

4. $125 \div (35 - 10)$ _____

5. $7ab - 15$ _____

Algebraic expressions are not *solved* as in computation, but instead are *evaluated*. The value of the variable, often given, is used to replace the variable in the expression.

For example, evaluate the expression $5 \cdot y + 12$ when y equals 12.

STEP 1: Replace y with 12. $5 \cdot 12 + 12$

STEP 2: Follow order of operations steps.

$$5 \cdot 12 = 60 \text{ (multiply first)}$$
$$60 + 12 = 72 \text{ (then add)}$$

The algebraic expression equals 72.

Evaluate the expression using substitution.

$$(4 + x) \times 2 + 15 \div 3 - x \quad \text{when} \quad x = 2.$$

We replace each occurrence of x with the number 2, and simplify by applying the usual order of operations rules: parentheses first, then exponents, multiplication and division third, and finally addition and subtraction.

$(4 + x) \times 2 + 15 \div 3 - x$	First, replace each x with 2 so that the expression becomes
$(4 + 2) \times 2 + 15 \div 3 - 2 =$	Next handle the parentheses.
$6 \times 2 + 15 \div 3 - 2 =$	Then multiply and divide.
$12 + 5 - 2 =$	Complete the addition and subtraction.
$17 - 2 = 15$	

Practice 16

Use substitution to evaluate these expressions. Let $a = 5$, $b = 4$, and $c = 1$.

1. $4a^2$

2. $5a^2b$

3. $2a + b^2c^0$

4. $7ca^2$

5. $3b - c^2$

Practice 17

Evaluate each expression.

1. $35 - \dfrac{(3 \cdot 7)}{4} =$

2. $\dfrac{(7 + 33)}{4 \div 2} =$

3. $\dfrac{3}{4}(10 - 4) =$

4. $\dfrac{1}{2}(8) + \dfrac{1}{4}(24) =$

Evaluate each expression when $x = 5$, $y = 10$, and $z = 15$.

5. $\dfrac{1}{2}(8y) =$

6. $\dfrac{3}{4}(6 - x) =$

7. $6z - y =$

8. $(z - x)(x + 5) =$

9. $\dfrac{(y - z)}{5} =$

10. $x(y + z - 4) =$

WRITING EXPRESSIONS FROM WORD PROBLEMS

The most important use of writing expressions is in real-life situations. Careful reading of the problem will help ensure that you use the correct mathematical operation.
Here are some key words to help guide you:

=	+	−	×	÷
is	add	subtract	multiply	divide
as	sum	difference	product	quotient
equals	plus	minus	times	split
equal to	total	remainder	"of"	per
	more than	less than		
	increased by	decreased by		

Reading word problems requires attention to detail. Sometimes there can be confusion over some expressions.

For instance, "five more than x", which is written $x + 5$, and "five is more than x", which is written $5 > x$, look very similar. The difference here is the word "is." "$x + 5$" is an expression, not an equation or inequality like "$5 > x$".

Here is another example: "four less than z", which should be written $z - 4$, not $4 - z$ or $4 < z$. "$4 - z$" would be written "four minus z." And the equation or inequality "$4 < z$" would be written "four is less than z."

For example, how would you write an expression to represent that you got twelve points higher on this anatomy test than on the last one?

First, choose and define your variable:
Let $x =$ the score you got on the last test.
So the expression to show twelve more is $x + 12$.

Here are some more examples:

a. There are twice the number of LPNs to the number of RNs on this shift. You could express this statement as $2p$.

b. The insurance rate for eye care has increased by $250.00. ($x + 250$)

c. The shift has ten fewer patients to care for. ($r - 10$)

d. This nursing supervisor has three more than twice as many years of experience as the former supervisor. ($2s + 3$)

Practice 18

Write an expression to represent each word problem.

1. Robert had two fewer cavities than I had. _____

2. I doubled my income after I finished the certificate program. _____

3. The stipend increased her income by 500 dollars. _____

4. Dr. Phil Berg has five more than twice the number of patients than any other dentist.

_____

5. He lost 12 pounds this month. _____

SOLVING EQUATIONS

To solve an equation, get the variable by itself on one side of the equal sign. Use inverse operations to do this:

- Addition is the inverse of subtraction and vice versa.
- Multiplication is the inverse of division and vice versa.

Here are some examples.

Solve the equation: $x + 1.5 = -5.2$

$x + 1.5 - 1.5 = -5.2 - 1.5$	To get x by itself on the left side of the equation, subtract 1.5 from both sides of the equation.
$x = -6.7$	Simplify each side.

Solve the equation: $z - 7 = 5$

$z - 7 + 7 = 5 + 7$	To get z by itself on the left side of the equation, add 7 to both sides of the equation.
$z = 12$	Simplify each side.

Solve the equation: $5a = 36$

$\dfrac{5a}{5} = \dfrac{36}{5}$	To get a by itself on the left side of the equation, divide both sides by 5.
$a = 7.2$ or $7\dfrac{1}{5}$	Simplify each side.

Solve the equation: $\dfrac{y}{2} = 3.8$

$\dfrac{y}{2} \cdot 2 = 3.8 \cdot 2$	To get y by itself on the left side of the equation, multiply both sides by 2.
$y = 7.6$ or $7\dfrac{3}{5}$	Simplify each side.

Practice 19

Solve the equations.

1. $x + 7.5 = 65$

2. $z - 13 = 42$

3. $k + 3\frac{1}{2} = 45$

4. $r - 5 = 17.4$

5. $b - 4.25 = -16.5$

6. $-6a = -4.5$

7. $\dfrac{t}{-8} = 16.2$

8. $12c = 60$

9. $\dfrac{m}{4} = -4.1$

10. $-50w = -14$

WRITING EQUATIONS FROM WORD PROBLEMS

An **algebraic equation** is an equation that contains one or more variables. There will also be algebraic expressions on both sides of the equation. So an equation is a mathematical sentence with an equal sign that illustrates that two expressions represent the same number. To understand word problems, you must be able to translate the words or other data into an equation.

For example, if the patient's temperature decreases by 2 degrees, it will be 99.4 degrees. What is the patient's temperature now?

Use t for the variable representing the patient's temperature.

temperature decreased by 2 degrees is 99.4 degrees

↓   ↓   ↓   ↓ ↓

t $-$ 2 $= 99.4$

Solve the equation: $t - 2 = 99.4$

$t - 2 + 2 = 99.4 + 2$ To get t by itself on the left side of the equation, add 2 to both sides of the equation.

$t = 101.4$ Simplify.

If a certified nurse's aid works a 12-hour shift, he or she will earn $165. How much will the aid earn in an hour?

Use x for the amount that the aid earns each hour.

12 hours times the amount earned per hour is $165.

12   times x $= \$165$

$12x = 165$

Solve the equation: $12x = 165$

$$\frac{12x}{12} = \frac{165}{12}$$ Divide both sides by 12.

$$x = 13.75$$ Simplify.

Practice 20

Write an equation to represent each word problem. Then solve it.

1. Sharon wants to donate 123 nursing books to the college library. The nursing collection has 1,357 books stored on the library shelves. How many books will be in the collection after Sharon's donation?

Equation: _____   Solution: _____

2. If a patient's pulse decreases by 8 beats, it will be 78 beats a minute. How many beats a minute is the pulse before the decrease?

Equation: _____   Solution: _____

3. If you double the cost of a dietitian's apron and then add $2, you will get the cost of a tailored dietitian's jacket. A dietitian's apron costs $16.50. How much will each dietitian's tailored jacket cost?

Equation: _____   Solution: _____

4. The cost of a polymer crown is $1,005. The insurance pays $\frac{1}{2}$ the cost plus $75. What part of the bill is left for the patient to pay?

Equation: _____   Solution: _____

5. Dinh has 7 more patients to care for than Juan. If Dinh has 18 patients to care for, how many does Juan have?

Equation: _____   Solution: _____

6. If you divide a number by 5 and add –8, the result is 3. What is the number?

Equation: _____   Solution: _____

7. If you multiply a number by 4 and add 7, the result is the 31 residents who work in the large city hospital. What is the number?

Equation: _____   Solution: _____

8. Together the surgical technicians spent $112.44 for lunch. There were 12 technicians. How much did each spend on lunch?

Equation: _____   Solution: _____

9. The cost of an eye appointment is $125 and imported frames are $325. If the patient paid a total of $625.35, what was the cost of the lens and the coatings?

Equation: _____   Solution: _____

10. The sum of a number and 3 times the same number is 100. What is the number?

Equation: _____   Solution: _____

UNIT REVIEW

◆◆◆◆ Critical Thinking With Pre-Algebra Basics

1. The cafeteria at the hospital had a checking account balance of $4,218.00 on Monday. On Tuesday, a check of $495 was written on the account. A deposit of $717 was made on Wednesday, and a check for $125 was written Thursday. What was the checking account balance after these transactions?

2. Write the algebraic expression for *one-half a number is then increased by 9.*

3. Write the algebraic expression for *five less than a number.*

4. Write the algebraic expression for *twice a number increased by 4.*

5. Solve: $12x = 84$

6. Solve: $0.36 + y = 2.5$

7. What number divided by 4 equals 60?

8. Solve: $4z + 5 = 21$

9. A clinic purchased ten dozen boxes of tissues. The total purchase cost $258.00. How much did 12 boxes of tissue cost?

10. Fifteen added to what number equals 97?

11. In the hospital, a pharmacy technician named Tia worked 12 more shifts a month than Sal. The total number of shifts that were worked by the two pharmacy technicians was 76. How many shifts did Tia work?

12. One paycheck is $250 less than another. The sum of the two checks is $1,628. How much is each check written for?

13. The sum of two consecutive numbers is 57. What is the smaller number?

14. What is the value of $2^4 - 1^6 + 4^3$?

15. What is $|17| + |-5|$ divided by 2?

◆◆◆◆ Professional Expertise

- Use PEMDAS to remember the order of operations.
- Always include the negative signs when needed.
- Read each problem carefully.
- Sketch out a picture or number line to help you visualize the problem.

PRE-ALGEBRA BASICS POST-TEST

1. $-6 + 5 =$ _____

2. $-12 - 12 =$ _____

3. $5 + 4 \times 8 - 16 \div 4 =$ _____

4. $12 - 40 \div 2 \div 5 + 2 =$ _____

5. $4^2 + 3^0 =$ _____

6. $12^3 \times 3^2 =$ _____

7. $\sqrt{121} =$ _____

8. $\sqrt{9} \times 20 =$ _____

9. $|-68| =$ _____

10. $10 - 8 \times 2 + 12 \div 3 =$ _____

11. The coefficient of $4abf$ is _____

12. Write as an expression: the quotient of some number y and 5 _____

13. Solve: $\dfrac{t}{-4} = 24.4$ _____

14. Beth has \$450 more than Fred. Together they have \$3,219. How much money does Fred have? _____

15. Subtract 10 from Thanh's age and double the result, and you get Xuyen's age. Xuyen is 22. How old is Thanh? _____

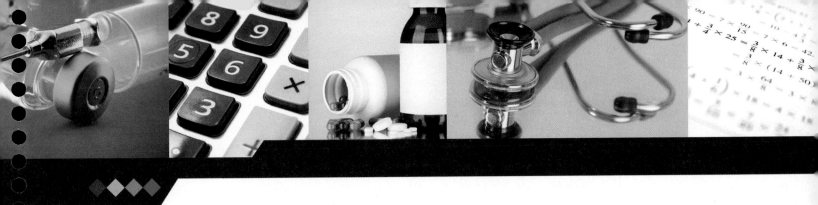

UNIT

8

The Metric System

STUDENT LEARNING OUTCOMES

After completing the tasks in this unit, you will be able to:

8-1 Name the units in the metric system

8-2 Convert metric units to standard units

8-3 Complete metric-to-metric conversions

8-4 Use ratio and proportion to make dental stone measurements

8-5 Identify how the metric system is used in the health care field

---

PRE-TEST

1. Look at the drug label.

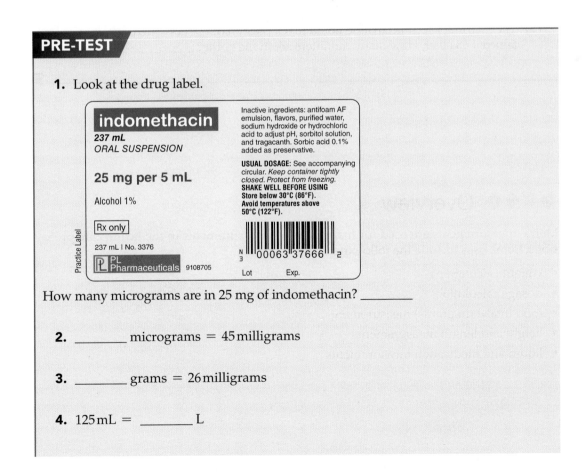

indomethacin
237 mL
ORAL SUSPENSION

25 mg per 5 mL

Alcohol 1%

Rx only

237 mL I No. 3376
PL Pharmaceuticals 9108705

Inactive ingredients: antifoam AF emulsion, flavors, purified water, sodium hydroxide or hydrochloric acid to adjust pH, sorbitol solution, and tragacanth. Sorbic acid 0.1% added as preservative.

USUAL DOSAGE: See accompanying circular. Keep container tightly closed. Protect from freezing.
SHAKE WELL BEFORE USING
Store below 30°C (86°F).
Avoid temperatures above 50°C (122°F).

Practice Label

N 3 00063 37666 2

Lot   Exp.

How many micrograms are in 25 mg of indomethacin? _____

2. _____ micrograms = 45 milligrams

3. _____ grams = 26 milligrams

4. 125 mL = _____ L

185

5. $0.45\,g =$ _____ mcg

6. $4.9\,mL =$ _____ L

7. _____ L $= 300\,mL$

8. $15\,mcg =$ _____ g

9. _____ mg $= 45\,g$

10. _____ mcg $= 25\,mg$

11. $84\,mcg =$ _____ g

12. $67\,kg =$ _____ g

13. The medical assistant was asked to measure the infant. The infant measured 0.361 meters or _____ centimeters.

14. A drug label notes that the client's medicine has 150 milligrams in 2.5 milliliters of syrup. How many milliliters would deliver 225 milligrams of medicine? _____

15. The pharmacy technician aide noted that a plastic container of medication contained 0.084 liter. How many milliliters are in the bottle? _____

◆◆◆◆ Overview

Metric measurements are used for many types of measurements in the health care professions. Some uses include the following:

- weight calculations
- dosage calculations
- food intake (in grams) measurements
- height and length measurements
- liquid and medication measurements

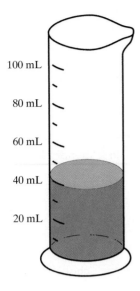

40 mL of 1:40
acetic acid (solution)

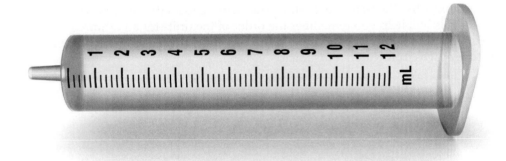

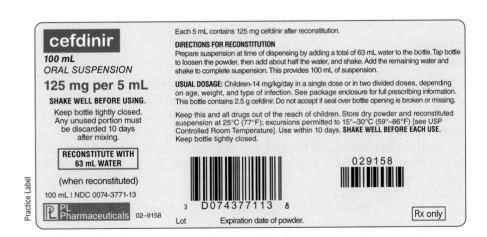

Metric units come in base units. These units measure different types of materials.

Base Unit	Measurement Type	Examples
Liter (l or L)	volume	liquids, blood, urine
Gram (g or G)	weight	an item's weight
		an amount of medicine
Meter (m)	length	height, length, instruments

The metric system uses units based on multiples of ten. For this reason, metric numbers are written in whole numbers or decimal numbers, but never as fractions. You can solve metric conversion problems by moving the decimal either to the left or to the right. So if you are moving from grams to milligrams, you must move the decimal three places to the right. This is the same as multiplying the number by 1000. So 1.5 grams × 1000 = 1500 milligrams.

Unit:	kilo-	hecto-	deka-	base	deci-	centi-	milli-	x	x	micro-
	thousand		ten	one	tenth	hundredth	thousandth			millionth
Value:	1000	100	10	1	0.1	0.01	0.001			0.000001
				meter (m)						
Symbol:	k	h	da	grams (g)	d	c	m			mc
				liter (l or L)						
Mnemonic Device:	kiss	hairy	dogs	but	drink	chocolate	milk,	m	o	m

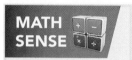

MATH SENSE

Decimals and metric measurements are based on units of ten.

Using a mnemonic device helps you keep the metric units in the correct sequence or order. Try something silly like "kiss hairy dogs but drink chocolate milk, mom." Knowing a device like this will help you remember the order of the units for an exam.

Note that the letters *mo* (in "mom") are placeholders. They help you remember to count three spaces from "milli-" to "micro-".

◆◆◆◆ Using the Metric Symbols

REVIEW

In the metric system, a unit of measurement (a prefix) and a base element (a root word) form the metric units. To form the abbreviation for *millimeter*, use the first letter of the prefix *milli*, which is *m*, and add it to the abbreviation for the root word *meter*, which is *m*, to form *mm*.

Together, the prefix and root indicate the type of measurement, as in volume, weight, or length. For example, in the word "kilogram," *kilo-* is the prefix and means thousand and *gram* is the root and means weight. The prefixes are the key to deciphering what number of units you have.

Prefix	Meaning	Symbol
kilo-	thousand	k
hecto-	hundred	h
deka-	ten	da
base	one	m, g, L
deci-	tenth	d
centi-	hundredth	c
milli-	thousandth	m
micro-	millionth	mc

Root	Use	Symbol
gram	weight	g
meter	length	m
liter	volume	L or l

Every metric prefix may be combined with every root. The application of these terms depends on the measurement being conveyed. Thus, liquids are measured in liters, and dry medications are measured in grams because this type of medication is measured by weight.

Practice 1

Supply the words or abbreviations.

1. kilogram _____

2. mL _____

3. gram _____

4. mg _____

5. centimeter _____

6. mm _____

7. kilometer _____

8. mcg _____

9. L _____

10. kg _____

11. km _____

12. meter _____

13. microgram _____

14. kL _____

15. cm _____

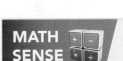

SET-UP HINT

k h d b d c m m o m

You can use the first letters of the metric units to recall their order by writing them on a piece of scratch paper or an answer sheet on examination days.

Writing metric notation correctly is important to avoid making medical errors. We add a leading zero before a decimal number that does not include a whole number. So, we write 0.65 milligrams, not .65 milligrams. Furthermore, the nonessential, trailing zeros are also dropped. So 1.500 grams becomes 1.5 grams because the trailing zeros do not add any value. The placement of the decimal is the key to the value of a number in the metric system: 1.5 grams is not 1500 grams.

Let's practice adding leading zeros and deleting trailing zeros.

MATH SENSE

Use leading zeros and drop the trailing zeros to avoid making careless errors and to ensure the creation of proper decimal numbers.

Practice 2

If the metric notation is correct, write OK on the line. If the metric notation is incorrect, write the correct form.

1. 4.80 milligrams _____

2. .35 grams _____

3. 1.09 liters _____

4. 12.420 micrograms _____

5. 5.7 milliliters _____

6. .9 liters _____

7. .500 milligrams _____

8. 7.12 kilograms _____

9. .160 milliliters _____

10. 90.059 grams _____

◆◆◆◆ Changing Unit Measures

REVIEW

In health care, sometimes a doctor's order comes in micrograms, but your supply on hand comes in milligrams. You need to convert from micrograms to milligrams to ensure accurate dosing. To change units within the metric system, count the spaces from the number you are starting with to the unit you are converting to.

$$45.5 \text{ grams} = \text{_____} \text{ milligrams}$$

SET-UP HINT kilo- ← 3 spaces → base unit* ← 3 spaces → milli- ← 3 spaces → micro-
(*gram, liters, meters)

Note that the *m* and *o* are placeholders and hold no value. They are included only to help you remember to count three spaces from milli- to micro-. Also note that most conversions in health care are between the unit kilo- (k) and the base (b) (gram, meter, and liter); between the base and the unit milli- (m); and between the units milli- and micro- (mc). As illustrated above, there are three spaces between each of these conversion pairs.

For example, from gram to milligram are three spaces. Note that the direction from gram to milligram is to the right. Move the decimal three places to the right, which is equivalent to multiplying the number by 1000. Thus,

$$45.5 \text{ grams} = 45\ 5\ 0\ 0 \text{ milligrams}$$
∪ ∪ ∪

Note that most health care conversions are done between kilogram and gram, gram and milligram, milligram and microgram, meter and centimeter, and liter and milliliter. With practice, you will discover that converting between units begins to feel natural. Practice making the conversion by moving the decimal from one unit to another. Use a pencil to draw the ∪ as you count the spaces. Start at the existing decimal and move to the right of each metric unit. Remember that "b" stands for the base units of meters, liters, or grams.

MATH SENSE Note that the units decrease or increase based on the direction from the base unit that one moves the decimal.

Units become larger kilo	Base Unit	Units become smaller and smaller ....micro
	grams	
⟵	meters	⟶
	liters	

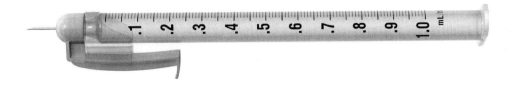

EXAMPLE

Use the workspace to write the mnemonic device.

50 milliliters = _____ liter   k h d b d c m m o m

0. 0 5 0
   ∪∪∪ = 0.05 liter

Moving three decimal places left is equivalent to dividing the number 50 by 1000.

Unit:	kilo-	hecto-	deka-	base	deci-	centi-	milli-	x	x	micro-
Value:	1000	100	10	1 meter (m)	0.1	0.01	0.001			0.000001
Symbol:	k	h	da	grams (g) liter (L)	d	c	m			mc or mc
Mnemonic Device:	kiss	hairy	dogs	but	drink	chocolate	milk,	m	o	m

Practice 3

Convert the following.

1. k h d b d c m m o m   8 grams = _____ kilogram

2. k h d b d c m m o m   120 grams = _____ milligrams

3. k h d b d c m m o m   4.25 kilograms = _____ grams

4. k h d b d c m m o m   220 milliliters = _____ liters

5. k h d b d c m m o m   _____ gram = 1000 micrograms

6. k h d b d c m m o m   _____ milligram = 426 micrograms

7. k h d b d c m m o m   _____ kilogram = 358.6 grams

8. k h d b d c m m o m   _____ centimeters = 3.97 meters

9. k h d b d c m m o m   37.5 micrograms = _____ milligrams

10. k h d b d c m m o m   _____ centimeter = 6.75 millimeters

Practice 4

Convert the following.

1. 10 liters = _____ milliliter

2. 2.5 liters = _____ milliliter

3. _____ milligram = 48 micrograms

4. 0.25 gram = _____ milligrams

5. 20.5 kilograms = _____ grams

6. 75 milligrams = _____ gram

7. _____ grams = 0.2 kilogram

8. 14.3 liters = _____ milliliters

9. 0.07 milligram = _____ micrograms

10. 4 kilograms = _____ milligrams

11. 14 centimeters = _____ meter

12. 0.001 kilogram = _____ gram

13. _____ liter = 250 milliliters

14. 3.8 milligrams = _____ gram

15. _____ milligrams = 0.6 gram

16. 56.75 milliliters = _____ liter

17. _____ milligrams = 36 grams

18. _____ gram = 10 milligrams

19. 7500 milliliters = _____ liters

20. _____ millimeters = 50 centimeters

21. 12.5 milligrams = _____ micrograms

22. 5.78 grams = _____ kilogram

23. 24 decimeters = _____ centimeters

24. 250 micrograms = _____ milligram

25. 12.76 kilograms = _____ grams

26. 45 meters = _____ millimeters

27. 23.5 centimeters = _____ millimeters

28. 750 micrograms = _____ milligram

29. 800 centimeters = _____ meters

30. 0.0975 milligram = _____ micrograms

31. 1000 milliliters = _____ liter

32. 3 kilograms = _____ grams

33. 12500 centimeters = _____ meters

34. 75.5 milligrams = _____ micrograms

35. 0.125 gram = _____ milligrams

36. 0.150 milligram = _____ microgram

37. 45250 milligrams = _____ gram

38. 9500 grams = _____ kilograms

39. 1000 micrograms = _____ gram

40. 25 micrograms = _____ milligram

41. 5524 grams = _____ kilograms

42. 45 milliliters = _____ liter

43. 1.25 meters = _____ centimeters

44. 550 micrograms = _____ milligram

45. 0.09 liter = _____ milliliters

46. 24.5 centimeters = _____ meter

47. 0.1 gram = _____ milligrams

48. 0.25 liter = _____ milliliters

49. 8500 micrograms = _____ milligrams

50. 0.625 gram = _____ micrograms

Practice 5

Solve the word problems using your knowledge of metric conversions.

1. The medical assistant was asked to measure the infant. The infant measured 0.4453 meters or _____ centimeters.

2. The physician asked the client in the cardiac unit to exercise on the treadmill. The physical therapy assistant recorded 0.5 kilometers for the first day of physical therapy. The next day the client walked 0.68 kilometers. How many more meters did the client walk on the second day? _____

3. The nutritional aide noted that a plastic container of cranberry juice contains 1.89 liters. How many milliliters are in the bottle? _____ If the nutritional aide was asked to pour 180 milliliter servings from this container, how many full servings could be poured? _____

4. The medical assistant asked the client's family to ensure adequate fluid intake, at least 2.2 liters of fluids. How many milliliters would that be? _____ How many full 240 milliliter (8 ounce glasses) portions should the client drink a day? _____

5. The certified nurse's aide measures the patient's output of urine to be 3100 milliliters. The patient is on a liquid diet and IV. In total today, the patient received 2.5 liters of dextrose water and drank a total of 1850 milliliters of juice, water, tea, and broth. What is the difference in the patient's intake from output in milliliters? _____

6. A drug label notes that the client's medicine has 250 milligrams in 5 milliliters of syrup. How many milliliters would deliver 125 milligrams of medicine? _____

7. A child claims to have grown 3.5 centimeters since his last checkup. His previous height was 1.2 meters. The medical assistant measures the child and discovers that he has grown 3.56 centimeters. What is the child's new height in centimeters that should be recorded in his medical record? _____ What is the child's new height in meters? _____

8. A can of pear halves weighs 425 grams. How many kilograms does the can weigh? _____

9. The pharmacy technician reads a prescription. The physician has ordered 0.03 grams of cevimeline hydrochloride for a client. The pharmacy has on hand 30 milligram capsules. Is the physician's order consistent with the supply on hand in the pharmacy? _____ How do you know this? _____
_____

10. Look at the following drug label.

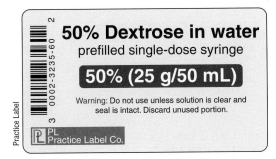

How many milligrams of dextrose are in this prefilled 50 mL syringe? _____

USING PROPORTIONS AND METRIC UNITS TO MEASURE DENTAL STONE

Sometimes dental assistants need to mix dental stone material for dental molds. The amount of stone and water varies according to the size of the mold needed. A dental assistant learns the importance of mixing a uniform and consistent material for the mold. This task uses the metric system: Dental stone is measured by weight in grams, and room temperature water is measured by volume in milliliters. Knowledge of the metric system coupled with the use of ratio and proportion help maintain the correct ratio of dental stone to water.

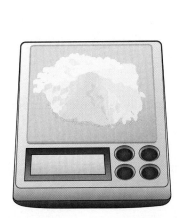

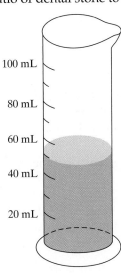

The typical ratio of dental stone to water is:

$$\frac{263 \text{ grams of dental stone powder}}{80 \text{ milliliters of room temperature water}}$$

Dental assistants use this ratio as the standard to solve variances in either stone or water to create the proper amount of material for the mold. On occasion, they may be asked to use other ratios of dental stone to water, depending on the type of material or the mold being created.

For example:

In Unit 6, we learned to use proportion to solve these conversion problems. We will set up the problems as proportions, cross multiply, and then divide by the leftover number. This will solve for the unknown.

If the dentist requests a smaller mold using 35 mL of water, how much stone should be used?

The setup is: $\dfrac{263 \text{ g}}{80 \text{ mL}} = \dfrac{? \text{ g}}{35 \text{ mL}}$

STEP 1: $263 \times 35 = 9205$

STEP 2: $9205 \div 80 = 115.0625$. Round to the nearest whole number.

The final answer is that 115 grams of stone to 35 milliliters of water should be used.

Practice 6

Solve the following using this ratio:

$$\frac{263 \text{ grams dental stone powder}}{80 \text{ milliliters of water}}$$

Round to the nearest whole number.

1. If you use 75 grams of stone, how many milliliters of room temperature water are needed?

2. If you use 125 milliliters of water, how many grams of dental stone are needed?

3. If you use 95 grams of stone, how many milliliters of room temperature water are needed?

4. If you use 75 milliliters of water, how many grams of dental stone are needed?

5. If you use 65 grams of stone, how many milliliters of room temperature water are needed?

6. If you use 55 grams of stone, how many milliliters of room temperature water are needed?

7. If you use 40 milliliters of water, how many grams of dental stone are needed?

8. If you use 35 grams of stone, how many milliliters of room temperature water are needed?

9. If you use 50 grams of stone, how many milliliters of room temperature water are needed?

10. If you use 60 milliliters of water, how many grams of dental stone are needed?

UNIT REVIEW

◆◆◆◆ Critical Thinking Using the Metric System

Circle the most logical answer.

1. The glass holds 240 (L, mL, mcg) of water.

2. The comb is 6 (cm, mm, m) long.

3. The hospital room is 20 (km, m, mm) wide.

4. The case of gloves weighs 4.5 (kg, g, mg).

Add one of the mathematical symbols $<$, $>$, or $=$ to make each statement true.

5. 5 m _____ 50 cm

6. 14.5 cm _____ 0.145 m

7. 0.25 mcg _____ 0.25 mg

8. 16 mL _____ 0.16 L

9. 12 kg _____ 12000 g

10. 4.8 L _____ 48 mL

11. A long-term care resident is on a sodium-restricted diet and is limited to 1500 mg of sodium (Na) each day. A whole-grain cracker has 0.16 g of sodium. How many crackers can she eat and stay below the 1500 mg of sodium?

12. Cough syrup has 5 mg of medication in a 1 mL solution. How many mg of medication are in 20 mL of solution?

13. A sleep medication is available as 0.125 milligram caplets. The patient is advised by his physician to take 500 mcg at bedtime. How many caplets will he take?

14. The physical therapists encouraged the runner to prepare slowly for the 5-K marathon. A 5-K marathon is _____ meters.

15. A child receives 2 teaspoons of a penicillin suspension every six hours. The label reads "125 milligrams of penicillin in 5 milliliters of suspension." What is the child's dose in milliliters for 24 hours?

◆◆◆◆ Professional Expertise

- Always double-check the placement of the decimal in conversions to ensure proper calculation of doses, weights, and measurements.
- Always include the unit of measure in the proper metric notation after the numeral.
- Metric abbreviations are singular and do not include periods.
- If the metric number is a decimal number without a whole number, always place a zero before the metric number as a placeholder: 0.45 mm, not .45 mm. Add leading zeros as needed.
- Drop trailing zeros, which have no value. So 9.500 grams should be written as 9.5 grams.
- When converting, double-check the number of places you have moved the decimal point for accuracy, using zeros as placeholders if needed.
- Do not use cc; use mL for milliliters.
- Do not use μ for microgram; use mcg.

METRIC SYSTEM POST-TEST

1. Look at the drug label. How many milligrams are in 2 milliliters of atropine?
_____

LOT
EXP

atropine
sulfate

Injection, USP

10 X 20 ,mL Multiple Dose Vials
FOR SC, IM OR IV USE

400 mcg/mL

(0.4 mg/mL)

PL Pharmaceuticals

Practice Label

Each mL contains atropine sulfate 400 mcg (0.4 mg), sodium chloride 9 mg and benzyl alcohol 0.015 mL in Water for Injection. pH 3.0-6.5; Sulfuric acid added, if needed, for pH adjustment.

POISON

Usual Dose: See package insert.
Store at controlled room temperature 15°-30°C (59°-86° F).
Caution: Federal law prohibits dispensing without prescription.
Product Code
2210-43   B-32210

2. _____ milligrams = 84 micrograms

3. _____ kilogram = 24.8 grams

4. 2.7 liters = _____ milliliters

5. 0.014 gram = _____ micrograms

6. 1.2 milliliters = _____ liter

7. 10 micrograms = _____ gram

8. _____ liter = 250 milliliters

9. _____ milligrams = 0.015 gram

10. _____ micrograms = 30 milligrams

11. 0.008 microgram = _____ milligram

12. The medical assistant was asked to measure the infant. The infant measured 0.345 meters or _____ centimeters.

13. A drug label notes that the client's medicine has 250 milligrams in 5 milliliters of syrup. How many milliliters would deliver 375 milligrams of medicine? _____

14. The pharmacy technician aide noted that a plastic container of medication contains 0.24 liter. How many milliliters are in the bottle? _____

15. 0.75 gram = _____ milligrams

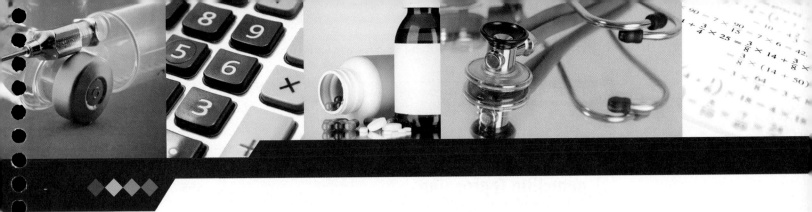

Reading Drug Labels, Medicine Cups, Syringes, and Intravenous Fluid Administration Bags

STUDENT LEARNING OUTCOMES

After completing the tasks in this unit, you will be able to:

9-1 Name the parts of drug labels

9-2 Label syringes and medicine cups for proper dosing

9-3 Read intravenous fluid administration bags

9-4 Use the drug label to find key dosing information

 ## Overview

Reading medication labels is part of the workplace skills for the allied health career. Most prescription drug labels contain certain information:

NAME	INFORMATION PRESENTED
Generic name	Indicates the chemical name of the drug and includes any drug marketed under its chemical name without advertising.
Trade name	Indicates the brand name; may have a ® or ™.
Manufacturer	Indicates the maker or manufacturer of the drug.
National Drug Code (NDC) number	Identifies the manufacturer, medication, and the container size.
Lot number (control number)	Placed on the label prior to shipping to identify the lot.
Drug form	Indicates cream, capsule, caplet, drop, tablet, suppository, syrup, etc.
Dosage strength	Provides the strength per dose as in tablet, milliliter, syrup, etc.
Usual adult dose	Indicates the usual adult dose for typical use.
Total amount in vial, packet, box	Indicates the total number of items in the container.
Prescription warning	Indicates that the medication is a prescription drug.
Expiration date	Provides the last date that the medication should be taken, applied, or used.

PRE-TEST

Read the label below.

NDC 0781-8153-94

penicillin G procaine for injection, USP

5,000,000 Units*

(5 million units)
For IM or IV use
Rx only

Practice Label

PL Pharmaceuticals

*Each vial contains Penicillin G sodium, equivalent to 5,000,000 units (5 million units) of penicillin G as the sodium salt with 1.68 mEq of sodium per million units of penicillin G, Store dry powder at 20°–25°C (68°–77°F) [see USP Controlled Room Temperture]. Sterile constituted solution may be kept in refrigerator (2° to 8°C) for 3 days without significant loss of potency

PREPARATION OF SOLUTION

Diluent added	Final Concentration
8 mL	500,000 units/mL
3 mL	1,000,000 units/mL

Exp: Lot:

Locate and identify seven different types of information that appear on this drug label.

1. _____

2. _____

3. _____

4. _____

5. _____

6. _____

7. _____

8. Shade the medicine cup to read 18 mL.

```
2 Tbsp — 30 mL
        — 25 mL
        — 20 mL
1 Tbsp — 15 mL
2 tsp — 10 mL
1 tsp — 5 mL
½ tsp
```

9. Shade the medicine cup to read $\frac{1}{3}$ ounce.

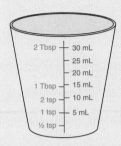

Look at the following label:

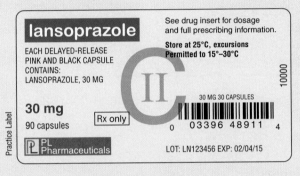

10. What is the generic name of this drug? _____

11. How many capsules are in the vial? _____

12. What is the form of this drug? _____

13. What is the strength of this drug? _____

14. Using the syringe below, mark a 6.4 mL dose.

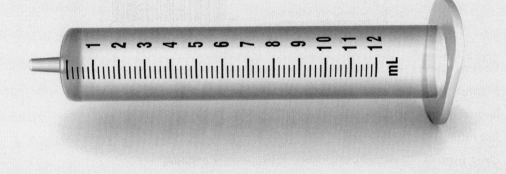

15.

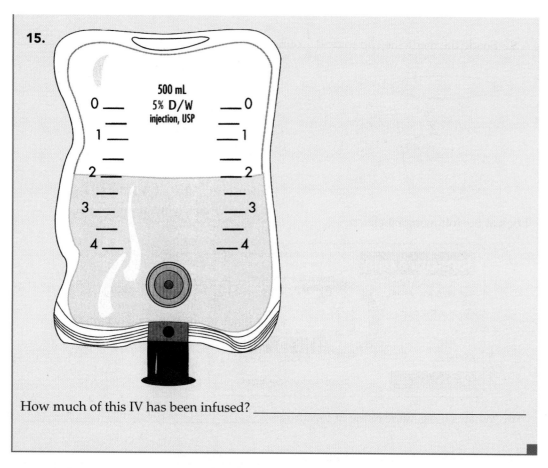

How much of this IV has been infused? _____

EXAMPLE

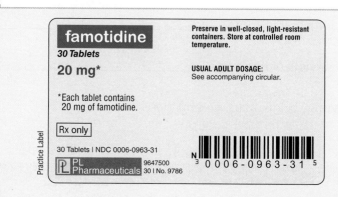

Generic name	famotidine
Manufacturer	PL Pharmaceuticals
National Drug Code (NDC) number	0006-0963-31
Lot number (control number)	Not shown*
Drug form	Tablet
Dosage strength	20 mg
Usual adult dose	See accompanying circular
Total amount in vial, packet, box	30 tablets
Prescription warning	Rx only
Expiration date	Not shown*

*The lot number and expiration date are added prior to shipment. The NDC number may also not appear on all labels. These labels are educational, so they do not show this information.

EXAMPLE

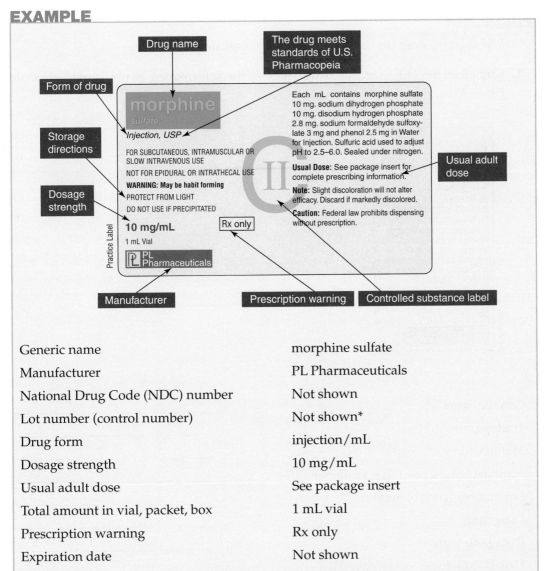

Generic name	morphine sulfate
Manufacturer	PL Pharmaceuticals
National Drug Code (NDC) number	Not shown
Lot number (control number)	Not shown*
Drug form	injection/mL
Dosage strength	10 mg/mL
Usual adult dose	See package insert
Total amount in vial, packet, box	1 mL vial
Prescription warning	Rx only
Expiration date	Not shown

*The lot number and expiration date are added prior to shipment. The NDC number may also not appear on all labels. These labels are educational, so they do not show this information.

Also, other information appears on the drug labels, such as a bar code, controlled substance schedule, notation about single- or multi-dose packages, mixing directions, and label alerts.

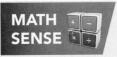

MATH SENSE A lot of information is presented on drug labels, so careful reading will ensure proper math calculations and accurate dosing.

Practice 1

Read the following drug labels, and then complete the missing information.

1. Complete the table for this drug label. If the information is not provided, write *not shown.*

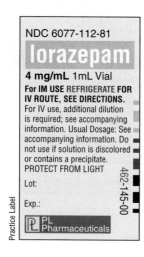

Generic name	_____
Trade name	_____
Manufacturer	_____
National Drug Code (NDC) number	_____
Lot number (control number)	_____
Drug form	_____
Dosage strength	_____
Usual adult dose	_____
Total amount in vial, packet, box	_____
Prescription warning	_____
Expiration date	_____

2. Complete the table for this drug label. If the information is not provided, write *not shown.*

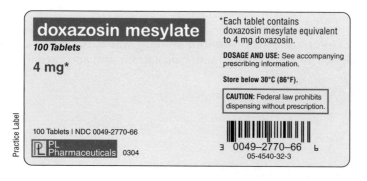

Generic name   _____

Trade name   _____

Manufacturer   _____

National Drug Code (NDC) number   _____

Lot number (control number)   _____

Drug form   _____

Dosage strength   _____

Usual adult dose   _____

Total amount in vial, packet, box   _____

Prescription warning   _____

Expiration date   _____

3. Complete the table for this drug label. If the information is not provided, write *not shown.*

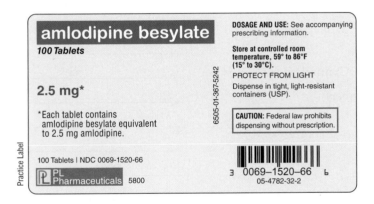

Generic name   _____

Trade name   _____

Manufacturer   _____

National Drug Code (NDC) number   _____

Lot number (control number)   _____

Drug form   _____

Dosage strength   _____

Usual adult dose   _____

Total amount in vial, packet, box   _____

Prescription warning   _____

Expiration date   _____

4. Complete the table for this drug label. If the information is not provided, write *not shown*.

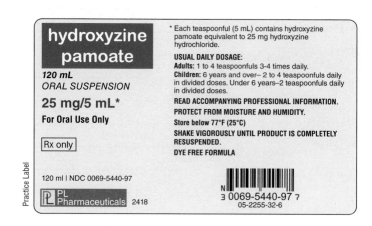

Generic name _____

Trade name _____

Manufacturer _____

National Drug Code (NDC) number _____

Lot number (control number) _____

Drug form _____

Dosage strength _____

Usual adult dose _____

Total amount in vial, packet, box _____

Prescription warning _____

Expiration date _____

5. Complete the table for this drug label. If the information is not provided, write *not shown*.

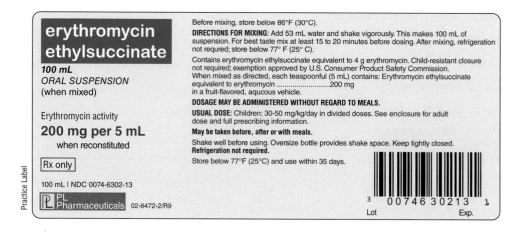

Generic name _____

Trade name _____

Manufacturer _____

National Drug Code (NDC) number _____

Lot number (control number) _____

Drug form _____

Dosage strength _____

Usual adult dose _____

Total amount in vial, packet, box _____

Prescription warning _____

Expiration date _____

◆◆◆◆ Medicine Cups

REVIEW

Medicine cups are used to dispense liquid medications such as cough syrup and Maalox (or milk of magnesia). To measure accurately, first pour the solution into the medicine cup. Next, place the cup on a level countertop to ensure the accuracy of the measurement.

For example, the nurse reads the order: Give 20 milliliters of cough syrup every 4 to 6 hours as needed. The nurse will pour 20 milliliters into the medicine cup for the client.

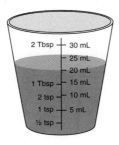

Practice 2

Read the following medicine cups and note the volume of medication in each.

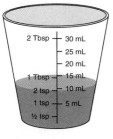
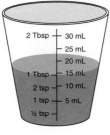
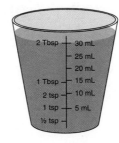
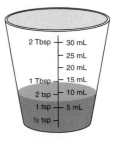

1. _____ **2.** _____ **3.** _____ **4.** _____

◆◆◆◆ Syringes

REVIEW

Parental medications are injected by a needle. These medications are absorbed by the body quickly and more completely than drugs taken orally. Syringes are sterile and are used to inject these medications. Syringes are labeled in tenths and hundredths, and the barrel of the syringe has markings in milliliters (mL) or other units indicating volume. Since using metric measurements has become the norm, cubic centimeter (cc) and minim (*m*) are no longer used. The metric units are based on units of ten, making them easy to measure. By having one standard for syringes, fewer medication errors will occur. Carefully read the syringe from the edge of the plunger closest to the needle.

EXAMPLE

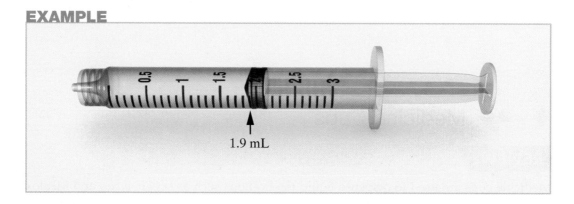

1.9 mL

Practice 3

Read the following syringes and indicate the total volume of the solution in each syringe.

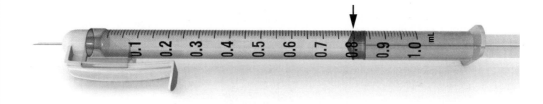

1. _____

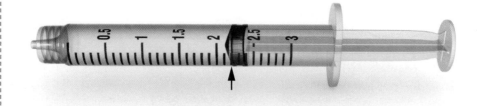

2. _____

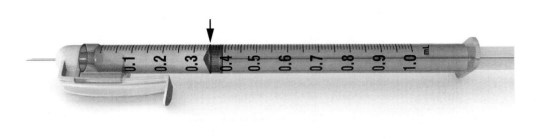

3. _____

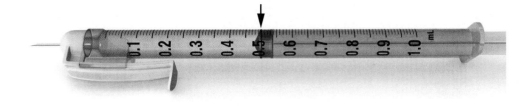

4. _____

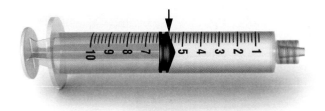

5. _____

◆◆◆◆ IV Bags

REVIEW

Intravenous infusions, or through-the-vein dosing, are used to provide a wide range of fluids: blood, medication, and nutritional and/or electrolyte-balanced water. Intravenous (IV) dosing goes directly into the vein and can be given to a client over time. Intravenous fluid administration bags are monitored by time, volume, and rate to ensure proper dosing. IV bags are made from durable plastic and are supplied in a variety of sizes: 250 mL, 500 mL, and 1000 mL. Smaller bags, which come in 100 mL, are available for mixing specific medications. The capacity is noted on the bag. Determining the amount of liquid remaining in an IV bag is straightforward. To read the IV bag, subtract the volume of the infused fluid from the capacity noted on the bag.

For example, look at this 500 milliliter bag. Observe that 200 milliliters has been infused.

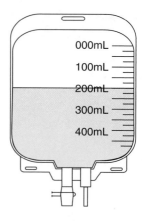

So, 500 milliliters − 200 milliliters = 300 milliliters remains to be infused.

Practice 4

Note the volume of IV fluid infused and the volume remaining to be infused in the following IV bags.

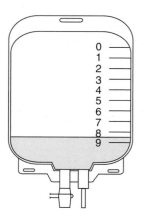

1. Volume infused _____
Volume remaining _____

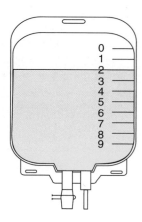

2. Volume infused _____
Volume remaining _____

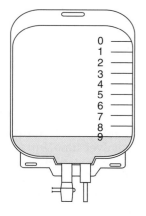

3. Volume infused _____
Volume remaining _____

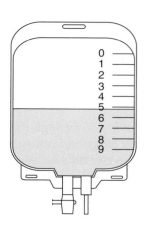

4. Volume infused _____
Volume remaining _____

UNIT REVIEW

◆◆◆◆ Critical Thinking with Reading Drug Labels, Medicine Cups, Syringes, and IV Fluid Administration Bags

1. If a medicine cup has 15 mL already poured into it and the dosage reads 24 mL, how many more mL must be added to the medicine cup to make a full dose?

2. The syringe is filled to 2.8 mL. The dosage reads 2.2 mL. The syringe is overfilled by _____ mL.

Use the following drug label to answer questions 3-5.

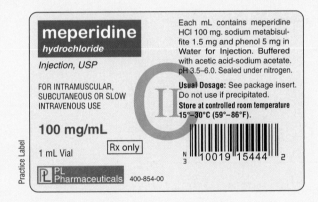

3. How many milliliters are in the entire vial?

4. What is the dosage strength?

5. What is the generic name of this medication?

6. What is the usual route that meperidine hydrochloride is normally given?

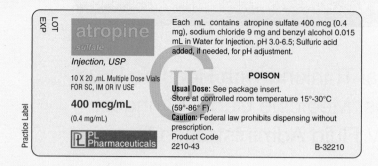

7. If the label reads 400 mcg/mL and the doctor orders 0.4 mg for the patient, how many mL will the patient receive?

8. Mark the syringe for the dosage to be given in problem number 7 above.

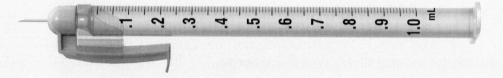

Use the following drug label to answer questions 9-15.

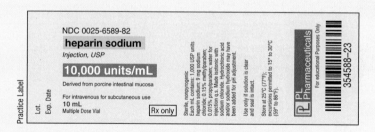

9. What is the manufacturer's name?

10. What is the national drug code for heparin sodium?

11. What is the route for this medication to be given?

12. What is the form of this drug?

13. What is the dosage strength?

14. If the doctor orders 5000 units of heparin sodium, the dosage given will be how many milliliters?

15. Can this vial be used more than once? How do you know?

◆◆◆◆ Professional Expertise

- Read labels carefully for accuracy.
- Always include the units of measure.
- Double-check the spelling of medications when reading and writing the drug names.
- When reading syringes, be sure to focus on the units of measure before filling the syringe with a medication dosage.

READING DRUG LABELS, MEDICINE CUPS, SYRINGES, AND IV FLUID ADMINISTRATION BAGS POST-TEST

1. Explain the difference between the generic name and the trade name of a prescription medication.

_____

_____

_____

_____

_____

Look at the label and provide the following information. If the information is not provided, write *not shown*.

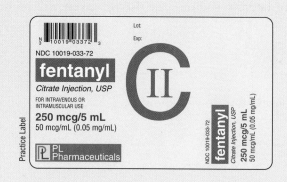

Generic name	2. _____
Trade name	3. _____
Manufacturer	4. _____
National Drug Code (NDC) number	5. _____
Lot number (control number)	6. _____
Drug form	7. _____
Dosage strength	8. _____
Usual adult dose	9. _____
Total amount in vial, packet, box	10. _____
Prescription warning	11. _____
Expiration date	12. _____

13. The medical assistants were asked to dispense 7.5 milliliters of a liquid medication. Shade the medicine cup to indicate this dosage.

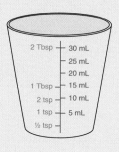

14. The physician has ordered an IM injection of 1.2 milliliters. Shade the syringe to indicate this volume of medication.

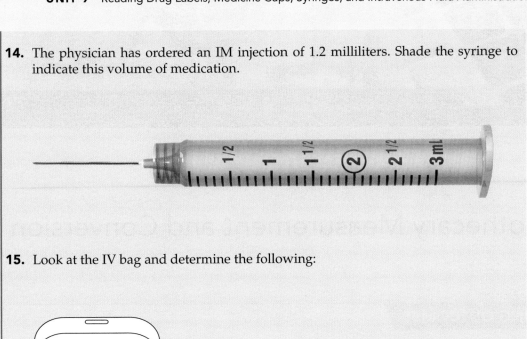

15. Look at the IV bag and determine the following:

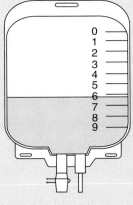

Volume infused _____
Volume remaining _____

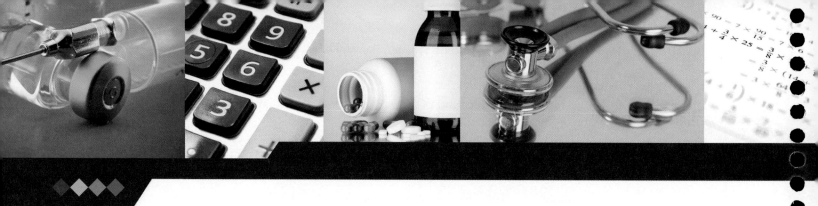

STUDENT LEARNING OUTCOMES

After completing the tasks in this unit, you will be able to:

10-1 Convert among apothecary, household, and metric measurement systems

10-3 Properly format the answers

10-2 Use the correct number formats for the measurement systems

◆◆◆◆ Overview

This unit brings together the fundamental skills of the previous units and applies these basics to health care situations. Although you will learn new information in this unit, the processes for arriving at the correct answers depend on your ability to compute using fractions, decimals, ratios, proportions, and, to a lesser degree, percents. This unit will cover apothecary measurements and two methods of converting among measurement systems. These fundamentals will help prepare you for math applications in the health care professions.

PRE-TEST

1. Write fifteen drops in medical notation. _____

2. 2.5 ounces = _____ teaspoons

3. $1\frac{1}{2}$ pints = _____ ounces

4. grains $4\frac{1}{6}$ = _____ mg

5. fluid ounces 8 = _____ mL

6. 24 kg = _____ pounds

7. 78 mL = _____ fluid ounces

8. grains $\dfrac{1}{400}$ = _____ mg

9. 75 mL = _____ fluid ounces

10. 5.4 mL = _____ drops

11. $3\dfrac{1}{2}$ teaspoons = _____ mL

12. The client weighs $122\dfrac{1}{4}$ pounds. How many kilograms does this client weigh? Round to the nearest tenth. _____

13. The physician's assistant prescribes 10 milliliters of cough syrup. How many teaspoons of cough syrup is that? _____

14. The participants in a weight reduction program are asked to drink six 8-ounce glasses of water daily. How many milliliters of water is this per day per person? _____

15. $4\dfrac{1}{3}$ cups = _____ milliliters

 Apothecary Measurement and Conversions

The **apothecary system** is an old measurement system that originated in England. This system, which uses grains for weight and minims for volume, is used by physicians and pharmacists to calculate drug amounts. It relies on several number systems to denote measurements: lowercase Roman numerals, Arabic numerals, and fractions. Although this system is being replaced by metric units to make the measuring system more uniform and avoid medication errors, we discuss this system because you may encounter the apothecary units of measure, as some physicians still use this system as a matter of habit. So until the apothecary system is completely converted over to metric units, you may see labels, prescriptions, and doctors' orders using some of these units. The apothecary system uses some basic rules that do not exist in other measurement systems. These rules include:

RULE 1: Fractions of $\frac{1}{2}$ may be written as *ss*.

The nurse will give grains iss of the medication to the patient.

RULE 2: Lowercase Roman numerals are used for apothecary amounts of ten or less and for the numbers 20 and 30.

The doctor prescribed grains x of the medication to be given immediately.

RULE 3: The symbol is placed before the quantity: Thus, grains $7\frac{1}{2}$ is written as *grains viiss* or *gr viiss*.

The pharmacist prepared grains ivss for the medication order.

In metric and household measurements, the symbol follows the quantity:

$$25 \text{ milligrams}, 3 \text{ cups}, 16\frac{1}{3} \text{ pounds}.$$

YOU MUST MEMORIZE TWO COMMON SYMBOLS THAT EXIST IN APOTHECARY:		
Term	**Symbol**	**Approximate Conversion**
fluid ounce	℥	fluid ounce 1 = 8 teaspoons
grain	gr	grain i = 60 or 65 milligrams*

*65 mg is the exact conversion from grain 1 and 60 mg is the rounded conversion

Once you are familiar with these terms, symbols, and their equivalents, you will be ready to use these apothecary units in your conversions. This is a new concept for health care students to learn. We think of science and measurement as exact, but apothecary is a measurement system of approximate equivalents. Approximate equivalents come into play when you are converting among the measurement systems. Metric-to-metric or household-to-household measurement conversions usually can be done in exact measurements. In general, metric- or household-to-apothecary measurement conversions are done through approximate measures. The equivalents are called approximate because they are rounded to the nearest whole number. In exact measures, 1 gram is equivalent to grains 15.432; however, the simple conversion in approximate equivalents used in health care is 1 gram = grains 15. To accomplish these conversions, you must memorize some of the approximate equivalents. With the ongoing movement away from the apothecary measurements, the health care industry is using the metric system more and more. Drug companies are responding and including both systems on labels as health care workers get accustomed to the change.

SET-UP HINT

Notice that the conversions in the table are set up so that the unit (1) elements are all on the left and that these will be placed on top of the known part of the ratio and proportion equation. This simplifies the learning process, expedites learning, and helps recall these conversions.

APPROXIMATE EQUIVALENTS	
1 teaspoon = 5 milliliters	1 kilogram = 2.2 pounds
grain i = 60 or 65 milligrams	1 teaspoon = 60 drops
grain i = 1 drop	1 pint = 2 cups
fluid ounce 1 = 8 teaspoons	1 quart = fluid ounces 32
fluid ounce 1 = 2 tablespoons	1 quart = 1 liter
fluid ounce 1 = 30 milliliters	1 cup = 240–250 milliliters
1 inch = 2.54 centimeters	

These conversions are accomplished by setting up the known and unknown quantities in proportion format or with dimensional analysis.

Use the following example as your guide:

EXAMPLE

How many milliliters are in $2\frac{1}{2}$ ounces?

To solve with proportion format:

a. Set up the known conversion on one side of the equal sign and the unknown on the other side of the equal sign.

$$\underset{\text{known}}{\frac{1\,\text{ounce}}{30\,\text{milliliters}}} = \underset{\text{unknown}}{\frac{2\frac{1}{2}\,\text{ounces}}{?\,\text{milliliters}}}$$

b. Cross multiply. $30 \times 2\frac{1}{2} = 75$

c. Shortcut—any number divided by 1 is itself. Thus, the answer is 75 milliliters.

EXAMPLE

Convert 48 milligrams to grains.

a. Set up the known conversion on one side of the equal sign and the unknown on the other side of the equal sign.

$$\underset{\text{known}}{\frac{\text{grain i}}{60\,\text{milligrams}}} = \underset{\text{unknown}}{\frac{?\,\text{ounces}}{48\,\text{milligrams}}}$$

b. Cross multiply. $1 \times 48 = 48 \rightarrow \dfrac{48}{60}$

c. Divide and/or reduce. $\dfrac{48}{60} \rightarrow$ reduces to grain $\dfrac{4}{5}$

The answer is grain $\dfrac{4}{5}$.

SET-UP HINT

Grains will be in whole numbers and/or fractions. Milliliters will be in whole numbers and decimals.

To solve with dimensional analysis:

How many milliliters are in $2\frac{1}{2}$ ounces?

a. Place the unit of measure of the unknown on one side of the equation.

$$?\,\text{milliliters} =$$

b. Use the conversion factor most appropriate to the problem. Place the factor of the answer's unit of measure on top and the units that you are converting to on the bottom as the denominator.

$$? \text{ milliliters} = \frac{30 \text{ milliliters}}{1 \text{ ounce}}$$

c. Multiply the first factor by the information given in the problem.

$$? \text{ milliliters} = \frac{30 \text{ milliliters}}{1 \text{ ounce}} \times \frac{2\frac{1}{2} \text{ ounces}}{1}$$

d. Cancel the like units and then solve by multiplication/division. Multiply straight across.

$$? \text{ milliliters} = \frac{30 \, \cancel{\text{milliliters}}}{1 \, \cancel{\text{ounce}}} \times \frac{2\frac{1}{2} \, \cancel{\text{ounces}}}{1} \rightarrow 30 \, \cancel{\text{milliliters}} \times 2\frac{1}{2}$$

$$= 75 \text{ milliliters}$$

The answer is 75 milliliters.

EXAMPLE

Convert 48 milligrams to grains.

a. Place the unit of measure of the unknown on one side of the equation.

$$? \text{ grains} =$$

b. Use the conversion factor most appropriate to the problem. Place the factor of the answer's unit of measure on top and the units that you are converting to on the bottom as the denominator.

$$? \text{ grain} = \frac{\text{grain i}}{60 \text{ milligrams}}$$

c. Multiply the first factor by the information given in the problem. Multiply straight across.

$$? \text{ grain} = \frac{\text{grain i}}{60 \text{ milligrams}} \times \frac{48 \text{ milligram}}{1}$$

d. Cancel the like units and then solve by multiplication/division.

$$? \text{ grain} = \frac{\text{grain i}}{60 \, \cancel{\text{milligrams}}} \times \frac{48 \, \cancel{\text{milligrams}}}{1} \rightarrow \frac{1 \times 48}{60 \times 1} =$$

e. Reduce if necessary.

$$\frac{48}{60} \rightarrow \text{ reduces to grain } \frac{4}{5}$$

The answer is grain $\frac{4}{5}$.

Practice 1

Conversions between metric and grains are dry equivalents. Use ratio and proportion or dimensional analysis. Show all of your work to the right of the problem.

1. 45 milligrams = grain _____

2. grain $\dfrac{1}{2}$ = _____ milligrams

3. 75 milligrams = grains _____

4. _____ milligram = grain $\dfrac{1}{150}$

5. grain $\dfrac{1}{6}$ = _____ milligrams

6. grain $\dfrac{1}{100}$ = _____ milligram

7. 15 milligrams = grain _____

8. 0.8 milligrams = grain _____

9. grain _____ = 0.30 milligram

10. 0.6 milligram = grain _____

11. grains iiiss = _____ milligrams

12. 0.05 milligram = grain _____

MULTIPLE CONVERSIONS

When completing multiple conversions, it is best to work within the same unit of measure before changing to another unit of measure. For example, do all of the metric conversions, and then move to the grain conversions; or make the grain-to-metric conversion into milligrams, and then convert from milligrams to grams or micrograms. By doing so, you will have only one math setup per problem. Use the standard conversion equivalents to make the conversions.

   You may need to convert twice to get to a known conversion.
   For example,

$$0.0001\,\text{grams} = \text{grains} \underline{\hspace{2cm}}$$

First, convert from grams to milligrams:

$$0.0001 \text{ grams becomes } 0.1 \text{ milligrams}$$

Then, set up with known equivalents for the conversion:

$$\frac{\text{gr i}}{60\,\text{mg}} = \frac{\text{gr ?}}{0.1\,\text{mg}}$$

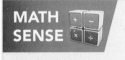

MATH SENSE

microgram = mcg, formerly seen as μg. Of note, mcg is the preferred form because μg may be misread, as listed in the Joint Commission Do Not Use List.

Convert the 0.1 mg to a fraction to ensure the proper format in the final answer:

$$\frac{\text{gr i}}{60\,\text{mg}} = \frac{\text{gr ?}}{\frac{1}{10}\,\text{mg}}$$

Work the problem:

STEP 1: $1 \times \dfrac{1}{10} = \dfrac{1}{10}$

STEP 2: $\dfrac{1}{10} \div 60 \rightarrow \dfrac{1}{10} \times \dfrac{1}{60} = \dfrac{1}{600}$

The final answer is grain $\dfrac{1}{600}$.

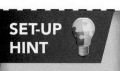

SET-UP HINT

Remember that grains are in fractions, not decimals.

Practice 2

Convert the following.

1. 1.5 grams = grains _____

2. 0.6 grams = grains _____

3. 2.5 grams = grains _____

4. 0.5 grams = grains _____

5. 0.2 grams = grains _____

6. 1.2 grams = grains _____

7. 1.4 grams = grains _____

8. 0.8 grams = grains _____

9. 0.3 grams = grains _____

10. 2.2 grams = grains _____

Once you have memorized the conversions and the steps for converting using ratio and proportion, practice is the best way to master the conversion among the systems.

Practice 3

Convert the following.

1. grains xv = _____ milligrams = _____ gram

2. 500 mg = grains _____ = _____ gram

3. 0.015 gram = grain _____ = _____ milligrams

4. 0.0005 gram = _____ milligram = grain _____

5. _____ milligram = _____ microgram = grain $\frac{1}{4}$

6. 0.3 milligram = grain _____ = _____ gram

7. grains iss = _____ milligrams = _____ gram

8. 400 micrograms = grain_____ = _____ milligram

9. grains viiiss = _____ milligrams = _____ gram

10. grain $\frac{1}{8}$ = _____ milligram

CONVERTING LIQUID EQUIVALENTS

You will convert liquid equivalents in the same manner, using ratio and proportion or dimensional analysis. You will need a wider range of conversions to convert liquid equivalents. Rely on the conversion charts, but work toward memorizing these equivalents so that you can efficiently apply them.

Practice 4

Make these liquid conversions.

1. fluid ounce 1 = _____ teaspoons

2. 15 milliliters = _____ fluid ounce

3. 1 tablespoon = _____ milliliters

4. 10 teaspoons = _____ milliliters

5. 6 teaspoons = _____ fluid ounce

6. fluid ounce $\frac{1}{2}$ = _____ teaspoons

7. 45 milliliters = _____ fluid ounce

8. 15 milliliters = _____ fluid ounce

9. 20 milliliters = _____ teaspoons

10. 3 tablespoons = _____ milliliters

11. $2\frac{1}{2}$ quarts = _____ milliliters

12. 45 milliliters = _____ fluid ounces

13. 1 teaspoon = _____ milliliters

14. $1\frac{1}{4}$ cups = _____ milliliters

15. 2 liters = _____ fluid ounces

16. 2 tablespoons = _____ fluid ounce

17. 15 teaspoons = _____ milliliters

18. 4 milliliters = _____ drops

19. 60 milliliters = _____ tablespoons

20. 2.5 milliliters = _____ teaspoon

Practice 5

Complete these mixed application conversions.

1. grain $\frac{1}{2}$ = _____ milligrams

2. 2 teaspoons = _____ milliliters

3. $12\frac{1}{2}$ teaspoons = _____ milliliters

4. grain $\frac{1}{400}$ = _____ milligram

5. $2\frac{1}{4}$ quarts = _____ milliliters

6. 12 teaspoons = _____ fluid ounces

7. fluid ounces 14 = _____ milliliters

8. 4.4 liters = _____ quarts

9. 35 milliliters = _____ teaspoons

10. 30 milliliters = _____ fluid ounce

11. grains viii = _____ milligrams

12. 4 kilograms = _____ pounds

13. 0.3 milligrams = grain _____

14. $39\frac{3}{5}$ pounds = _____ kilograms

15. $2\frac{1}{2}$ cups = _____ fluid ounces

16. 250 milliliters = _____ pint

17. fluid ounces 4 = _____ cup

18. 15 milliliters = _____ fluid ounce

19. grains v = _____ milligrams

20. 120 milligrams = grains _____

21. grain $\frac{1}{150}$ = _____ milligram

22. fluid ounce $\frac{1}{8}$ = _____ teaspoon

23. $\frac{1}{4}$ cup = _____ fluid ounces

24. fluid ounces 6 = _____ milliliters

25. grains vii = _____ milligrams

26. 16 tablespoons = _____ fluid ounces

27. fluid ounces 6 = _____ tablespoons

28. 0.3 liter = _____ fluid ounces

29. 14 inches = _____ centimeters

30. 90 milligrams = grains _____

31. 40 teaspoons = _____ fluid ounces

32. 16 tablespoons = _____ milliliters

33. fluid ounces 3 = _____ tablespoons

34. grain $\frac{1}{100}$ = _____ micrograms

35. fluid ounces 64 = _____ pints

36. 0.4 milligram = grain _____

37. 5 teaspoons = _____ milliliters

38. 75 milliliters = _____ tablespoons

39. $4\frac{1}{2}$ cups = _____ fluid ounces

40. 90 milliliters = _____ fluid ounces

Practice 6

Make these conversions.

1. 600 milligrams = grains _____

2. 180 milliliters = _____ tablespoons

3. 24 teaspoons = _____ fluid ounces

4. fluid ounce $\frac{1}{2}$ _____ teaspoons

5. 5 tablespoons = _____ milliliters

6. fluid ounces 48 = _____ cups

7. 20 milliliters = _____ teaspoons

8. fluid ounces 20 = _____ cups

9. grains xv = _____ milligrams

10. 750 milliliters = _____ pints

11. 240 milliliters = _____ fluid ounces

12. 0.3 milligram = _____ gram

13. $4\frac{1}{2}$ quarts = _____ milliliters

14. $6\frac{1}{2}$ teaspoons = _____ milliliters

15. 0.1 milligram = grain _____

16. 1500 milliliters = _____ cups

17. 4.5 liters = _____ quarts

18. fluid ounces 96 = _____ liters

19. $2\frac{1}{3}$ cups = _____ milliliters

20. 5 tablespoons = _____ teaspoons

21. fluid ounces 4 = _____ milliliters

22. 500 milligrams = grains _____

23. 120 milliliters = _____ teaspoons

24. $2\frac{1}{4}$ cups = _____ milliliters

25. $3\frac{1}{2}$ cups = _____ milliliters

◆

◆◆◆◆ Rounding in Dosage Calculations

REVIEW

The metric system is used to measure liquids, weights, and medicine. Rounding is used to ensure proper dosing. To assist in this process, follow these five guidelines:

1. Any decimal number that stands alone without a whole number must have a 0 placed in the whole number place. This is the standard way of noting a decimal number that does not have a whole number with it. It also helps ensure reading and interpreting the number correctly.

EXAMPLES

> 0.5 gram   0.25 milligram   0.125 microgram

2. Round decimals to the correct place value. This is somewhat dependent on your profession; however, some general guidelines exist. For example, kilograms and degrees in Celsius and Fahrenheit are placed in tenths.

3. Multi-step problems require that you convert between number systems, especially between fractions and decimals. If the drug measurement is in metrics (milligram, gram, microgram), the solution to the problem must be in decimals. There are no fractions in the metric system. Therefore, $\frac{1}{4}$ milligram is stated as 0.25 milligram.

4. Do not over-round. In medications, a small amount of medication can be critical in dosing. If you begin to round as you set up the problem, you may round again when you finalize the problem, and this can skew the dosage amount. A good rule of thumb is to round only when you reach your final answer. Of note are pediatric doses, which are rounded down, not up, to avoid overdosing. The same principle is used with adults for high-alert drugs.

5. In some cases, it is important to place a 0 at the end of the number. The trailing zero is used to show the exact level of a value such as a lab result, the size of a lesion, or a catheter size.

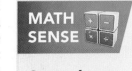

MATH SENSE

Correct formats mean correct answers!

Practice 7

Write the following in proper medical notation.

1. 25.89 kilograms _____

2. 2.7759 milliliters of liquid medicine _____

3. 12.54 milligrams of a tablet _____

4. $5\frac{1}{4}$ kilograms _____

5. $50\frac{1}{2}$ milligrams of pain medication _____

Practice 8

Make the conversion and ensure that your answer has the accurate format.

1. 650 milliliters = _____ pints

2. 20 drops = _____ teaspoon

3. _____ teaspoon = 30 drops

4. grains v = _____ milligrams

5. $8\frac{1}{2}$ ounces = _____ milliliters

6. 750 milliliters = _____ quarts

7. grains 15 = _____ gram

8. _____ milligrams = grain $\frac{1}{20}$

9. grains x = _____ milligrams

10. $7\frac{1}{2}$ teaspoons = _____ milliliters

11. grain $\frac{1}{6}$ = _____ milligrams

12. 98 pounds 8 ounces = _____ kilograms

13. 2 teaspoons = _____ drops

14. 400 milligrams = grains _____

15. $1\frac{1}{4}$ teaspoons = _____ drops

UNIT REVIEW

◆◆◆◆ Critical Thinking in Apothecary System

1. Why are a drop and a grain considered approximately equivalent?

2. Write $\dfrac{4}{10}$ in proper medical notation for milligrams.

3. Mr. Sythe has a circular wound. It is $1\dfrac{1}{5}$ inches or _____ mm.

4. 15 ounces = _____ tablespoons

5. 200 mg/day = _____ g/week

6. 75 mg/day = _____ mcg/week

7. If a patient drank 16 ounces of tea, how many mL did he drink?

8. A child weighs $97\dfrac{3}{4}$ pounds or _____ kg.

9. The incision is $2\dfrac{1}{2}$ inches or _____ cm.

10. A child is drinking $\dfrac{1}{4}$ cup of milk every 2 hours. At this rate, how many mL will he ingest in 6 hours?

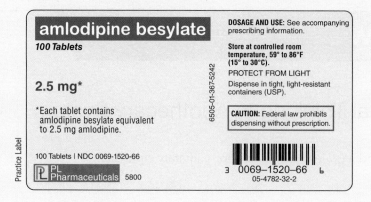

11. How many milligrams are in 3 tablets of amlodipine besylate?

12. If the doctor ordered 100 mg of fenofibrate, how many tablets would you administer? Explain why this is the correct number of tablets.

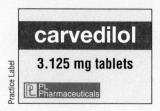

13. How many mcg are in each tablet of carvedilol?

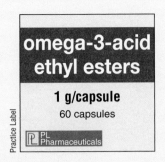

14. How many milligrams are in two capsules of omega-3-acid ethyl esters?

15. Ten milliliters or _____ teaspoons of an oral suspension are given a child every six hours. That is _____ tablespoons in a 24-hour period.

◆◆◆◆ ## Professional Expertise

- Equivalents are not exact answers. They are approximates.
- Memorize the common equivalents.
- Metric measures are considered industry standard, and apothecary measures are being phased out.
- Use fractions and whole numbers for household and apothecary units.
- Use decimals and whole numbers for metric units.
- Remember to use an initial 0 if no whole number is included with a decimal number.

APOTHECARY SYSTEM POST-TEST

1. Write seven and a half centimeters in medical notation. _____

2. 380 mL = _____ cups

3. 0.3 mg = grain _____

4. grain iiss = _____ milligrams

5. fluid ounces 4 = _____ milliliters

6. 48 kilograms = _____ ounces

7. 95 milliliters = _____ tablespoons

8. grain $\dfrac{1}{100}$ = _____ milligram

9. 75 milliliters = _____ fluid ounces

10. 1.5 milliliters = _____ drops

11. 12 fluid ounces = _____ pints

12. The client weighs $68\dfrac{1}{2}$ pounds. How many kilograms does this client weigh? _____

13. The physician assistant prescribes 12 milliliters of cough syrup. How many teaspoons of cough syrup is that? _____

14. The participants in a weight reduction program are asked to drink eight 8-ounce glasses of water daily. How many milliliters of water is this per day? _____

15. Three ounces equals _____ drops.

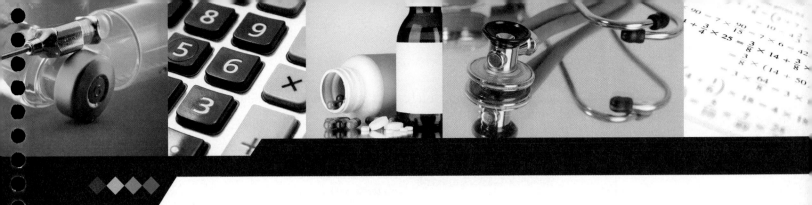

STUDENT LEARNING OUTCOMES

After completing the tasks in this unit, you will be able to:

11-1 Calculate dosages with the dosage formula and/ or dimensional analysis

11-2 Use drug labels to gather dosage information to calculate the supply on hand

11-3 Convert among systems to calculate dosages

11-4 Convert a drug order to the format of the supply on hand

 Overview

This unit pulls together all the math skills you have reviewed and practiced previously in this text. Your task will be to determine the individual dose of medication a client will receive. This is a common task for nurses.

PRE-TEST

1. The doctor's order is for 20 milligrams. You have 30 milligrams in 5 milliliters. Round to the nearest tenth. Give: _____

2. Order: 150 milligrams of a drug by mouth. You have scored tablets in 100 milligrams. Give: _____

3. Order: pain medication 0.3 gram orally every 4 hours. In the supply are tablets labeled grains v of the pain medication. Give: _____

4. Order: 1.25 milligrams. You have 0.75 milligrams in 5 milliliters. Round to the nearest tenth. Give: _____

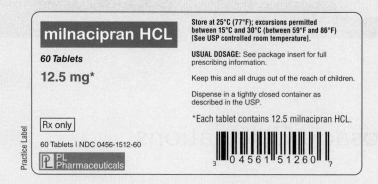

milnacipran HCL

60 Tablets

12.5 mg*

Rx only

60 Tablets I NDC 0456-1512-60

PL Pharmaceuticals

Store at 25°C (77°F); excursions permitted between 15°C and 30°C (between 59°F and 86°F) [See USP controlled room temperature].

USUAL DOSAGE: See package insert for full prescribing information.

Keep this and all drugs out of the reach of children.

Dispense in a tightly closed container as described in the USP.

*Each tablet contains 12.5 milnacipran HCL.

5. Look at the drug label for milnacipran HCL. The doctor has ordered 25 milligrams of milnacipran HCL. The patient will receive _____ tablets.

6. Order: Zocor 60 milligrams per day divided into 3 equal doses of 20 milligrams, 20 milligrams, and an evening dose of _____ milligrams.

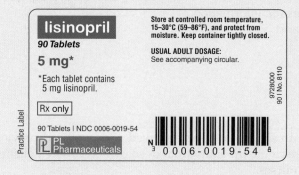

lisinopril

90 Tablets

5 mg*

*Each tablet contains 5 mg lisinopril.

Rx only

90 Tablets I NDC 0006-0019-54

PL Pharmaceuticals

Store at controlled room temperature, 15–30°C (59–86°F), and protect from moisture. Keep container tightly closed.

USUAL ADULT DOSAGE:
See accompanying circular.

9728000
90 I No. 8110

7. Order: lisinopril 15 milligrams once daily.
Give: _____

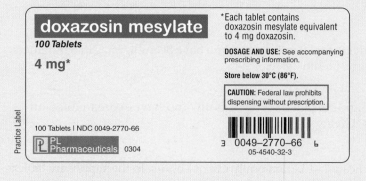

doxazosin mesylate

100 Tablets

4 mg*

100 Tablets I NDC 0049-2770-66

PL Pharmaceuticals   0304

*Each tablet contains doxazosin mesylate equivalent to 4 mg doxazosin.

DOSAGE AND USE: See accompanying prescribing information.

Store below 30°C (86°F).

CAUTION: Federal law prohibits dispensing without prescription.

0049–2770–66
05-4540-32-3

8. The physician orders doxazosin mesylate 8 milligrams once daily at bedtime.
   Give: _____

9. The doctor orders 200 milligrams of a drug by mouth every 4 hours. The vial
   contains 250 milligrams in 5 milliliters. Give _____ milliliters.

10. Order: grains ii
    Have: 60 milligram tablets
    Give: _____

11. Order: 30 milligrams orally
    Have: 12.5 milligrams in each 5 milliliters
    Give: _____

12. Order: grain $\frac{1}{150}$
    Have: 100 micrograms per tablet
    Give: _____

13. Order: grains v orally
    Have: 1.25 grains per tablet
    Give: _____

14. Dr. Brown orders 0.3 grams of zidovudine in tablets every 4 hours for an HIV
    patient. The pharmacy carries this medication in 100 milligram tablets. How many
    tablets will the patient receive? _____

15. The nurse has 30 milligram scored tablets in her medicine cabinet. Dr. Smith orders
    15 milligrams of phenobarbital. She will give _____.

◆◆◆◆ Performing Dosage Calculations

REVIEW

In order to calculate an individual dose, you must know three important pieces of information: the desired dose, the dosage strength, and the medication's unit of measure. These
three items are given in each dosage calculation.

TERM	SYMBOL	MEANING	EXAMPLE
dosage ordered or desired dose	D	the amount of medication that the physician has ordered for the client	Give 500 milligrams Give grains v Give 1.2 milliliters
dosage strength or supply on hand	H	the amount of drug in a specific unit of measure	250 milligrams grains v
unit of measure or quantity of unit	Q	the unit of measure for the specific dosage strength or supply on hand	_____ per 2 mL _____ per capsule _____ per tablet

We can see how these are used in this medication order:

The physician ordered sertraline HCL 50 milligrams once a day for his client.

The nurse looks at her medication label:

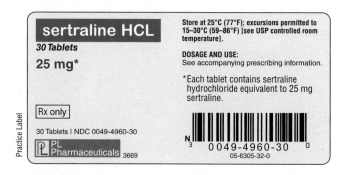

The drug label reads sertraline HCL 25 milligrams per tablet.

The three essential pieces of information are:

D = 50 milligrams

H = 25 milligrams

Q = 1 tablet

This problem will be calculated using the dosage formula:

$$\frac{\text{desired or dosage ordered}}{\text{supply on hand}} \times \text{quantity} = \text{unknown dosage}$$

This problem is set up like this:

$$\frac{50 \text{ mg}}{25 \text{ mg}} \times 1 \text{ tablet} = 2 \text{ tablets}$$

When using the dosage formula provided in this unit, you must ensure that the medication information is in the correct place, which is true for any math formula. This formula can be used for most medication orders and is useful to memorize.

The formula is abbreviated as:

$$\frac{D}{H} \times Q = x$$

RULE 1: The dosage ordered/desired and the have/supply must be in the same unit of measure.

RULE 2: The quantity and the unknown dosage will be in the same unit of measure.

Use the formula:

$$\frac{\text{dosage (D)}}{\text{supply on hand (H)}} \times \text{quantity (Q)} = \text{medication given}$$

The *dosage* is the amount of the medication that the doctor orders. The *supply on hand* is the available form of the drug: milligrams, grams, caplets, tablets, and so on. This is what the pharmacy or the medication cabinet has on hand. The *quantity* is the amount of medication per tablet, milliliter, milligram, and so on.

It is important that the dosage and the supply on hand have the same unit of measure. Thus, if the doctor's order is for milligrams, and you have the medication only in grams, you will need to convert the order to grams to match the supply that you have on hand.

You can apply this formula in two steps:

EXAMPLE

The doctor orders 250 milligrams. The supply in the medicine cabinet is in 125 milligram tablets.

To solve with the dosage calculation formula:

$$\frac{D}{H} \times Q = x \qquad \begin{aligned}\text{Order} &= 250 \text{ milligrams} \\ \text{Have} &= 125 \text{ milligrams}\end{aligned} \quad \text{quantity} = \begin{cases} \text{solid form of} \\ \text{medication, and} \\ \text{Q is 1, so Q can be} \\ \text{eliminated as a math} \\ \text{step in this problem.} \end{cases}$$

a. Put the information into the format

$$\frac{D}{H} \times Q = x \quad \frac{250 \text{ milligrams}}{125 \text{ milligrams}} \times 1 \text{ tablet} = x$$

b. Calculate. Remember that the horizontal line indicates division, and divide 250 by 125. The result will be 2 tablets.

EXAMPLE

The doctor orders 60 milligrams of liquid cough syrup. The liquid cough syrup has a label that reads 100 milligrams in 5 milliliters.

a. Put the information into the format:

$$\frac{D}{H} \times Q = x \rightarrow \frac{60 \text{ milliliters}}{100 \text{ milliliters}} \times 5 \text{ milliliters} = \underline{\qquad} \text{ milliliters}$$

b. Multiply and divide.

$$\frac{60 \times 5}{100} = \frac{300}{100} =$$

c. Reduce to solve.

$$\frac{300}{100} = 3 \text{ milliliters}$$

The answer is 3 milliliters.

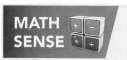

EXAMPLE

The doctor orders Zithromax 500 milligrams. The supply in the medicine cabinet is Zithromax 250 milligrams per tablet.

a. Put the information into the format:

$$\frac{D}{H} \times Q = x \rightarrow \frac{500 \text{ milligrams}}{250 \text{ milligrams}} \times 1 \text{ tablet} = \underline{\hspace{2cm}} \text{ tablets}$$

b. Multiply and divide.

$$\frac{500 \text{ milligrams}}{250 \text{ milligrams}} = 2 \text{ tablets}$$

DIMENSIONAL ANALYSIS

A detailed section on using dimensional analysis is in Appendix D for your reference, and other applications of dimensional analysis occur in Units 10 and 12.

To solve the above example with dimensional analysis:

a. Place the unknown's unit of measure on one side of the equation.

$$? \text{ tablets} =$$

b. The first factor is the unit of measure over the dosage strength.

$$? \text{ tablets} = \frac{1 \text{ tablet}}{250 \text{ milligrams}}$$

c. Multiply the first factor by the second, which is the dosage placed over the number 1.

$$? \text{ tablets} = \frac{1 \text{ tablet}}{250 \text{ milligrams}} \times \frac{500 \text{ milligrams}}{1}$$

d. Cancel like units and multiply and divide.

$$? \text{ tablets} = \frac{1 \text{ tablet} \times 500}{250 \times 1} = \frac{500}{250} = 2 \text{ tablets}$$

The final answer is 2 tablets.

EXAMPLE

The doctor orders 60 milligrams of liquid cough syrup. The liquid cough syrup has a label that reads 100 milligrams in 5 milliliters.

a. Place the unknown's unit of measure on one side of the equation.

$$? \text{ milliliters} =$$

The first factor is the unit of measure over the dosage strength.

$$? \text{ milliliters} = \frac{5 \text{ milliliters}}{100 \text{ milligrams}}$$

b. Multiply the first factor by the second, which is the dosage placed over the number 1.

$$? \text{ milliliters} = \frac{5 \text{ milliliters}}{100 \text{ milligrams}} \times \frac{60 \text{ milligrams}}{1}$$

c. Cancel like units and multiply and divide.

$$? \text{ milliliters} = \frac{5}{100} \times \frac{60}{1} = \frac{300}{100} = 3 \text{ milliliters}$$

The final answer is 3 milliliters.

Practice 1

Use the dosage formula or dimensional analysis to calculate dosage and complete the following dosage calculations.

1. Order: 30 milligrams
     Have: 10 milligrams per tablet
     Give: _____

2. Order: 1 milligram
     Have: 5 milligrams per milliliter
     Give: _____

3. Order: 1500 milligrams
     Have: 500 milligrams per tablet
     Give: _____

4. Order: 15 milligrams
     Have: 7.5 milligrams per tablet
     Give: _____

5. Order: 10 milligrams
     Have: 20 milligrams per milliliter
     Give: _____

6. Order: 0.25 gram
     Have: 50 milligrams in 2 milliliters
     Give: _____

7. Order: 1.5 milligrams
     Have: 3.0 milligrams per milliliter
     Give: _____

8. Order: 0.1 gram
     Have: 25 milligrams in 2 milliliters
     Give: _____

9. Order: 0.15 gram
     Have: 25 milligrams per tablet
     Give: _____

10. Order: 10 milligrams
     Have: 2.5 milligrams per capsule
     Give: _____

Now that the formula is familiar to you, the next step is to apply the metric and apothecary conversions you learned in Unit 10.

Convert the unit of measure of the "order" and "have" to the same unit of measure. One guideline is that it is often easier to convert the order unit to the have unit. This also helps in being able to compute the answer. Once the units are identifiable, it is easy to make the conversion. To review conversions among systems see Unit 10.

Practice 2

Use the dosage formula or dimensional analysis to calculate dosage and complete the following dosage calculations.

1. Order: 1 gram
   Have: 50 milligrams in 2 milliliters
   Give: _____

2. Order: 0.5 gram
   Have: 200 milligrams per tablet
   Give: _____

3. Order: 0.15 gram
   Have: 300 milligrams per caplet
   Give: _____

4. Order: grains x
   Have: 180 milligrams per milliliter
   Give: _____

5. Order: 0.06 gram
   Have: 15 milligrams per tablet
   Give: _____

6. Order: 1.5 gram
   Have: 125 milligrams per 2 milliliters
   Give: _____

7. Order: 1.5 grams
   Have: 1000 milligrams per tablet
   Give: _____

8. Order: grains iss
   Have: 30 milligrams per tablet
   Give: _____

9. Order: 1.5 gram
   Have: 750 milligrams per tablet
   Give: _____

10. Order: grain $\frac{1}{8}$

Have: 7.5 milligrams per tablet
Give: _____

11. Order: 25 milligrams/orally
Have: 10 milligram scored tablets
Give: _____

12. Order: 125 milligrams
Have: 100 milligrams in 4 milliliters
Give: _____

13. Order: grains iss
Have: 50 milligrams per caplet
Give: _____

14. Order: 75 milligrams
Have: 25 milligrams in 2 milliliters
Give: _____

15. Order: 25 milligrams/orally
Have: 10 milligram caplets
Give: _____

16. Order: 300 milligrams
Have: grains v in each tablet
Give: _____

17. Order: 12.5 milliliters orally after meals
Have: 25 milliliters
Give: _____

18. Order: 0.25 milliliter by mouth
Have: 0.125 milliliter
Give: _____

19. Order: 120 milligrams by mouth
Have: grain ss per tablet
Give: _____

20. Order: 1500 milligrams
Have: 500 milligrams per caplet
Give: _____

USING DRUG LABELS TO CALCULATE DOSAGES

Practice 3

Use the medication labels to complete these calculations. The drug label will supply the dosage strength and the unit.

1. The physician orders glipizide extended release tablets 10 milligrams once a day.

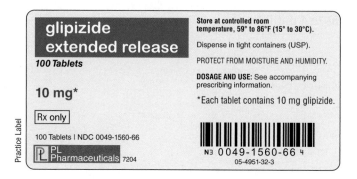

Give: _____

2. The client has a medication order for rosuvastatin calcium 20 milligrams once a day without food.

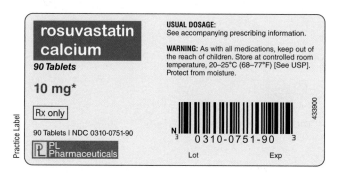

Give: _____

3. The order is for piroxicam 20 milligrams per day.

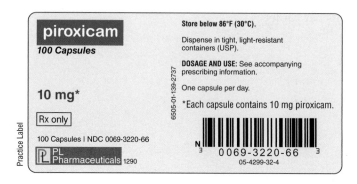

Give: _____

4. The physician writes an order for sertraline HCL 25 milligrams per day.

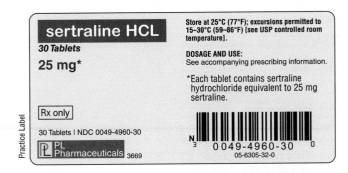

Give: _____

5. Dr. Ballard writes an order for quinapril HCL 20 milligrams once daily.

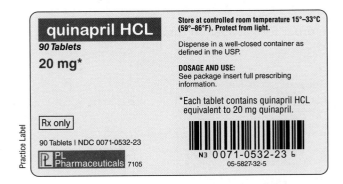

Give: _____

6. The patient will receive a new order for famotidine 40 milligrams to control stomach acid upset.

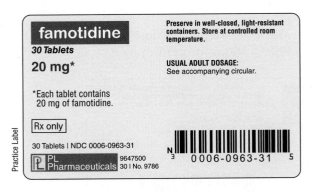

The patient will take: _____

7. The physician has written an order for phenytoin 100 milligrams chewable tablets.

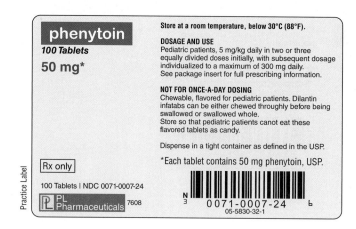

Give: _____

8. The client has a medication order for gabapentin (oral solution) 500 milligrams per dose three times a day.

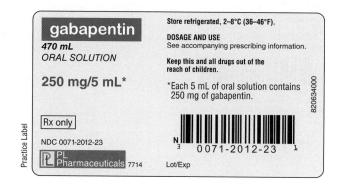

Each dose gives: _____

9. The pharmacy technician is asked to prepare a dose for a client of losartan potassium-hydrochlorothiazide 50 milligrams per day.

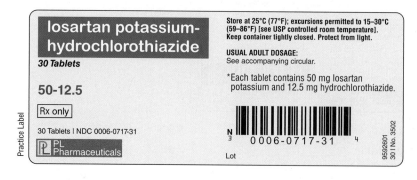

The client will take: _____

10. The physician writes an order for montelukast sodium 5 milligrams once a day in the morning.

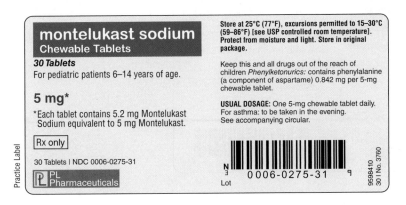

Give: _____

UNIT REVIEW

◆◆◆◆ Critical Thinking in Dosage Calculations

1. If a pint of cough syrup contains 473 mL of medication, how many full 10 mL doses are in the bottle?

2. If a pint of cough syrup contains 473 mL of medication, how many full teaspoons are in the bottle?

3. The patient is ordered Coumadin gr $\frac{1}{6}$. Coumadin is supplied in 5 mg tablets. How many tablets will the patient receive?

4. A child is prescribed acetaminophen 160 mg by mouth every 6 hours for pain reduction. Acetaminophen is supplied in liquid form at 80 mg per 2.5 mL. How many teaspoons will the child receive per dose?

5. The doctor orders Lactulose 25 g. The drug label reads 10 g/15 mL. The proper dose in tablespoons is _____.

Use the following drug label for problems 6 and 7.

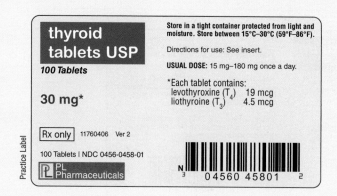

thyroid tablets USP
100 Tablets

30 mg*

Practice Label

Rx only 11760406 Ver 2

100 Tablets | NDC 0456-0458-01

PL Pharmaceuticals

Store in a tight container protected from light and moisture. Store between 15°C–30°C (59°F–86°F).

Directions for use: See insert.

USUAL DOSE: 15 mg–180 mg once a day.

*Each tablet contains:
levothyroxine (T₄) 19 mcg
liothyroine (T₃) 4.5 mcg

N₃ 04560 45801 2

6. The doctor has ordered $\frac{1}{2}$ grain once a day. How many milligrams will this be in a week?

7. If the doctor ordered 90 milligrams a day, does the bottle of medication have enough tablets for a 30-day supply?

8. The resident was reading the drug label for Nitrostat, which read Nitrostat $\frac{1}{200}$ grains. How many milligrams are in two tablets of this medication?

9. A medication label provides the following dosage strength: 125 mg per 5 mL. If the ordered dosage is 100 mg, shade the syringe for the proper dosage.

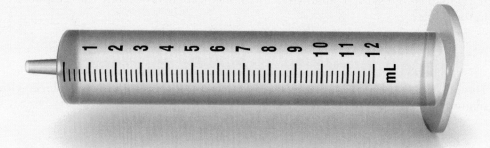

10. A drug is available in 1.5 g caplets. The physician has ordered 3 g orally four times a day. How many caplets will the patient receive in one day?

Use this information to answer problems 11 and 12.

Phenobarbital is supplied in 15 mg, 30 mg, and 60 mg scored tablets. Your patient has a medication order that reads: Phenobarbital gr $\frac{1}{4}$ orally each day.

11. Which dosage strength best meets the patient's prescription?

12. How many tablets will the patient receive at that dosage strength?

13. The physician assistant in Villa Care is reading the drug label for Levothroid, which reads: Levothroid 25 mcg per tablet. The doctor has prescribed Levothroid 0.1 mg orally per day.

She will administer _____ tablets.

Use the label below for problems 14 and 15.

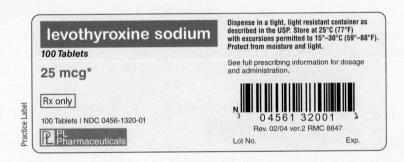

14. If the doctor prescribes the patient 50 mcg levothyroxine by mouth daily, how many milligrams of this medication will the patient receive each day?

15. Does the bottle contain a 90-day supply?

◆◆◆◆ Professional Expertise

- Include the proper form of the drug in the final answer.
- Be consistent in your use of a computation method to ensure proper calculation of the dosage. Practice perfects your calculations, so choose one method and use it each time.
- Use the label to find the dosage strength such as 25 mg/1 mL or 50 mcg tablets.

DOSAGE CALCULATIONS POST-TEST

1. The doctor's order is for 20 milligrams. You have 10 milligrams in 5 milliliters. Give: _____

2. Order: 250 milligrams of a drug by mouth. You have scored tablets in 100 milligram dosages. Give: _____

3. Order: pain medication 0.6 gram orally every 4 hours. In the supply are tablets labeled grains v of the pain medication. Give: _____

4. Order: 1.25 milligrams. You have 0.25 milligrams in 5 milliliters. Give: _____

5. Order: piroxicam 20 milligram capsules once a day for osteoarthritis. How many milligrams are ordered for a ten-day supply?

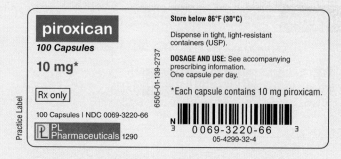

6. Order: simvastatin 60 milligrams per day in the evening.

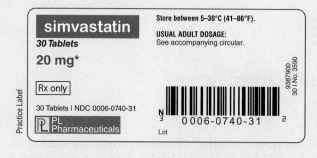

Give: _____

7. Order: The patient has fibromyalgia. The doctor prescribed lisinopril as follows: one dose of 12.5 mg for day 1, 12.5 mg twice for days 2 and 3, 25 mg for day 4 through day 7, and 50 mg beyond day 7. If the patient takes this medication as prescribed, how many tablets are needed for a 30-day supply? Round to the nearest whole number.

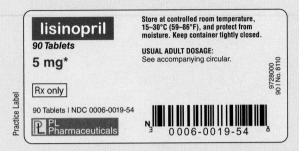

8. The physician orders nebivolol 5 milligrams once daily for high blood pressure.

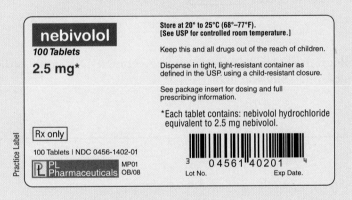

Give: _____

9. The doctor orders 200 milligrams of a drug by mouth every 4 hours. The vial contains 125 milligrams in 5 milliliters. Give _____ milliliters.

10. Order: grains iii
    Have: 60 milligram tablets
    Give: _____

11. Order: 50 milligrams orally

      Have: 12.5 milligrams in each 5 milliliters

      Give: _____

12. Order: grain $\dfrac{1}{150}$

      Have: 200 micrograms per tablet

      Give: _____

13. Order: grains v orally

      Have: $2\dfrac{1}{2}$ grains per tablet

      Give: _____

14. Dr. Brown orders 0.2 grams of zidovudine in tablets every 4 hours for an HIV patient. The pharmacy carries this medication in 100 milligram tablets. How many tablets will the patient receive? _____

15. The nurse has 15 milligram tablets in her medicine cabinet. Dr. Smith orders 30 milligrams of phenobarbital. She will give _____.

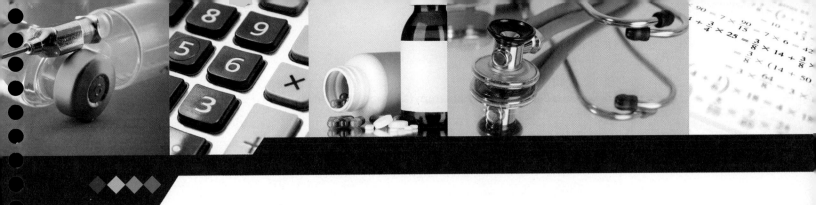

STUDENT LEARNING OUTCOMES

After completing the tasks in this unit, you will be able to:

12-1 Calculate dosages using the dosage formula and/or dimensional analysis

12-2 Use drug labels to gather dosage information to calculate the supply on hand

12-3 Shade syringes to the proper dosage per the doctor's order

12-4 Convert among systems to calculate dosages

12-5 Convert a drug order to the format of the supply on hand

◆◆◆◆ Overview

Parenteral medications are not taken orally. Instead, these medications may be in the form of injections, inhalants, patches, or suppositories. The common parenteral routes are shown in the following table:

ROUTE	ABBREVIATION	ENTRY POINT
intradermal	ID	between the layers of skin
intramuscular	IM	into a muscle
intravenous	IV	into a vein
subcutaneous	sub-Q	under the skin

PRE-TEST

1. The physician orders gabapentin 125 milligrams with a full glass of water.

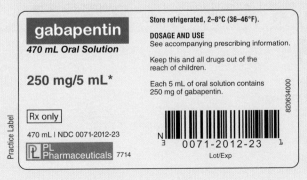

gabapentin
470 mL Oral Solution

250 mg/5 mL*

Rx only

470 mL | NDC 0071-2012-23

PL Pharmaceuticals 7714

Practice Label

Store refrigerated, 2–8°C (36–46°F).

DOSAGE AND USE
See accompanying prescribing information.

Keep this and all drugs out of the reach of children.

Each 5 mL of oral solution contains 250 mg of gabapentin.

820634000

N 3   0071-2012-23   1
Lot/Exp

How many mL will be given? _____

2. Give Dilaudid 0.25 milligram IM from a vial that is labeled 2 milligrams per milliliter.
Give: _____

3. Order: Atropine 0.4 milligrams IV
Have: Atropine 0.8 milligram per milliliter
Give: _____

4. The physician has ordered calcitonin 100 units IM for the client. The calcitonin vial reads 200 units in 1 milliliters.

Give: _____. Shade the syringe.

5. The physician has ordered adrenalin 0.5 milligram sub-Q stat. The adrenalin label reads 2 : 2000 solution.
Give: _____

6. Order: Cefazolin Sodium 250 milligrams IM every 8 hours
Have: Cefazolin Sodium 300 milligrams in 5 milliliters
Give: _____ mL (Round to the nearest tenth.)

7. The physician has ordered magnesium sulfate 250 milligrams stat. The magnesium sulfate vial is labeled 20% solution.
Give: _____

8. Give Butorphanol 0.75 milligrams IV for the client every 3 to 4 hours. The Butorphanol drug label reads 2 milligrams per milliliter.
Give: _____ Round to the nearest hundredth.

9. The physician orders Imitrex 4 milligrams sub-Q as needed for headache every 4 to 6 hours for the client. The Imitrex drug label on the vial reads 10 milligrams per milliliter.

Give: _____. Shade the syringe.

10. Order: Zemplar 4 micrograms IM
Have: Zemplar 2.5 micrograms per milliliter

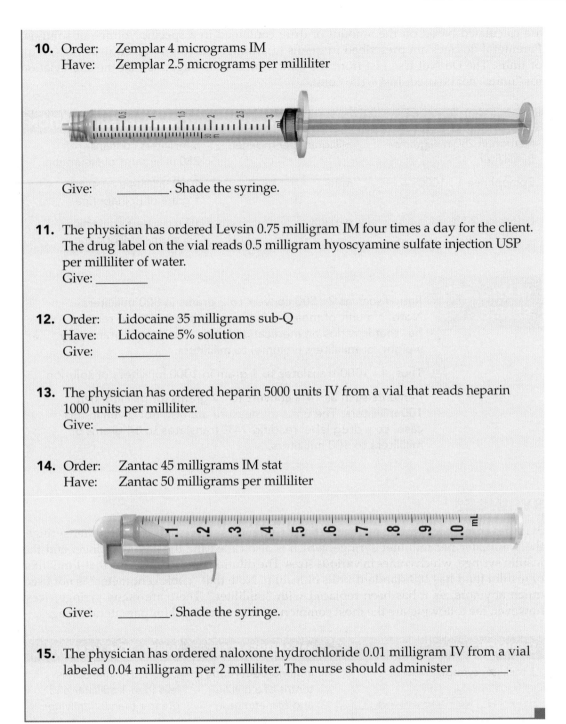

Give: _____. Shade the syringe.

11. The physician has ordered Levsin 0.75 milligram IM four times a day for the client. The drug label on the vial reads 0.5 milligram hyoscyamine sulfate injection USP per milliliter of water.
Give: _____

12. Order: Lidocaine 35 milligrams sub-Q
Have: Lidocaine 5% solution
Give: _____

13. The physician has ordered heparin 5000 units IV from a vial that reads heparin 1000 units per milliliter.
Give: _____

14. Order: Zantac 45 milligrams IM stat
Have: Zantac 50 milligrams per milliliter

Give: _____. Shade the syringe.

15. The physician has ordered naloxone hydrochloride 0.01 milligram IV from a vial labeled 0.04 milligram per 2 milliliter. The nurse should administer _____.

◆◆◆◆ Injections

REVIEW

Injections are mixtures of pure drug dissolved in an appropriate liquid. The dosage or solution strength will be provided on the medication label and will be given in milligrams per milliliter as a ratio or as a percent. It is important to remember that parenteral doses are calculated based on the amount of drug contained in a specific volume of solution. Parenteral dosages are prescribed in grams (g), milligrams (mg), milliequivalents (mEq), or units. The Do Not Use List from the Joint Commission suggests that the abbreviation for "units" not be used. Just write "unit."

EXAMPLE OF DOSAGE	GIVEN FORM	DOSAGE INTERPRETATION
Neurontin 250 milligrams/ 5 milliliter	milligram per milliliter	5 milliliters contains 250 milligrams of Neurontin
Epinephrine 1 : 1000	ratio	1000 milliliters contains 1 gram of Epinephrine
Lidocaine 2.5%	percent	100 milliliters contains 2.5 grams of Lidocaine

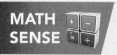

MATH SENSE

Ratios such as 2 : 500 convert to 2 grams in 500 milliliters. Note: No unit of measure is given, so it is critical to remember that in ratios on medication labels, the ratio is grams (dry weight) or milliliters (volume) to milliliters.

Thus, 1 : 1000 translates to 1 gram in 1000 milliliters of solution.

Percents such as 14% convert to 14 grams (or milliliters) in 100 milliliters. The units of measure are also not given in this case, so a drug label reading 14% translates to 14 grams or milliliters to 100 milliliters.

SYRINGES

Syringes administer parenteral medications. Common syringes are the 3 milliliter syringe; the 1 milliliter per milliliter syringe, which is also called the tuberculin syringe; and the insulin syringe, which comes in various sizes. The dilution of insulin is such that 1 milliliter of insulin fluid has 100 standard units of insulin. Note that "cubic centimeter" is not used much anymore, as it has been replaced with "milliliter." There are many syringe sizes; however, the following are the most common syringe sizes used for parenteral dosages.

SYRINGE	MEASUREMENT	WHEN IT IS USED
1 milliliter syringe	in hundredths and tenths of a milliliter and sometimes in minims, but rarely	Used if the injection is less than 1 milliliter and greater than 0.5 milliliter.
insulin syringe	in hundredths and units	Used for insulin units. 1 milliliter of insulin fluid is 100 units of insulin. Used for insulin of at least 50 units but less than 100 units.
3 milliliter syringe	in tenths	Used when the injection is less than 3 milliliters.

IM INJECTION GUIDELINES

For IM injections, there are guidelines for maximum volumes given in injection sites. This is important for accurate dosage calculation and consideration of multiple syringes. Any dosage larger than the recommended amount is usually checked and verified with the physician, and the dosage is then divided equally or as close to equally as possible and given in two separate injection sites.

CLIENT	AGE	MAXIMUM DOSE PER SITE
Adult	12+	3 milliliters IM or 1 milliliter deltoid arm
Child	6–12 years	2 milliliters
Child	0–5 years	1 milliliter
Infant	Premature	0.5 milliliter

UNITS OF MEASURES

In addition to the apothecary, metric, and household measures, health care has two other units of measure commonly used in client medication orders.

Medications are also prescribed in milliequivalents (mEq) and units (U). One milliequivalent equals one-thousandth $\left(\dfrac{1}{1000}\right)$. Sodium, potassium, sodium bicarbonate, and potassium chloride are commonly prescribed in milliequivalents. A unit is a standardized amount needed to produce a certain desired effect of a medication. Units are used to prescribe medications such as heparin, insulin, and penicillin. No conversions are used because these medications are prescribed in milliequivalents per milliliter (mEq/mL) or units per milliliter (U/mL), and the labeling matches these measures.

To calculate the dosage, there are several means of getting to the correct dose. One may use the dosage formula, ratio and proportion, or dimensional analysis. Choose the method that you are most comfortable with and use it consistently. An example of each follows.

EXAMPLE

The doctor has ordered that 500 milligrams of Ampicillin be given. On hand is a vial labeled Ampicillin 250 milligrams in 5 milliliters.

To solve with the dosage formula:

$$\frac{\text{ordered dosage}}{\text{supply on hand}} \times \text{quantity} = \text{dosage to be given}$$

Set up:

$$\frac{500 \text{ milligrams}}{250 \text{ milligrams}} \times 5 \text{ milliliters} = \text{dosage to be given}$$

Solve:

$$\frac{500 \text{ milligrams}}{250 \text{ milligrams}} \times 5 \text{ milliliters} = \frac{2}{1} \times 5 \text{ milliliters}$$

$$= 10 \text{ milliliters}$$

To solve with ratio and proportion:

Set up:

500 milligrams : ? milliliters :: 250 milligrams : 5 milliliters

(continued on next page)

Solve:

a. $\dfrac{500 \text{ milligrams}}{? \text{ milliliters}} = \dfrac{250 \text{ milligrams}}{5 \text{ milliliters}}$

b. $500 \times 5 = 2500$

c. $\dfrac{2500 \text{ milligrams}}{250 \text{ milligrams}} = 10 \text{ milliliters}$

To solve with dimensional analysis:

a. Place the unknown unit on the left side of the equation (what you are solving).

$$? \text{ milliliters} =$$

b. The dosage unit of measure is 5 milliliters. The dose on hand is 250 milligrams. Use this known information to form the first factor.

$$? \text{ milliliters} = \frac{5 \text{ milliliters}}{250 \text{ milligrams}}$$

c. The physician has ordered 500 milligrams. Place the 500 milligrams over 1 to form the second factor of the equation.

$$? \text{ milliliters} = \frac{5 \text{ milliliters}}{250 \text{ milligrams}} \times \frac{500 \text{ milligrams}}{1}$$

d. Cancel like units and solve.

$$? \text{ milliliters} = \frac{5 \text{ milliliters}}{250 \; \cancel{\text{milligrams}}} \times \frac{500 \; \cancel{\text{milligrams}}}{1} \rightarrow \frac{5}{1} \times \frac{2}{1}$$

$$= 10 \text{ milliliters}$$

Practice 1

Solve the following parenteral dosages. Round to the nearest tenth.

1. Order: Ephedrine sulfate 12.5 milligrams subcutaneously
   Have: Vial labeled ephedrine sulfate 25 milligrams per milliliter
   Give: _____

2. Order: Diazepam 2 milligram IM
   Have: Vial labeled Diazepam 5 milligrams per milliliter
   Give: _____. Shade the syringe.

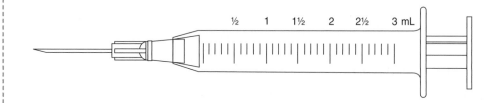

3. Order: Kefzol 500 milligram IM every 6 hours
Have: Label reads Kefzol 225 milligrams per milliliter
Give: _____

4. Order: Colchicine IV 0.5 milligram
Have: Vial labeled colchicine IV 500 micrograms per milliliter
Give: _____

5. Order: Amitriptyline 25 milligrams IM
Have: Vial labeled amitriptyline 10 milligrams per milliliter
Give: _____. Shade the syringe.

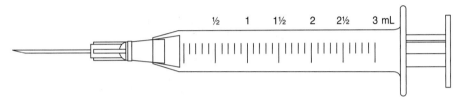

6. Order: Add to IV: Bretylium 500 milligrams
Have: Bretylium 50 milligrams per milliliter
Give: _____

7. Order: Furosemide 20 milligrams IV
Have: Furosemide 10 milligrams per milliliter
Give: _____

8. Order: Nafcillin 500 milligrams IM
Have: When 3.4 milliliters of diluent is added to 1 gram vial, 250 milligrams = 1 milliliter
Give: _____. Shade the syringe.

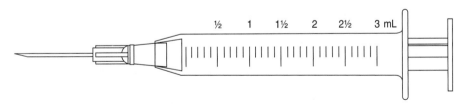

9. Order: Phenergen 25 milligrams
Have: Phenergen 50 milligrams per milliliter
Give: _____. Shade the syringe.

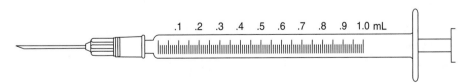

10. Order: As pre-op, give morphine 8 milligrams
Have: Morphine grain $\frac{1}{6}$ in 2 milliliters
Give: _____

11. The physician orders heparin 5000 units. The heparin label reads 10,000 units per milliliter.
Give: _____

12. Give penicillin G 100,000 units from a vial labeled 1,000,000 units in 5 milliliters.
Give: _____

13. The physician has ordered Decadron 3 milligrams from a vial labeled 4 milligrams per milliliter.
Give: _____. Shade the syringe.

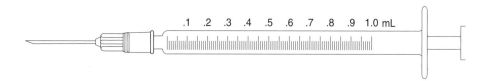

14. Give heparin 15,000 units IV. The vial is labeled heparin 1000 units per milliliter.
Give: _____

15. Give lidocaine 200 milligrams IM stat from a vial labeled lidocaine 10%.
Give: _____

16. The physician has ordered lanoxin 125 micrograms IM daily. The drug label reads 250 micrograms (25 milligrams) per milliliter.
Give: _____

17. The client is in pain. The physician's order is for Demerol 75 milligrams every 4 hours IM as needed for pain. The Demerol label reads 100 milligrams in 2 milliliter.
Give: _____. Shade the syringe.

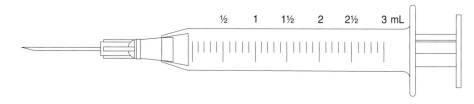

18. The drug order reads Prostigmin 0.5 milligram IM stat. The drug label reads Prostigmin 1 : 2000 solution.
Give: _____

19. The physician has ordered phenylephrine 2.5 milligrams sub-Q for the client. The drug label on the vial reads 10 milligrams per milliliter.
Give: _____

20. Dr. Smith has ordered morphine sulfate grain $\frac{1}{12}$. The morphine sulfate vial is labeled 10 milligrams per milliliter.
Give: _____

UNIT REVIEW

◆◆◆◆◆ Critical Thinking in Parenteral Dosages

1. The physician orders hydroxyzine pamoate 50 milligrams by mouth every 12 hours.

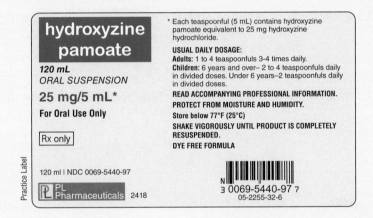

You will administer _____ teaspoons every 12 hours.

Use the label for lorazepam for problems 2 and 3.

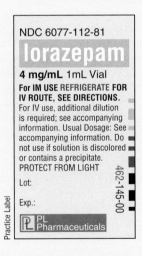

2. How many milligrams of lorazepam are in 3 milliliters of this drug?

3. How many grams of lorazepam are in 0.5 milliliters of this drug?

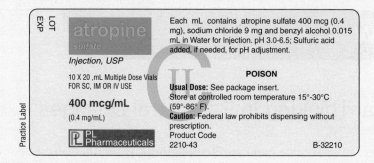

4. If the dose is for 0.2 milligrams of atropine sulfate, how many milliliters will be given?

5. If the dose is for 0.3 milligrams of atropine sulfate, how many milliliters will be given?

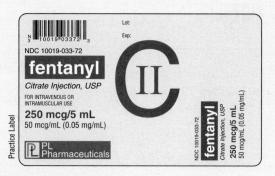

6. How many milligrams of fentanyl are in 7.5 mL of this medication? Round to the nearest tenth.

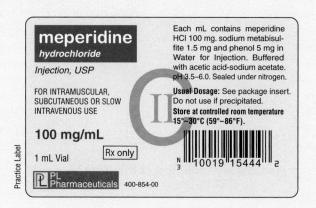

7. The physician ordered 0.5 milliliters of meperidine hydrochloride. The medication's drug label reads 100 mg per milliliter. The patient will receive _____.

8. Mrs. Van was ordered Demerol 65 milligrams every three hours for pain. Demerol is supplied 75 mg/1.5 mL. Shade the syringe that Mrs. Van will receive.

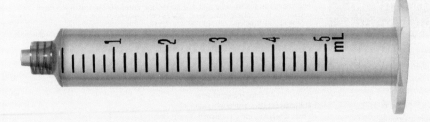

9. A patient is to receive heparin 5500 USC every 12 hours. Heparin is available in 10,000 units per milliliter. The patient will receive _____.

10. Cleocin 300 mg IM every day appears in the patient's chart. The Cleocin label reads 0.6g/mL. The patient will receive _____.

11. Mr. Nguyen is to receive Atropine gr $\frac{1}{100}$ IM. The Atropine label reads 0.4 mg/mL. Mr. Nguyen will receive _____.

12. A patient is ordered morphine sulfate gr $\frac{1}{10}$ as needed for pain every three hours. The morphine sulfate label reads 10 mg/ampule. How many mL will the patient receive?

13. The client is to receive Vitamin B$_{12}$ 0.75 mg IM every day. The label reads Vitamin B$_{12}$ 1000 mcg per 1 mL. The client will receive _____.

Use the following label for problems 14 and 15.

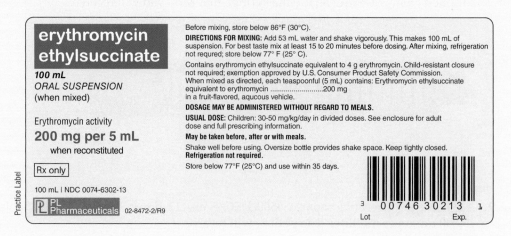

14. Erythromycin ethylsuccinate is used to treat and prevent bacterial infections. Fruit-flavored suspensions are used for pediatric patients. Why is erythromycin ethylsuccinate not considered a parenteral medication?

15. If 5 mL contains erythromycin ethylsuccinate 200 mg, then 1.5 mL contains how many mg of erythromycin ethylsuccinate?

◆◆◆◆ Professional Expertise

- Match all drug labels carefully with the physician's order.
- Use metric measures such as mL because cc is on the Joint Commission's Recommended to Be Replaced List.
- Review the syringe sizes with the dosage to be given to ensure proper measurement.
- Double-check the metric conversions and decimal placement for syringe doses.

PARENTERAL DOSAGE POST-TEST

1. The physician orders Loxitane 30 milligrams IM every 12 hours. The Loxitane label reads 50 milligrams per milliliter.
Give: _____. Shade the syringe.

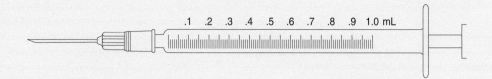

2. Give Dilaudid 0.5 milligram IM from a vial that is labeled 2 milligrams per milliliter.
Give: _____

3. Order: Atropine 0.6 milligrams IV
  Have: Atropine 0.8 milligram per milliliter
  Give: _____

4. The physician has ordered calcitonin 100 units IM for the client. The calcitonin vial reads 400 units in 2 milliliters.
  Give: _____. Shade the syringe.

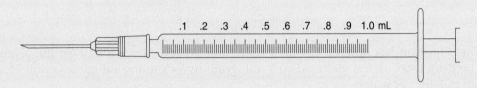

5. The physician has ordered adrenalin 0.5 milligram sub-Q stat. The adrenalin label reads 1 : 1000 solution.
  Give: _____

6. Order: Cefazolin Sodium 250 milligrams IM every 8 hours
  Have: Cefazolin Sodium 500 milligrams in 5 milliliters
  Give: _____. Shade the syringe.

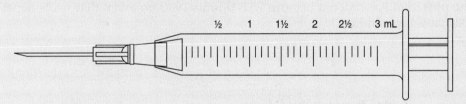

7. The physician has ordered magnesium sulfate 550 milligrams stat. The magnesium sulfate vial is labeled 20% solution.
  Give: _____

8. Give Butorphanol 0.5 milligrams IV for the client every 3 to 4 hours. The Butorphanol drug label reads 2 milligrams per milliliter.
  Give: _____

9. The physician orders Imitrex 4 milligrams sub-Q as needed for headache every 4 to 6 hours for the client. The Imitrex drug label on the vial reads 12 milligrams per milliliter.
  Give: _____. Shade the syringe.

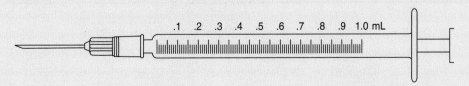

10. Order: Zemplar 3 micrograms IM
     Have: Zemplar 5 micrograms per milliliter
     Give: _____. Shade the syringe.

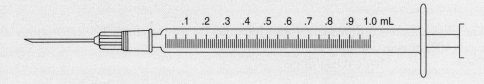

11. The physician has ordered Levsin 1 milligram IM four times a day for the client. The drug label on the vial reads 0.5 milligram hyoscyamine sulfate injection USP per milliliter of water.
     Give: _____

12. Order: Lidocaine 25 milligrams sub-Q
     Have: Lidocaine 5% solution
     Give: _____

13. The physician has ordered heparin 25,000 units IV from a vial that reads heparin 1000 units per milliliter.
     Give: _____

14. Order: Zantac 35 milligrams IM stat
     Have: Zantac 25 milligrams per milliliter
     Give: _____. Shade the syringe.

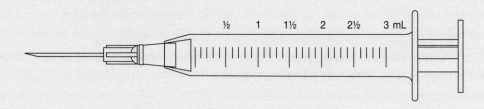

15. The physician has ordered naloxone hydrochloride 0.01 milligram IV from a vial labeled 0.02 milligram per milliliter. The nurse should administer _____.

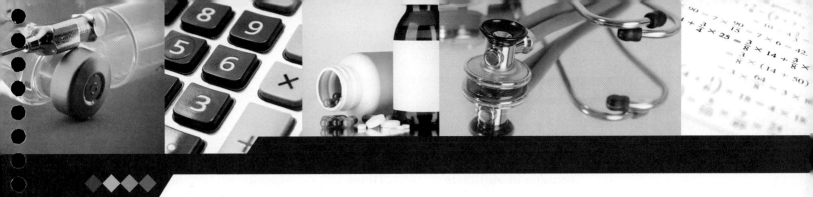

After completing the tasks in this unit, you will be able to:

13-1 Calculate intravenous flow rate, time, and volume

13-2 Calculate amount infused versus amount remaining to be infused

13-3 Use the language that is used for intravenous infusion

 ## Overview

Intravenous (IV) fluids and medications are solutions that are placed directly into the bloodstream via a vein. This is called infusion. Because intravenous medications and solutions have a very quick effect, they are used for critical care situations when a patient needs medication immediately. Moderate to large doses of fluids or medications are given this way. An IV medication may be prepared by a physician, nurse, pharmacist, or a pharmacy technician. IV solutions are also used to maintain and to replace fluids, to keep a vein open for further treatment, and to provide therapy.

The following are the common abbreviations used in IV administration.

TERM	ABBREVIATION
Intravenous	IV
Piggy-back	PB
Drop/drops	gtt/gtts
Hour	hr
Minutes	min
Drops per minute	gtts/min
Drops per milliliter	gtts/mL
Milliliters per hour	mL/hr
Water	H_2O, W
5% dextrose water	D_5W
10% dextrose water	$D_{10}W$
Normal Saline (0.9%)	NS
One-half normal saline (0.45%)	$\frac{1}{2}$ NS
Ringer's lactate solution	RL
Lactated Ringer's solution	LR

PRE-TEST

Calculate the drops per minute for each of the following:

	Total Volume for Infusion in Milliliters	Time in Hours	Drop Factor	Answer (drops per minute)
1.	250	8	15	_____
2.	500	6	20	_____
3.	1200	10	60	_____
4.	125	8	20	_____
5.	750	12	60	_____

Find the milliliters per hour rate for each of the following:

	Total Volume in Milliliters	Total Infusion Time	Answer (milliliters per hour)
6.	1500	12 hours	_____
7.	550	8 hours	_____
8.	1250	12 hours	_____
9.	1500	24 hours	_____
10.	75	30 minutes	_____

Calculate the total infusion time for each of the following:

	Total Volume in Milliliters	Infusion Rate (milliliters per hour)	Answer (time in hours)
11.	500	83	_____
12.	750	100	_____
13.	1500	60	_____
14.	1000	100	_____
15.	450	33	_____

Find the total volume to be infused for each of the following:

	Flow Rate in Milliliters per Hour	Time in Hours	Total Volume in Milliliters
16.	75	6	_____
17.	83	12	_____
18.	75	3	_____
19.	125	8	_____
20.	75	$2\frac{1}{2}$	_____

IV INFUSION SETS

An IV infusion set is used to administer fluids and medications and has several parts: a sealed plastic bag or a bottle, a drip chamber, tubing, and a needle or catheter at the insertion site into the patient. Infusion or flow rates are adjusted to the desired drops per minute by a clamp on the tubing. The infusion set tracks the number of drops being delivered. It should be noted that the larger the tubing, the larger the drop.

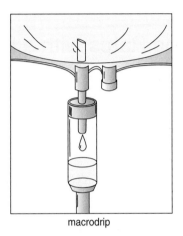
macrodrip

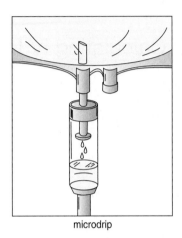
microdrip

Both manual and electronic infusion pumps are in use today. Electronic infusion pumps require less computation on the part of the nurse because these machines have a controller that measures the drops or volume for a preset flow rate. However, the nurse must still monitor the equipment and the client to ensure proper and safe use. For manual IV sets, the health care professional must calculate the flow rate in drops per minute (gtts/min). Like many medical terms, "gtt" is derived from the Latin, in this case the Latin term "gutta," which means drop. To calculate the flow rate, you must know the administration set's drop factor. Larger, macrodrip tubing administers a larger drop and may be used for 10 drops per milliliter, 15 drops per milliliter, or 20 drops per milliliter. Smaller, microdrip tubing administers 60 drops per milliliter.

Nurses often need to use the information on drug orders to calculate IV infusion rates. The drug order will include the type of fluid, the amount of fluid, and the number of hours that the fluid is to be infused. IV administration sets are predetermined by the manufacturer to deliver a certain number of drops per minute per milliliter of fluid that is given. If nurses are unfamiliar with the type of administration set, they should read the label on the infusion set. In general, the following drip rates are used:

Microdrip administration	60 drops per milliliter
Standard administration/macrodrip administration	10, 15, 20 drops per milliliter
Blood administration	10 drops per milliliter

These are called **drop factors**. The drop factor is the number of drops contained in 1 milliliter. Large volumes of fluid require a macrodrip administration. Macrodrip sets run 125 milliliters per hour or more, whereas microdrip sets run 50 milliliters per hour or less. These rates are often specified by the facility to ensure proper drug administration. Nurses are responsible for ensuring that the IV flow is regular, in addition to monitoring flow rate and ensuring needle placement, condition of the vein, and patient safety and comfort.

Health care professionals see flow rates expressed in a variety of ways. You will need to solve these calculations using the information that is presented in each problem, which will require the application of literal equations

$$\text{Rate (flow rate)} = \frac{\text{Volume}}{\text{Time}} \rightarrow R = \frac{V}{t}$$

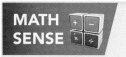

MATH SENSE

Solve literal equations by performing the inverse operations (V, t, or R) until you have solved the equation.

◆◆◆◆ Calculating IV Infusion Rates with a Formula

REVIEW

We can use a formula to calculate infusion rates. Such a formula uses key pieces of information about the amount or volume to be infused, the time in minutes, and what the infusion or administration set drop factor is.

$$\frac{\text{Amount of fluid in milliliters (mL)}}{\text{Total time of infusion in minutes}} \times \text{Administration set drop factor}$$

$$= \text{Drops per minute}$$

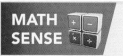

MATH SENSE

A shortcut can be used to handle the hours to minutes conversion. Then, cancellation is used to reduce the amount of calculation needed.

EXAMPLE

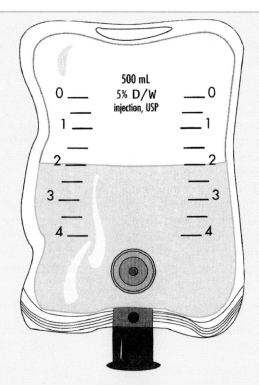

500 mL
5% D/W
injection, USP

0 — — 0
1 — — 1
2 — — 2
3 — — 3
4 — — 4

To administer 500 milliliters of IV fluid over 12 hours using a microdrip administration set, how many drops per minute would the nurse administer? (Hint: Microdrip has a drop factor of 60 drops per minute.)

Set up:

$$\frac{500 \text{ milliliter}}{12 \text{ hours} \times 60 \text{ minutes}} \times 60 \text{ drop factor} = \underline{\hspace{1.5cm}} \text{ drops per minute}$$

WORKING THROUGH THE FORMULA

Do not multiply 12 × 60 because cross-cancellation will reduce or eliminate the 60.

$$\frac{500 \text{ milliliter}}{12 \times \cancel{60}} \times \cancel{60} = \text{drops per minute}$$

$$500 \div 12 = 41.6666$$

The answer is 42 drops per minute.

CALCULATING IV INFUSION RATES WITH DIMENSIONAL ANALYSIS

To administer 500 milliliters of IV fluid over 12 hours using a microdrip administration set, how many drops per minute would the nurse administer? (Hint: Microdrip has a drop factor of 60 drops per minute.)

a. Set up the unknown quantity on one side of the equation. We are solving drops per minute.

$$z \text{ drops per minute} =$$

b. The first factor is the total amount to be administered in milliliters over the time in hours.

$$z \text{ drops per minute} = \frac{500 \text{ milliliters}}{12 \text{ hours}}$$

c. The second factor is the hours to minutes conversion. This is multiplied by the first factor.

$$z \text{ drops per minute} = \frac{500 \text{ milliliters}}{12 \text{ hours}} \times \frac{1 \text{ hour}}{60 \text{ minutes}}$$

d. Multiply this by the drop factor.

$$z \text{ drops per minute} = \frac{500 \text{ milliliters}}{12 \text{ hours}} \times \frac{1 \text{ hour}}{60 \text{ minutes}} \times \frac{60 \text{ drops}}{1 \text{ milliliter}}$$

e. Cancel like units and then solve. (Convert values to like units where appropriate.)

$$z \text{ drops per minute} = \frac{500 \cancel{\text{ milliliters}}}{12 \cancel{\text{ hours}}} \times \frac{1 \cancel{\text{ hour}}}{60 \text{ minutes}} \times \frac{60 \text{ drops}}{1 \cancel{\text{ milliliter}}}$$

$$z \text{ drops per minute} = 500 \div 12 = 41.6666$$

The answer is 42 drops per minute.

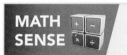

MATH SENSE

Drops must be rounded up or down to ensure a whole number of drops. There are no partial drops. Thus, drops per minute and drops per hour will be whole numbers.

Practice 1

Use one of the above methods to complete the following calculations of IV flow rates. Round your answers to the nearest whole number.

	Amount of Fluid in Milliliters	Time in Hours	IV Set Drop Factor	Drops per Minute
1.	300	3	60	_____
2.	1000	12	60	_____
3.	125	3	10	_____
4.	350	4	60	_____
5.	2500	24	60	_____
6.	450	8	20	_____
7.	24	1	60	_____
8.	1000	24	15	_____
9.	600	12	20	_____
10.	250	8	60	_____
11.	1600	12	60	_____
12.	48	3	15	_____
13.	1800	18	15	_____
14.	1500	12	60	_____
15.	150	24	60	_____
16.	675	8	60	_____
17.	320	5	15	_____
18.	200	$1\frac{1}{2}$	20	_____
19.	1400	8	15	_____
20.	900	12	60	_____

Practice 2

Find the drops per minute for each of the following problems.

1. The physician has ordered D_5W 1500 milliliters in 12 hours using a 15 drops per milliliter infusion rate. Infuse at _____ drops per minute.

2. The registered nurse is to infuse 1 unit of whole plasma (500 milliliters) over 4 hours using a blood administration rate of 10 drops per milliliter. Infuse at _____ drops per minute.

3. The nurse reads the physician's order for 1000 milliliters of $D_5\frac{1}{4}$NS over 12 hours at 15 drops per milliliters. Infuse at _____.

4. Infuse 325 milliliters D$_5$ $\frac{1}{2}$ NS over 4 hours. Use 60 drops per milliliter. Infuse at _____.

5. The nurse receives a physician's order for 300 milliliters plasma over 8 hours at 10 drops per milliliter. Infuse at _____.

6. Infuse 1200 milliliters D$_5$ LR over 24 hours at 15 drops per milliliter. Infuse at _____.

7. The nurse is asked to infuse D$_5$ $\frac{1}{3}$ NS 500 milliliters over 4 hours using microdrip tubing. Infuse at _____.

8. The physician prescribes Ionosol MB 750 milliliters over 12 hours using microdrip tubing. Infuse at _____.

9. The registered nurse received client Howard's medication order for 250 milliliters of packed red cells over 4 hours using a blood administration rate of 10 drops per milliliter. Infuse at _____.

10. An order reads D$_5$W 1000 milliliters infused over 24 hours at 20 drops per milliliter. Infuse at _____.

◆◆◆◆ Modified Setup

REVIEW

These types of calculations are straightforward when all parts of the calculation are given. However, you will encounter situations when you must calculate the missing part of the problem. In this case, a modified setup may be required. The possible unknowns may be flow rate, infusion time, or total volume.

To find the mL/hr, use this basic formula:

$$\frac{V}{t} = F$$

V = volume in milliliters

t = time in hours

F = flow rate in milliliter per hour to nearest whole number

EXAMPLE

The doctor has prescribed 750 milligrams of Ampicillin in 125 milliliters NS to infuse over 45 minutes. What is the milliliter per hour infusion rate?

To solve with the formula method:

Set up:

$$\frac{V}{t} = F \qquad \frac{1 \text{ hour}}{60 \text{ minutes}} = \frac{x \text{ hour}}{45 \text{ minutes}} \rightarrow 1 \times 45 = 45$$

$$\text{Then} \rightarrow 45 \div 60 = 0.75 \text{ hour}$$

(continued on next page)

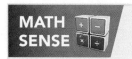

Drops are rounded to the nearest whole number.

$$\frac{125 \text{ milliliters}}{45 \text{ minutes}} \rightarrow 45 \text{ minutes is } \frac{45}{60} \text{ or } 0.75 \text{ hour}$$

Solve:

$$\frac{125 \text{ milliliters}}{0.75 \text{ hour}} = 166.666 \text{ milliliters per hour}$$

The answer is 167 milliliters per hour.

To solve using dimensional analysis:

a. The unknown to be solved is the flow rate, which is placed on the left side of the equal sign.

$$? \text{ milliliters per hour } =$$

b. The first factor is $\dfrac{\text{volume}}{\text{time}}$, and it is placed in the equation.

$$? \text{ milliliters per hour } = \frac{125 \text{ milliliters}}{45 \text{ minutes}}$$

c. Multiply the first factor by the second factor, which is the conversion of minutes to parts of an hour.

$$? \text{ milliliters per hour } = \frac{125 \text{ milliliters}}{45 \text{ minutes}} \times \frac{60 \text{ minutes}}{1 \text{ hour}}$$

(Note: This step will not be necessary if the problem uses hours instead of minutes.)

d. Cancel like units of measure and solve.

$$? \text{ milliliters per hour } = \frac{125 \text{ milliliters}}{45 \text{ \sout{minutes}}} \times \frac{60 \text{ \sout{minutes}}}{1 \text{ hour}} \rightarrow \frac{7500}{45}$$

$$= 166.66 \text{ milliliters per hour}$$

$$\text{or } 167 \text{ milliliters per hour}$$

Practice 3

Choose a method and calculate these problems to find milliliters per hour.

1. 1 liter of D_5W IV to infuse in 12 hours by infusion pump. Infuse at _____ milliliters per hour.

2. Infuse 50 milliliters of antibiotic in D_5W in 30 minutes. Infuse at _____ milliliters per hour.

3. The nurse is asked to infuse 150 milliliters NS IV PB in 30 minutes. Infuse at _____ milliliters per hour.

4. Infuse 1800 milliliters NS IV in 24 hours. Infuse at _____ milliliters per hour.

5. Infuse 2000 milliliters D$_5$W IV in 18 hours. Infuse at _____ milliliters per hour.

6. Infuse 650 milliliters D$_5$ 0.45% NaCl IV for 5 hours. Infuse at _____ milliliters per hour.

7. The physician orders 1000 milliliters D$_{10}$W to infuse over 8 hours. Infuse at _____ milliliters per hour.

8. The physician's order is for D$_5$NS 1200 milliliters to infuse over 24 hours. Infuse at _____ milliliters per hour.

9. The nurse receives an order for 600 milliliters Normosol R over 8 hours. Infuse at _____ milliliters per hour.

10. Infuse 1400 milliliters of medication over 6 hours. Infuse at _____ milliliters per hour.

◆

◆◆◆◆ Infusion Duration

REVIEW

Sometimes the infusion time in hours (a specific duration) is not given. The following formula will help solve the problem.

$$t = \frac{V}{F}$$

t = specific time in hours
V = volume in milliliters (mL)
F = flow rate in milliliters per hour

EXAMPLE

The physician orders D$_5$ $\frac{1}{2}$ NS 1000 milliliters at 175 milliliters per hour.

To solve using the formula method:

Set up:

$$t = \frac{V}{F} \rightarrow t = \frac{1000 \text{ milliliters}}{175 \text{ milliliters per hour}}$$

Solve:

$$t = \frac{1000 \text{ milliliters}}{175 \text{ milliliters per hour}} \rightarrow 1000 \div 175$$

$$= 5.71428 \text{ hours for infusing 1000 milliliters}$$

(continued on next page)

Round to the nearest hundredth: 5.71 hours. Note that the decimal portion of the answer must be in minutes.

To convert the decimal number to hours and minutes:

a. Separate the whole number from the decimal number—5 hours and 0.71

b. Multiply the decimal number—0.71 × 60 minutes.

0.71 × 60 = 42.6 minutes. Round to the nearest minute: 43 minutes

c. Place the hours and minutes together.

5 hours 43 minutes

The answer is 5 hours 43 minutes.

To solve using dimensional analysis:

a. The unknown is the unit of time (t) in hours (h). Place this on the left side of the equation.

$$t\,h =$$

b. Place the first factor, which is the total number of milliliters to be infused, over the number 1.

$$t\,h = \frac{1000 \text{ milliliters}}{1}$$

c. Then multiply the first factor by the inverse of the flow rate.

$$t\,h = \frac{1000 \text{ milliliters}}{1} \times \frac{1 \text{ hour}}{175 \text{ milliliters}}$$

d. Cancel like units and then solve.

$$t\,h = \frac{1000}{175} \rightarrow 5.71428$$

e. To convert the decimal number to hours and minutes:

STEP 1: Separate the whole number from the decimal number—5 hours and 0.71.

STEP 2: Multiply the decimal number—0.71 × 60 minutes.

0.71 × 60 = 42.6 minutes. Round to the nearest minute: 43 minutes

STEP 3: Place the hours and minutes together.

5 hours 43 minutes

Practice 4

Solve the following by calculating the infusion times in hours.

1. The nurse receives an order that reads 500 milliliters D_5W IV at 50 milliliters per hour. Infuse for _____.

2. A baby is to receive 300 milliliters D_5NS at 25 milliliters per hour. Infuse for _____.

3. Infuse 2000 milliliters at 125 milliliters per hour. Infuse for _____.

4. The patient is to receive LR 1000 milliliters at 140 milliliters per hour. Infuse for _____.

5. A nurse is requested to infuse 600 milliliters Normosol R at 125 milliliters per hour. Infuse for _____.

6. Ordered: 1000 milliliters NS at 200 milliliters per hour. What is the total time of infusion? _____

7. Ordered: 650 milliliters D₅W at 83 milliliters per hour. What is the total time of infusion? _____

8. Ordered: 800 milliliters NS at 75 milliliters per hour. What is the total time of infusion? _____

9. Ordered: 750 milliliters RL at 83 milliliters per hour. What is the total time of infusion? _____

10. Ordered: 1800 milliliters 0.45% NS at 75 milliliters per hour. What is the total time of infusion? _____

◆◆◆◆ Calculating Total Volume

Sometimes the total volume of fluid to be infused must be calculated.

To calculate how much fluid will be infused, you may use a formula or dimensional analysis:

$$V = t \times F$$

| V = volume in milliliters (mL) |
| t = time in hours |
| F = flow rate in milliliters per hour |

EXAMPLE

What is the total volume infused in 8 hours if the infusion rate is 65 milliliters per hour?

To solve with the formula:

$V = t \times F$, where t = 5 hours and F = 65 milliliters per hour

5 hours × 65 milliliters per hour = 325 milliliters in total volume

To solve with dimensional analysis:

a. Determine the unit of measure for the unknown volume and place it on the left side of the equation.

$$V \text{ milliliter} =$$

b. The first factor is the length of time over 1.

$$V \text{ milliliter} = \frac{5 \text{ hours}}{1}$$

(continued on next page)

c. Multiply the first factor by the flow rate, which is the second factor.

$$\text{V milliliter} = \frac{5 \text{ hours}}{1} \times \frac{65 \text{ milliliters}}{1 \text{ hour}}$$

d. Cancel like units and solve.

$$\text{V milliliter} = \frac{5 \; \cancel{\text{hours}}}{1} \times \frac{65 \text{ milliliters}}{1 \; \cancel{\text{hour}}} \rightarrow \frac{5 \times 65}{1}$$

$$= 325 \text{ milliliters to be infused in 5 hours}$$

Practice 5

Solve to find the total volume to be infused.

1. Ordered: $D_5\frac{1}{2}$ NS IV at 125 milliliters per hour for 12 hours. What is the total volume to be infused? _____

2. Ordered: Penicillin IV over 4 hours at a rate of 75 milliliters per hour. What is the total volume to be infused? _____

3. The nurse will administer an IV solution at 83 milliliters per hour for 6 hours. What is the total volume to be infused? _____

4. The patient will receive an IV therapy that runs at 120 milliliters per hour for 12 hours. What is the total volume to be infused? _____

5. The physician has ordered a therapeutic IV solution at 31 milliliters per hour for 18 hours. What is the total volume to be infused? _____ .

6. The nurse will administer $\frac{1}{2}$ NS IV at 50 milliliters per hour for 6 hours. What is the total volume to be infused? _____

7. Ordered: D_5 RL IV at 67 milliliters per hour for 4 hours. What is the total volume to be infused? _____

8. The physician has ordered an antibiotic IV solution at 125 milliliters per hour for a total of 12 hours. What is the total volume to be infused? _____

9. Ordered: 100 milliliters of 0.45% NS IV for 4 hours. What is the total volume to be infused? _____

10. The nurse will prepare to administer D_{10}W IV at 33 milliliters per hour for 24 hours. What is the total volume to be infused? _____

UNIT REVIEW

◆◆◆◆ Critical Thinking with Intravenous Fluid Administration

1. The doctor orders 250 mL of dextrose water to be infused over two hours by infusion pump set at a drop factor of 60. Every thirty minutes the patient should receive _____ mL of dextrose water.

2. If the patient's chart has a drug order for 500 mg of medication in 150 mL of Normal Saline to be infused at 20 gtts/mL for 45 minutes, what is the drop rate?

3. True or False: When the IV has a drop factor of 60 gtts/mL, then the flow rate in gtt/min is the same as mL/hr. Explain your answer.

4. True or False: A nurse should never round gtt/min to the nearest whole number.

5. True or False: $\dfrac{\text{(total volume)}}{\text{(mL/minute)}} = \text{total hours}$

6. True or False: mL/hour $\times$ total hours = total volume

7. Infuse D_5W IV at 250 mL/hr for 4 hours. What is the total volume to be infused in liters?

8. Infuse 1 L Normal Saline IV at 60mL/hr. The drop factor is 15 gtt/mL. The flow rate is _____.

9. Infuse 0.5 L of D_5W 0.33 NaCL IV for 12 hours at a drop factor of 60 gtt/mL. How many milliliters will be infused per hour?

10. Infuse 2500 mL of D_5LR IV at 125 mL/hr. The drop factor is 15 gtt/mL. What is the flow rate?

11. If D_5W means that there are 5 grams of dextrose per 100 milliliters of sterile water, then D_5W is a 5% dextrose solution. How many grams of dextrose are in 1 quart of water?

12. If D_5W means that there are 5 grams of dextrose per 100 milliliters of sterile water, then D_5W is a 5% dextrose solution. How many grams of dextrose are in 750 mL of water?

13. If Normal Saline (NS) has 0.9% sodium chloride, how many grams of sodium chloride are in 500 mL NS?

14. If Normal Saline (NS) has 0.45% sodium chloride (NaCL), how many grams of sodium chloride are in 1250 mL of solution? Round to the nearest whole number.

15. The doctor orders 1 L of $D_{10}W$ to run from 1000 to 1800 via infusion pump. What is the flow rate?

◆◆◆◆ Professional Expertise

- Round gtt to the nearest whole number.
- Read the problem carefully to locate the information that you know and what you are trying to calculate: flow rate, volume, or time.
- $\% = \dfrac{\text{grams}}{\text{milliliters}}$
- If you get a flow rate of over 300 mL, double-check it to be sure your calculations were correct.

THE BASICS OF INTRAVENOUS FLUID ADMINISTRATION POST-TEST

Calculate the drops per minute rate for each of the following:

	Total Volume for Infusion in Milliliters	Time in Hours	Drop Factor	Answer (drops per minute)
1.	500	8	15	_____
2.	250	6	20	_____
3.	1500	12	60	_____
4.	125	4	10	_____
5.	750	8	60	_____

Find the milliliters per hour rate for each of the following:

	Total Volume in Milliliters	Total Infusion Time	Answer (milliliters per hour)
6.	1200	6 hours	_____
7.	750	12 hours	_____
8.	250	4 hours	_____
9.	1800	24 hours	_____
10.	100	30 minutes	_____

Calculate the total infusion time for each of the following:

	Total Volume in Milliliters	Infusion Rate (milliliters per hour)	Answer (time in hours)
11.	500	125	_____
12.	650	133	_____
13.	1200	60	_____
14.	1000	100	_____
15.	250	83	_____

Find the total volume to be infused for each of the following:

	Flow Rate in Milliliters per Hour	Time in Hours	Total Volume in Milliliters
16.	135	6	_____
17.	83	8	_____
18.	25	3	_____
19.	125	12	_____
20.	65	$2\frac{1}{2}$	_____

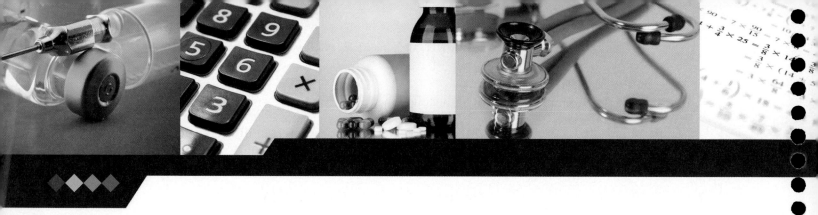

Basic Dosage by Body Weight

STUDENT LEARNING OUTCOMES

After completing the tasks in this unit, you will be able to:

14-1 Calculate dosage by body weight

14-2 Convert weights between pounds and kilograms

14-3 Calculate individual and daily dosages

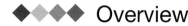 ## Overview

Many over-the-counter (OTC) medications for children, such as pain relievers, cold medications, and fever reducers, come in containers that have printed dosing instructions. Manufacturers know that parents know the weight of their children in pounds; thus, the printed dosing instructions come in teaspoons per age and pound limits. In a clinical setting, the body weight used is in kilograms and the recommended doses come in mg/kg, mcg/kg, and mL/kg.

Special population drug orders such as pediatric and geriatric medications are often calculated based on weight. These drug orders will state a medication amount per patient weight for a specific amount of time. For example, the drug order reads Methotrexate sodium IV 2.5 milligrams per kilogram every 14 days. The nurse will calculate the dose by multiplying 2.5 milligrams by the patient's weight in kilograms to compute the intravenous dose to be given every 14 days.

PRE-TEST

Convert the following pounds to kilograms:

Weight in Pounds and Ounces	Weight in Kilograms
1. 18 pounds 4 ounces	_____
2. 102 pounds	_____
3. 9 pounds 12 ounces	_____
4. 22 pounds 6 ounces	_____
5. 35 pounds 10 ounces	_____
6. 9 pounds 5 ounces	_____

Calculate the dosages:
Read the following client information and medication order.

Weight: 20 pounds 6 ounces
Ordered dose: 1.5 milligrams per kilogram per day
Recommended dosage from drug label: 3 milligrams every 8 hours

7. What is the daily dose? _____

8. What is the individual dose? _____

9. Does the dose ordered match the recommended dosage? _____

Read the following client information and medication order.

Weight: 44 pounds 8 ounces
Ordered dose: 0.5 milligrams per kilogram every 4 hours prn
Recommended dosage from drug label: dosages vary, not to exceed 45 milligrams over 24 hours

10. What is the daily dose? _____

11. What is the individual dose? _____

12. Does the ordered dose meet the recommended dosage guidelines? _____

Read the following client information and medication order.

Weight: 25 pounds
Ordered dose: 0.75 micrograms per kilogram every 8 hours
Recommended dosage from drug label: no more than 80 micrograms over 24 hours

13. What is the daily dose? _____

14. What is the individual dose? _____

15. Does the ordered dose meet the recommended dosage guidelines? _____

◆◆◆◆ Conversion to Kilograms

REVIEW

Converting a patient's weight to kilograms requires knowledge of basic math and the metric system. The first step is to convert the weight from pounds and ounces into kilograms.

EXAMPLE

The client weighs 32 pounds. What is his weight in kilograms?

To convert pounds to kilograms with a formula:
Set up:

$$\frac{1 \text{ kilogram}}{2.2 \text{ pounds}} = \frac{? \text{ kilograms}}{32 \text{ pounds}}$$

Solve:

a. 1 kilogram $\times$ 32 = 32

b. $\dfrac{32}{2.2} = 14.5454545$

c. Round to the nearest hundredth.

The answer is 14.55 kilograms.

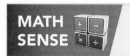

MATH SENSE

For calculating accurate dosages, the kilogram weight is rounded to the nearest hundredth for dosage by weight calculations.

USING DIMENSIONAL ANALYSIS

To convert pounds to kilograms with dimensional analysis:

The client weighs 32 pounds. What is his weight in kilograms?

a. Place the unknown weight on the left side of the equation.

$$? \text{ kilograms} =$$

b. Then the first factor is the conversion rate.

$$? \text{ kilograms} = \frac{1 \text{ kilogram}}{2.2 \text{ pounds}}$$

c. Multiply the first factor by the weight in pounds over 1.

$$? \text{ kilograms} = \frac{1 \text{ kilogram}}{2.2 \text{ pounds}} \times \frac{32 \text{ pounds}}{1} =$$

d. Cancel like units and solve.

$$? \text{ kilograms} = \frac{1 \text{ kilogram}}{2.2 \text{ \sout{pounds}}} \times \frac{32 \text{ \sout{pounds}}}{1} \rightarrow \frac{32}{2.2} = 14.54545$$

e. Round to the nearest hundredth.

The answer is 14.55 kilograms.

Practice 1

Convert the weight in pounds to weight in kilograms. Round to the nearest hundredth.

	Weight in Pounds	**Weight in Kilograms**
1.	14	_____
2.	55	_____
3.	27	_____
4.	98	_____
5.	40	_____
6.	110	_____
7.	16	_____
8.	8	_____
9.	30	_____
10.	105	_____

CONVERTING POUNDS AND OUNCES

When a pound weight includes ounces, use the same method but first convert the ounces to a decimal.

For example: Convert 14 pounds 4 ounces to kilograms.

$$14 \text{ pounds } 4 \text{ ounces} = 14\frac{4}{16}$$

$$= 14\frac{1}{4} \text{ or } 14.25 \text{ pounds.}$$

Convert 25 pounds 10 ounces to kilograms.

Separate the ounces and place them in fraction form over 16.

25 pounds and $\frac{10}{16}$. When $\frac{10}{16}$ is divided and made into a decimal, the result is 0.625.

Thus, the pound weight becomes 25.625 and is then ready to be converted with either method of conversion. Once the math is completed, round the kilogram to the nearest hundredth.

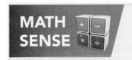

MATH SENSE

Remember that 1 pound has 16 ounces.

Practice 2

Convert the pounds to kilograms.

	Weight in Pounds and Ounces	**Decimal Number to Be Converted to Kilograms**	**Kilograms**
1.	14 pounds 8 ounces	_____	_____
2.	22 pounds 5 ounces	_____	_____
3.	16 pounds 4 ounces	_____	_____
4.	31 pounds 6 ounces	_____	_____
5.	42 pounds 2 ounces	_____	_____

Weight in Pounds and Ounces	Decimal Number to Be Converted to Kilograms	Kilograms
6. 9 pounds 8 ounces	_____	_____
7. 12 pounds 12 ounces	_____	_____
8. 109 pounds 8 ounces	_____	_____
9. 124 pounds 14 ounces	_____	_____
10. 7 pounds 10 ounces	_____	_____

◆◆◆◆ Calculating Dosage

REVIEW

Once you have converted the patient's weight from pounds to kilograms, your next step is to calculate the dosage by multiplying the dose ordered by the weight in kilograms.

EXAMPLE

The nurse receives a medication order for a child: Vancomycin hydrochloride 40 milligrams per kilogram per day in four divided doses for 10 days, not to exceed 2 grams a day. The child weighs 34 pounds 6 ounces. What is the total daily dose? What is the individual dose?

To solve with the proportional method:

1. Convert 34 pounds 6 ounces to kilograms.

   a. 34 pounds and $\frac{6}{16} \rightarrow 6 \div 16 = 0.375$ or 0.38

   34.38 pounds

   b. Set up:

   $$\frac{1 \text{ kilogram}}{2.2 \text{ pounds}} = \frac{? \text{ kilograms}}{34.38 \text{ pounds}}$$

   c. Solve:

   $$1 \times 34.38 = 34.38$$
   $$34.38 \div 2.2 = 15.6272 \text{ or } 15.63 \text{ kilograms}$$

2. Carefully reread the math problem.
   40 milligrams per kilogram per day in four divided doses for 10 days

   Set up:

   $$40 \times 15.63 =$$

   Solve:

   $$40 \times 15.63 = 625.2 \text{ milligrams per day in four divided doses for 10 days}$$

   625.2 divided into four doses ($625.2 \div 4 = 156.3$)

   Thus, the individual dose is 156.3 milligrams and the daily dose is 625.2 milligrams.

EXAMPLE

The nurse receives a medication order for a child: Vancomycin hydrochloride 40 milligrams per kilogram per day in four divided doses for 10 days, not to exceed 2 grams a day. The child weighs 34 pounds 6 ounces. What is the total daily dose? What is the individual dose?

To solve with the dimensional analysis:

1. Convert the 34 pounds 6 ounces to kilograms.

$$34 \text{ pounds and } \frac{6}{16} \rightarrow 6 \div 16 = 0.375 \text{ or } 0.38$$

$$34.38 \text{ pounds}$$

   a. Place the unknown on the left side of the equation and the conversion as the first factor that is multiplied by the decimal weight.

$$? \text{kilograms} = \frac{1 \text{ kilogram}}{2.2 \text{ pounds}} \times 34.38 \text{ pounds}$$

   b. Cancel like units and solve.

$$? \text{kilograms} = \frac{34.38}{2.2} = 15.63 \text{ kilograms}$$

2. Calculate the dosage.

   a. Set up the unknown on the left side of the equation.

$$? \text{milligrams per day} =$$

   b. Add the first factor, which from the problem is 40 milligrams per kilogram per day.

$$? \text{milligrams per day} = \frac{40 \text{ milligrams per day}}{1 \text{ kilogram}}$$

   c. Multiply the first factor by the weight in kilograms.

$$? \text{milligrams per day} = \frac{40 \text{ milligrams per day}}{1 \text{ kilogram}} \times 15.63 \text{ kilograms}$$

   d. Cancel like units and solve.

$$? \text{milligrams per day} = \frac{40 \text{ milligrams per day}}{1 \text{ kilogram}} \times 15.63 \text{ kilograms}$$

$$\rightarrow 40 \text{ milligrams} \times 15.63 = 625.2 \text{ milligrams per day}$$

   e. Solve for the individual dose.

   1. Place the dose per day on the left side of the equation.

$$? \text{individual dose} =$$

   2. Place the first factor, which is the daily dose over 1 day.

$$? \text{individual dose} = \frac{625.2 \text{ milligrams}}{1 \text{ day}}$$

   3. Multiply the first factor by the second factor, which is the number of doses or $\frac{1 \text{ day}}{4 \text{ doses}}$ because 4 doses are to be administered in a day.

$$? \text{individual dose} = \frac{625.2 \text{ milligrams}}{1 \text{ day}} \times \frac{1 \text{ day}}{4 \text{ doses}} =$$

(continued on next page)

4. Cancel like units and solve.

$$? \text{individual dose} = \frac{625.2 \text{ milligrams}}{1 \text{ \cancel{day}}} \times \frac{1 \text{ \cancel{day}}}{4 \text{ doses}}$$

$$\rightarrow \frac{625.2 \text{ milligrams}}{4 \text{ doses}} = 156.3 \text{ milligrams}$$

The answer is 156.3 milligrams per individual dose.

MATH SENSE

When weights consist of pounds and ounces, the ounces must be converted to a decimal number and then rounded to the nearest hundredth before the weight can be divided by 2.2 to be converted to kilograms.

Remember that for these dosages, kilograms are rounded to the nearest hundredth before calculating the individual and daily doses.

Practice 3

Find the dosage by solving the weight conversion problems.

1. Weight: 8 pounds 10 ounces
Recommended dose from drug label: 15 milligrams per kilogram over 24 hours
What is the weight in kilograms? _____
What is the daily dose? _____

2. Weight: 12 pounds 4 ounces
Recommended dose from drug label: 100 milligrams per kilogram every 12 hours
What is the weight in kilograms? _____
What is the individual dose? _____

3. Weight: 18 pounds
Recommended dose from drug label: 0.25 milliliter per kilogram per dose
What is the weight in kilograms? _____
What is the individual dose? Round to the nearest whole number. _____

4. Weight: 40 pounds 6 ounces
Ordered dose: Aspirin 300 milligrams not to exceed 1200 milligrams a day
Recommended dose from drug label: 65 milligrams per kilogram over 24 hours
Does the doctor's order fit within the recommended safe dosage guidelines of not exceeding 1200 milligrams per day? _____ What is the daily dose? _____

5. Weight: 22 pounds
Ordered dose: Ampicillin 30 milligrams per kilogram per day
Recommended dose from drug label: 25–50 milligrams per kilogram per day in equally divided doses every 8 hours
Does the doctor's order fit within the recommended safe dosage guidelines? _____
What is the daily dose? _____
What is the individual dosage? _____

6. The physician orders a medication at 1.5 milligrams per kilogram over 24 hours, divided into three doses. The client weighs 78 pounds.
   What is the weight in kilograms? _____
   What is the daily dose? Round to the nearest whole number. _____
   What is the individual dose? Round to the nearest whole number. _____

7. The nurse is to administer the recommended dose of Garamycin 2 milligrams per kilogram every 6 hours. The child weighs 42 pounds.
   What is the weight in kilograms? _____
   What is the daily dose? Round to the nearest whole number. _____
   What is the individual dose? _____

8. The physician orders Kantrex. The recommended dose is 2.5 milligrams per kilogram every 8 hours. The client weighs 38 pounds 4 ounces.
   What is the weight in kilograms? _____
   What is the daily dose? Round to the nearest whole number. _____
   What is the individual dose? Round to the nearest whole number. _____

9. The physician has ordered Proventil syrup orally at 0.1 milligrams per kilogram three times a day. The client weighs 28 pounds 8 ounces.
   What is the weight in kilograms? _____
   What is the daily dose? _____
   What is the individual dose? Round to the nearest whole tenth. _____

10. The physician orders a therapeutic IV medication at 2 milliliters per kilogram per dose. The client weighs 108 pounds.
    What is the weight in kilograms? _____
    What is the individual dose? _____

UNIT REVIEW

◆◆◆◆ Critical Thinking with Basic Dosage by Body Weight

Use your knowledge of basic dosage by body weight to solve the following problems.

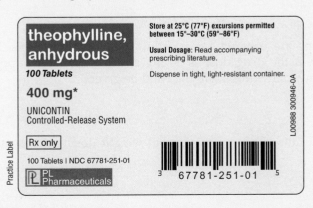

theophylline, anhydrous
100 Tablets
400 mg*
UNICONTIN
Controlled-Release System
Rx only
100 Tablets | NDC 67781-251-01
PL Pharmaceuticals
Practice Label

Store at 25°C (77°F) excursions permitted between 15°–30°C (59°–86°F)
Usual Dosage: Read accompanying prescribing literature.
Dispense in tight, light-resistant container.
L00988 300946-0A
3 67781-251-01 5

1. The pediatrician has ordered 5 mg/kg of theophylline anhydrous for a child weighing 54 pounds. How many tablets would be administered to this child?

2. The doctor orders morphine sulfate 7.5 mg subcutaneously every 4 hours as needed for pain for a female weighing 78 pounds. The recommended maximum dose for a child is 0.1 to 0.2 mg/kg/dose. Is this within a safe dosage range?

3. The doctor orders morphine sulfate 7.5 mg subcutaneously every 4 hours as needed for pain for a female weighing 78 pounds. The recommended maximum dose for a child is 0.1 to 0.2 mg/kg/dose. Morphine sulfate is available in 15 mg per 1 mL. How many milliliters would be drawn for this dosage?

4. Reading a drug label is important. If a child's cough syrup label says that the bottle contains 237 milliliters, how many full teaspoons are available in this bottle?

5. Convert 16 pounds to kilograms. Round to the nearest tenth if necessary.

6. Convert 34 pounds 3 ounces to kilograms. Round to the nearest tenth if necessary.

7. True or False: Weight in pounds is approximately twice the metric weight in kilograms.

8. True or False: Weight in kilograms is approximately half the weight in pounds.

9. True or False: A safe dosage is determined by comparing the ordered dose to the physician's ordered dose.

10. Ceclor is a common pediatric medication. It is available in oral suspension at 125 mg/5 mL. Two teaspoons has how many milligrams of medication?

11. Amoxicillin pediatric drops are ordered for a child. The drug label says 20 to 40 milligrams per kg/day. If the drug dose is 30 mg and the available supply is Amoxicillin 50 mg/mL, how many drops will the child be given?

Over-the-counter pediatric medications often use age and weight dosing. Look at this portion of a label.

AGE	WEIGHT	DOSE
Under 2 years	Under 24 pounds	Consult physician
2–5 years	24–48 pounds	1 teaspoon
6–11	49–95 pounds	2 teaspoons
12 years and older	96 pounds and over	4 teaspoons

12. Using the above label, what would be a dose in tablespoons for a 5-year-old child weighing 35 pounds?

13. Using the above label, what would be a dose in mL for an $8\frac{1}{2}$-year-old child weighing 78 pounds?

14. The nurse reads a medication chart: Order: Augmentin 350 mg p.o. q 8 hours for a 30-pound child with an upper respiratory infection. Augmentin is available in 125 mg/5 mL. What is the daily dosage?

15. Using the information in problem 14, what is the total volume of Augmentin required for a 10-day supply for the child?

◆◆◆◆ Professional Expertise

- Include the complete units of measure: mg/kg, mcg/kg, etc.
- Verify whether a dose is safe by comparing the ordered dose to the recommended dose on the drug label.
- Ensure that the child's weight is in kilograms for clinical settings.
- Do not round dosing for a child unless absolutely necessary.
- Verify any out-of-range medication orders with the physician.

BASIC DOSAGE BY BODY WEIGHT POST-TEST

Convert the following pounds to kilograms:

Weight in Pounds and Ounces	Weight in Kilograms
1. 14 pounds 2 ounces	_____
2. 82 pounds	_____
3. 7 pounds 15 ounces	_____
4. 8 pounds 12 ounces	_____
5. 12 pounds 10 ounces	_____
6. 33 pounds 8 ounces	_____

Calculate the dosages:
Read the following client information and medication order.

Weight: 77 pounds
Ordered dose: 1.2 milligrams per kilogram per day
Recommended dosage from drug label: 3 milligrams every 8 hours

7. What is the daily dose? _____

8. What is the individual dose? _____

9. Does the dose ordered match the recommended dosage? _____

Read the following client information and medication order.

Weight: 32 pounds 8 ounces
Ordered dose: 0.5 milligrams per kilogram every 4 hours prn
Recommended dosage from drug label: dosages vary, not to exceed 45 milligrams over 24 hours.

10. What is the daily dose? _____

11. What is the individual dose? _____

12. Does the ordered dose meet the recommended dosage guidelines? _____

Read the following client information and medication order.

Weight: 19 pounds
Ordered dose: 0.25 micrograms per kilogram every 8 hours
Recommended dosage from drug label: no more than 6 micrograms over 24 hours

13. What is the daily dose? _____

14. What is the individual dose? _____

15. Does the ordered dose meet the recommended dosage guidelines? _____

◆■◆◆ Whole Number Skills

1. Find the mean of the set of numbers: 16, 4, 25, 9, 10, 9, 3, 20 _____

2. 345 + _____ + 37 = 658

3. 1846 − 979 = _____

4. 324 × 87 = _____

5. $27)\overline{654}$ = _____

6. The heights of Michele's family members are 66 inches, 81 inches, 69 inches, 70 inches, and 64 inches. Find the range in heights of Michele's family members. _____

7. Convert from 8:15 P.M. standard time to Universal time. _____

◆◆■◆ Fraction Skills

8. Order the fractions from smallest to largest: $\dfrac{2}{3}, \dfrac{6}{7}, \dfrac{6}{21}, \dfrac{13}{21}$ _____

9. $20\dfrac{3}{5} + 6 + 3\dfrac{5}{6} =$ _____

10. $56\dfrac{1}{3} - 17\dfrac{11}{12} =$ _____

11. $2\dfrac{4}{5} \times \dfrac{2}{7} \times 5 =$ _____

12. $4\dfrac{1}{6} \div \dfrac{3}{8} =$ _____

13. Solve: $\dfrac{\frac{1}{10}}{\frac{1}{200}} =$ _____

◆■◆◆ Decimal Skills

14. Express as a fraction: 4.06 _____

15. Express as a decimal: $12\dfrac{5}{8}$ _____

16. $10.6 + 6 + 2.09 = $ _____

17. $65.7 - 12.68 = $ _____

18. $0.9 \times 41.2 = $ _____

19. $248.06 \div 0.8 = $ _____

◆◆◆◆ Ratio and Proportion Skills

20. A container holds 34 milliliters of medication. How many *full* 1.25 milliliter doses can be administered from this container? _____

21. Solve: $12 : 75 :: 2.5 : x$. Round to the nearest hundredth.
$x = $ _____

22. Solve: $8 : x :: 42 : 50$
$x = $ _____ Answer should be a mixed number.

23. Solve: $\dfrac{1}{2} : 8 :: x : 32$ $x = $ _____

24. Solve: $\dfrac{1}{50} : 10 :: \dfrac{10}{250} : x$ $x = $ _____

25. Simplify the ratio to the lowest terms: $9\dfrac{3}{8} : 5$ _____

◆◆◆◆ Percent Skills

26. What is $3\dfrac{2}{3}\%$ of 125? Write the answer as a mixed number. _____

27. What percent is 22 of 144? _____ Round to the nearest hundredth.

28. 24% of 250 is what number? _____

29. The original price minus a $45 discount is the sale price of a new desk. The sale price is $350. What was the original price? _____

30. There are 8 grams of pure drug in 75 milliliters of solution. What is the percent strength of solution? Round to the nearest hundredth. _____

◆◆◆◆ Combined Applications

31. $5\dfrac{1}{4}$ feet = _____ inches

32. _____ quarts = $7\dfrac{1}{2}$ pints

33. 36 pounds = _____ kilograms

34. _____ teaspoons = 70 milliliters

35. Convert 0.7% to a fraction = _____

36. Convert $4\frac{1}{2}$ to a percent = _____

37. Convert 9 to a percent = _____

38. Write 0.002 as a fraction = _____

39. Write 0.03% as a decimal = _____

◆◆◆◆ Pre-Algebra

40. $75 + (-8) =$ _____

41. $-15 - 22 =$ _____

42. $-72 \div 9 =$ _____

43. $-124 \times (-3) =$ _____

44. $21 + \sqrt{169} =$ _____

45. $(100 - 40) \div 4 =$ _____

◆◆◆◆ Drug Labels

46. Complete the table for this drug label. If the information is not provided, write *not shown*.

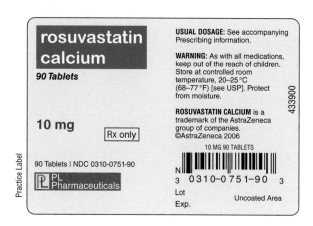

Generic name   _____

Trade name   _____

Manufacturer   _____

National Drug Code (NDC) number   _____

Lot number (control number)   _____

Drug form   _____

Dosage strength   _____

Usual adult dose   _____

Total amount in vial, packet, box   _____

Prescription warning   _____

Expiration date   _____

47. The medical assistant was asked to dispense 23 milliliters of a liquid medication. Shade the medicine cup to indicate this dosage.

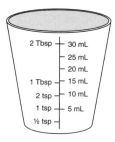

48. The physician has ordered an IM injection of 0.6 milliliters. Shade the syringe to indicate this volume of medication.

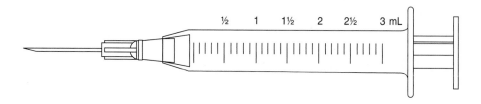

◆◆◆◆ Metric Measurements

49. 9.43 micrograms = _____ milligram

50. 193 grams = _____ kilogram. Round to the nearest tenth.

◆◆◆◆ Apothecary Measurements

51. 12 fluid ounces = _____ milliliters

52. $4\frac{1}{4}$ teaspoons = _____ milliliters

53. $6\frac{1}{2}$ pints = _____ milliliters

54. 0.2 milligrams = grain _____

55. grain $\frac{1}{100}$ = _____ milligram

56. 45 grams = grain _____

57. $4\frac{3}{4}$ teaspoons = _____ milliliters

◆◆◆◆ Oral Medications

58. Desired: Aspirin 0.5 grams every 4 hours
     Available: Aspirin 500 milligrams scored tablets
     Give: _____

59. The patient is ordered Vistaril 12 milligrams orally every 6 hours for nausea relief. You have on hand Vistaril oral suspension 5 milligrams per 2.5 milliliters.
You administer _____.

◆◆◆◆ Dosage Calculations

60. Ordered: Zocor 50 milligrams
     Have: Zocor 12.5 milligrams per tablet
     Desired dose: _____

61. The doctor has ordered Zyloprim 0.5 gram orally twice a day. On hand is Zyloprim 100 milligrams scored tablets. The nurse should give _____.

62. The client receives an order for Augmentin 250 milligrams. The Augmentin is labeled 100 milligrams in 5 milliliters. The client will be given _____.

◆◆◆◆ Parenteral Dosages

63. The physician orders megestrol acetate 600 milligrams per day. The megestrol acetate label reads oral suspension 40 milligrams per milliliter. Give: _____

64. Give Dilaudid 0.5 milligrams IM from a vial that is labeled 5 milligrams per milliliter. Give: _____

65. Ordered: Atropine sulfate 0.5 milligrams IM
Have: Atropine sulfate 0.25 milligrams per milliliter
Give: _____

66. The doctor prescribes heparin 4000 units sub-Q four times a day. You have heparin 1500 units per milliliter. You give _____.

67. Ordered: Quinidine 0.4 gram orally every 4 hours. Quinidine is supplied in 100 milligram tablets. How many tablets will you give? _____

◆◆◆◆ Calculating IV Dosages

68. The patient with oliguria has an order for 125 milliliters of 0.9% NS over 2 hours. The drop factor is 15 drops per milliliter. How many drops per minute should be given? _____

69. The nurse receives an order that reads 1200 milliliters D_5W IV at 60 milliliter per hour. Infuse for _____.

70. The nurse will administer an IV solution at 125 milliliters per hour for 6 hours. What is the total volume infused? _____

◆◆◆◆ Basic Dosages by Body Weight

Perform the calculations to determine whether the following is a therapeutic dosage for this child.
Ordered medication XYZ 5 milligrams orally every 12 hours for a child weighing 14 pounds.

You have medication XYZ 10 milligrams per milliliter. The recommended daily oral dosage for a child is 1.5 milligrams per kilogram per day in divided doses every 8 hours.

```
┌─────────────────────────────┐
│       Medication XYZ        │
│       Oral Solution         │
│         10 mg/mL            │
└─────────────────────────────┘
```

71. This child's weight is _____ kilograms.

72. What is the recommended dosage for this child? _____ milligrams per day

Weight: 24 pounds 4 ounces
Ordered dose: 1.6 milligrams per kilogram per day

Recommended dosage from drug label: 3 milligrams every 8 hours

73. What is the daily dose? _____

74. What is the individual dose? _____

75. Does the dose ordered match the recommended dosage? _____

Answers for the Post-Test

1. 12

2. 276

3. 867

4. 28,188

5. 24.22, or 24 R 6, or $24\frac{2}{9}$

6. 17

7. 2015

8. $\frac{6}{21}, \frac{13}{21}, \frac{2}{3}, \frac{6}{7}$

9. $30\frac{13}{30}$

10. $38\frac{5}{12}$

11. 4

12. $11\frac{1}{9}$

13. 20

14. $4\frac{3}{50}$

15. 12.625

16. 18.69

17. 53.02

18. 37.08

19. 310.075

20. 27 doses

21. 15.63

22. $9\frac{11}{21}$

23. 2

24. 20

25. 15 : 8

26. $4\frac{7}{12}$

27. 15.28

28. 60

29. $395.00

30. 10.67

31. 63

32. $3\frac{3}{4}$ pints

33. 16.4

34. 14

35. $\frac{7}{1000}$

36. 450%

37. 900%

38. $\frac{1}{500}$

39. 0.0003

40. 67

41. −37

42. −8

43. 372

44. 34

45. 15

46.

Generic name	rosuvastatin calcium
Trade name	Not shown
Manufacturer	PL Pharmaceuticals
National Drug Code (NDC) number	0310-0751-90
Lot number (control number)	Not shown
Drug form	Tablet
Dosage strength	10 milligrams
Usual adult dose	See accompanying prescribing information.
Total amount in vial, packet, box	90 tablets
Prescription warning	Rx only
Expiration date	Not shown

47. 23 milliliters

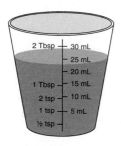

48. 0.6 milliliter

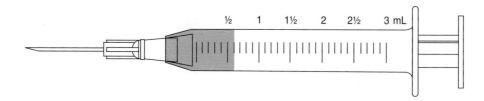

49. 0.00943 milligram

50. 0.2 kilogram

51. 360 milliliters

52. 21.25 milliliters

53. 3250 milliliters

54. grain $\dfrac{1}{300}$

55. 0.6 milligram

56. grain $7\dfrac{1}{2}$ or grain viiss

57. 23.75 milliliters

58. 1 tablet

59. 6 milliliters

60. 4 tablets

61. 5 tablets

62. 12.5 milliliters

63. 15 milliliters

64. 0.1 milliliter

65. 2 milliliters

66. 2.67 milliliters

67. 4 tablets

68. 16 drops per minute

69. 20 hours

70. 750 milliliters

71. 6.36 kilograms

72. 9.54 milligrams per day

73. 17.63 mg/day or 17.64 mg/day if kg is not rounded prior to multiplying by 1.6

74. 5.88 mg every 8 hours or 5.89 mg every 8 hours if kg is not rounded prior to multiplying by 1.6

75. No, contact the physician for clarification.

◆◆◆◆ Unit 1 Practice Exam

Name _____

Solve each problem below. Place your answer on the blank line.

1. $968 + 45 + 19 =$ _____

2. $529 + 3,456 =$ _____

3. The heights of the people in Michele's family are 68 inches, 65 inches, 73 inches, 74 inches, and 84 inches. Find the range of the people in Michele's family. _____

4. $709 +$ _____ $+ 49 = 1,670$

5. $2,852 - 1,418 =$ _____

6. $2,003 -$ _____ $= 907$

7. _____ $- 95 = 896$

8. $1,455 - 509 =$ _____

9. Write 1322 in standard time. _____

10. The dental office ordered 8 jackets for its staff. The jackets cost $37.00 each. What is the total cost for the 8 jackets? Write a number statement to solve this problem. Include the answer. _____

11. The heights of Michele's family members are 69 inches, 75 inches, 70 inches, 85 inches, and 76 inches. Find the median height of Michele's family members. _____

12. $14 \times 3 \times 12 =$ _____

13. $45 \times 138 =$ _____

14. Divide 932 by 8 = _____

15. $5,860 \div 14 =$ _____

16. $12\overline{)907} =$ _____

17. Heather's math tests had the following scores: 98, 75, 92, 98, 76, 87, 75, and 80. What is the mode of her scores? _____

18. Each gram of fat contains 9 calories. How many grams of fat are in 144 calories of fat in a piece of steak? _____

19. Bette was working hard to get a good grade. Her test scores were 68%, 79%, 100%, 85%, and 88%. What is the mean or average of her grades? _____

20. Round 12,885 to the nearest ten. _____

21. Use one of the symbols =, >, <, ≤, or ≥ to complete the number statement: 285 + 17 _____ 51 × 6

22. Write the Roman numeral xixss as an Arabic numeral. _____

23. After a heart attack, Bob spent two days in the coronary care unit. His bill was $4,596.00. What was his daily room rate? Write a number statement that represents this problem. _____

24. Write a number statement using the symbol >. _____

25. Find the prime factorization of 80. _____

◆◆◆◆ **Unit 2** Practice Exam

Name _____

Solve each problem. Put your answer on the blank line. Correct format is necessary.

1. Make into an equivalent fraction: $\dfrac{1}{4} = \dfrac{}{36}$ _____

2. Reduce to the lowest/simplest terms: $\dfrac{3}{129} =$ _____

3. Write as an improper fraction: $12\dfrac{3}{4} =$ _____

4. Write as a mixed number: $\dfrac{235}{9} =$ _____

5. $\dfrac{4}{5} + \dfrac{3}{8} =$ _____

6. $14\dfrac{3}{4} + \dfrac{5}{6} + 2\dfrac{7}{12} =$ _____

7. $22\dfrac{1}{5} + 1\dfrac{7}{9} =$ _____

8. $48\dfrac{2}{7} - 21\dfrac{5}{21} =$ _____

9. $676 - \dfrac{3}{11} =$ _____

10. $42\dfrac{5}{12} - 17\dfrac{5}{6} =$ _____

11. $\dfrac{3}{8} \times \dfrac{5}{7} =$ _____

12. $\dfrac{7}{12} \times 8 =$ _____

13. $7\dfrac{3}{4} \times 2\dfrac{1}{3} =$ _____

14. A bottle of medicine contains 12 doses of medication. How many full doses are in $4\dfrac{1}{4}$ bottles? _____

15. $\dfrac{3}{14} \div \dfrac{1}{5} =$ _____

16. $7\dfrac{1}{8} \div 10 =$ _____

17. How many full grain $\frac{3}{4}$ doses can be obtained from a grains $9\frac{1}{2}$ vial? _____

18. $35°C =$ _____ $°F$

19. $68°F =$ _____ $°C$

20. $\dfrac{\frac{2}{5}}{\frac{1}{7}} =$ _____

21. $\dfrac{\frac{1}{200}}{\frac{1}{6}} =$ _____

22. Order the following fractions by writing them in order from smallest to largest—do not just put the number of the order on top of each fraction. $\dfrac{1}{2}, \dfrac{3}{4}, \dfrac{4}{9}, \dfrac{17}{36}$. _____

23. One cup holds 8 ounces. If a cup is $\frac{2}{5}$ full, how many ounces are in the cup? _____

24. The nurse gave the patient a tablet of grain $\frac{1}{20}$ of medicine followed by a second tablet of grain $\frac{5}{80}$. How many total grains of the medication did the patient receive? _____

25. The physical therapist suggested that Bob begin a series of stretches. He told Bob to work out for $\frac{1}{3}$ of an hour. How many minutes is $\frac{1}{3}$ of an hour? _____ minutes.

◆◆◆◆ **Unit 3** Practice Exam

Name _____

1. Write the words in decimal numbers: seven-hundredths. _____

2. Write the decimal number of 17.005 in words. _____

3. Round 25.075 to the nearest hundredth: _____

4. Which is larger: 10.07 or 10.7? = _____

5. 0.4 + 12 + 0.11 = _____

6. 36.05 + 1.7 + 0.009 = _____

7. One medication is labeled 48.5 milliliters and another is labeled 0.5 milliliters. What is the total dosage in milliliters given of these two medications? _____

8. 8.008 − 0.98 = _____

9. 0.9 − 0.007 = _____

10. Patient Smith was on a diet. At the start of the diet, he weighed 122.6 kilograms. After one month he weighed 112.8 kilograms. What was his total weight loss in one month? _____

11. 0.596 × 2.3 = _____

12. 405 × 3.02 = _____

13. $16)\overline{42.98}$ Round to the nearest tenth = _____

14. $1.9)\overline{28.09}$ Round to the nearest hundredth = _____

15. Change 2.85 to a fraction. Reduce if necessary. _____

16. Write $\frac{7}{8}$ as a decimal. _____

17. 98.5°F = _____ °C

18. 14°C = _____ °F

19. $\dfrac{12.50}{0.50} \times 4.5 =$ _____

20. Something was wrong with Tu. He felt sick, and he had a fever. At 3:00 P.M. his temperature was 101.8°F. By 5:00 P.M. it was 102.3°F. How many degrees had his temperature gone up? _____

21. Valley Vista uses a 45.6 ounce can of kidney beans in a chili casserole recipe. If each portion gets an equal amount of the beans and the recipe serves 9 people, how many ounces of beans will each serving contain? Round to the nearest whole number. _____

22. On my way to an interview at the dental clinic for a dental assistant post, I had to stop to get gas. I put 7 gallons of gas in my car. Each gallon cost me $2.86. How much did I spend on gas? _____

23. The farm raises its own produce and meat. Will has a cow that produces milk. She gives 2.3 gallons of milk a day. How many gallons does she give in a month that has 30 days? _____

24. Bradley Benjamin heard that the nursing staff at Sky View earns $13.93 per hour. He is currently earning $12.46 per hour. How much more could he earn a week at Sky View than he currently earns if he calculates the rate for a 40-hour week? _____

25. Sally is trying to increase her dietary fiber intake. She eats 20.8 grams of fiber a day. If her goal is to eat 32 grams of dietary fiber a day, how many more grams of fiber does she need to eat? _____

◆◆◆◆ **Unit 4** Practice Exam

Name _____

Solve the ratio and proportion problems. Remember that ratios should be reduced to their simplest form.

1. Write 8 days out of 15 as a ratio: _____

2. Is this an example of a proportion? Check the appropriate box.

$2 : 3 :: 20 : 15$ ☐ Yes ☐ No

3. $5 : 30 = 12 : ?$? = _____

4. $\frac{1}{4} : 5 = ? : 70$? = _____

5. $82 : ? = \frac{1}{2} : 18$? = _____

6. $\frac{2}{4} = \frac{?}{98}$? = _____

7. $\dfrac{\frac{1}{2}}{\frac{1}{4}} = \dfrac{90}{?}$? = _____

8. $\frac{1}{12} : 28 = ? : 84$? = _____

9. If eggs cost $2.10 a dozen, how much do 16 eggs cost? _____

10. If Jerry makes $13.10 an hour, what is his pay for 15 hours? _____

11. A mouthwash costs $4.36 for 32 ounces. How much does each ounce cost? _____

12. Each calendar for the nursing home fund raiser costs $8.75. What is the cost for 25 calendars? _____

13. Simplify the following ratio $12\frac{1}{4} : 8$ _____

14. Simplify the following ratio $15 : \frac{1}{3}$ _____

15. Solve $\dfrac{1.7}{x} = \dfrac{8.2}{0.8}$. Round to the nearest tenth. _____

16. A set of three surgical masks costs $1.39. How many complete sets of masks can you buy with a budget of $10? Do not worry about tax or shipping. _____

17. 17 teaspoons = _____ tablespoons

18. 1 inch = 2.5 centimeters, so 17.8 inches = _____ centimeters. Round to the nearest tenth.

19. 1 kilogram = 2.2 pounds, so 49 kilograms = _____ pounds.

20. $\dfrac{5}{7\frac{2}{4}} = \dfrac{?}{12\frac{1}{2}}$? = _____

Theresa's Roasted Red Tomato Soup

Nutrition facts	Amount/serving	%DV*	Amount/serving	%DV*
Serving size ½ cup	Total fat 0 gram	0%	Total carbohydrates 20 grams	7%
(120 milliliters)	Saturated fat 0 gram	0%	Fiber 1 gram	4%
Condensed soup	Cholesterol 0 milligram	0%	Sugars 15 grams	
Servings about 2.5	Sodium 610 milligrams	30%	Protein 2 grams	
Calorie 90				
Fat calorie 0	Vitamin A 10% · Vitamin C 10% · Calcium 0% · Iron %			

*Percent daily values (%DV) are based on a 2,000 calorie diet.

21. If $\dfrac{1}{2}$ cup of soup equals 120 milliliters, how many milliliters are in $3\dfrac{1}{4}$ cups of soup? _____

22. If a can has 2.5 servings, how many cans are needed to serve 12 people? Round to the nearest full can. _____

23. One serving contains 90 calories; how many calories are in $4\dfrac{1}{2}$ servings? _____

24. 1 gram of fiber constitutes 4% of a daily dietary value. How many grams of fiber would be present in 25% of the daily value? _____

25. How many grams of carbohydrates are present if the portion meets 30% of the daily value of carbohydrates? Round to the nearest tenth if necessary. _____

◆■◆◆ **Unit 5** Practice Exam

Name _____

1. Convert $3\frac{1}{4}$ to a percent. _____

2. Convert 0.625 to a percent. _____

3. Convert 453 to a percent. _____

4. Convert $\frac{2}{5}$ to a percent. _____

5. Convert $4\frac{1}{5}$ to a percent. _____

6. Convert $\frac{\frac{2}{5}}{75}$ to a percent. _____

7. Convert 45% to a decimal. _____

8. Convert $5\frac{1}{4}\%$ to a decimal. _____

9. Convert $\frac{3}{4}\%$ to a fraction. _____

10. What is 12% of 233? _____

11. Find 56% of 250. _____

12. What is $22\frac{1}{2}\%$ of 400? _____

13. What percent of 80 is 14? _____

14. Find 32% of 360. _____

15. What is $12\frac{2}{3}\%$ of 120? _____

16. $15\frac{1}{4}\%$ of what number is 45.75? _____

17. What is 0.9% of 34? _____

18. Write the ratio of pure drug to solution: 16% _____

19. Write the ratio of pure drug to solution: 1.08% _____

20. Write the ratio of pure drug to solution: $2\frac{2}{5}\%$ _____

21. There are 3 grams of pure drug in 45 milliliters of solution. What is the percent strength of the solution? _____

22. There are 35 milliliters of pure drug in 100 milliliters of solution. How many milliliters of pure drug are needed to make 85 milliliters of this solution? _____

23. Take an 8% discount on a final sales price of $120.00. The final sales price would now be _____.

24. Write a simplified ratio of the pure drug form: $6\frac{1}{4}$% solution. _____

25. Write a simplified ratio of the pure drug form: 9% solution. _____

◆◆◆◆ **Unit 6** Practice Exam

Name _____

1–15. *Complete the table below:*

FRACTION	DECIMAL	RATIO	PERCENT
$\dfrac{1}{100}$	1. _____	2. _____	3. _____
4. _____	0.08	5. _____	6. _____
7. _____	8. _____	2 : 5	9. _____
10. _____	11. _____	12. _____	$5\dfrac{1}{4}\%$
13. _____	0.1	14. _____	15. _____

16. If 1 tablespoon is equivalent to 3 teaspoons, how many tablespoons are in 13 teaspoons? _____

17. One inch equals approximately 2.54 centimeters. If an infant is measured at 48 centimeters, how long is the infant in inches? Round to the nearest tenth. _____

18. One cup has 8 ounces. So $14\dfrac{1}{4}$ cups equals _____ ounces.

19. One teaspoon contains 5 milliliters. Nine and one-half teaspoons contains _____ milliliters.

20. If one pound contains 16 ounces, how many ounces are in 24 pounds? _____

21. If 1 kilogram equals 2.2 pounds, how many kilograms are in 70 pounds? _____

22. $3\dfrac{1}{4}$ feet = _____ inches

23. _____ quarts = 12 pints

24. 15 pounds = _____ kilograms. Round to the nearest tenth.

25. _____ teaspoons = 30 milliliters

◆◆◆◆ **Unit 7** Practice Exam

Name _____

Write integers for the following situations:

1. 30 degrees below 0 _____

2. A gain of 6 yards _____

Put the following sets of integers in order from least to greatest:

3. 9, −68, 53, −19 _____, _____, _____, _____

4. 0, −34, 12, 50 _____, _____, _____, _____

Find the absolute value:

5. $|\,26\,| =$ _____

6. $|-132\,| =$ _____

Solve:

7. $5 + (-10) =$ _____

8. $-8 - 52 =$ _____

9. $-36 \div 9 =$ _____

10. $-25 \times (-4) =$ _____

11. $6 \div (-3) =$ _____

12. $-3 + 28 =$ _____

13. $-19 \times (-1) =$ _____

14. $6 + (-9) =$ _____

15. $5 - (-2) =$ _____

16. $|-5 - 4| =$ _____

17. $|-2| \times 2 =$ _____

18. $18^2 =$ _____

19. $1^0 + (6)^2 =$ _____

20. $75 + (15)^2 =$ _____

21. $3^2 + 21^0 + 7^2 =$ _____

22. $2 + \sqrt{169} =$ _____

23. $\sqrt{25} + \sqrt{9} =$ _____

24. $\left(\sqrt{144} - \sqrt{64}\right)^2 =$ _____

25. $\left(9^2 - 4^2\right) \div 5 =$ _____

◆◆◆◆ Unit 8 Practice Exam

Name _____

1. The numerical value for centi- is _____.

2. The numerical value for micro- is _____.

3. The numerical value for milli- is _____.

4. Gram and milligram are metric measures for measuring _____.

5. Liter and milliliter are metric measures for measuring _____.

Circle the correct metric notation for each:

6. Twelve and one-half kilograms

    a. $12\frac{1}{2}$ kg   **b.** 12.5 KG   **c.** 12.5 kg   **d.** $12\frac{1}{2}$ KG

7. One hundred five micrograms

    a. 105 mg   **b.** 0.105 mcg   **c.** 105 mcg   **d.** 100.5 mcg

8. Write the correct metric notation for six hundredths of a milliliter. _____

9. Write the correct metric notation for two tenths of a milligram. _____

10. Write the correct metric notation for ninety-three milligrams. _____ _____

11. Write the correct metric notation for twelve hundredths of a kilogram. _____

12. 2.76 milligrams = _____ micrograms

13. 25 centimeters = _____ millimeters

14. 120.8 grams = _____ kilogram

15. _____ milligram = 4.7 micrograms

16. _____ liter = 95 milliliters

17. 12 grams = _____ milligrams

18. 9.05 milliliters = _____ liter

19. _____ gram = 10000 micrograms

20. _____ centimeters = 54 millimeters

21. 0.5 gram = _____ micrograms

22. 1200 milliliters = _____ liters

23. _____ kilogram = 23.8 grams

24. 33.7 meters = _____ millimeters

25. A newborn weighs 3090 grams. How many kilograms does he weigh? _____

◆◆◆◆ **Unit 9** Practice Exam

Name _____

1. Look at the IV bag.

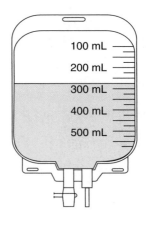

How many milliliters have been infused? _____

2. Look at the label and provide the following information. If the information is not provided, write *not shown*.

NDC 0781-8153-94	*Each vial contains Penicillin G sodium, equivalent to 5,000,000 units (5 million units) of penicillin G as the sodium salt with 1.68 mEq of sodium per million units of penicillin G, Store dry powder at 20°–25°C (68°–77°F) [see USP Controlled Room Temperture]. Sterile constituted solution may be kept in refrigerator (2° to 8°C) for 3 days without significant loss of potency
penicillin G procaine for injection, USP	
5,000,000 Units*	
(5 million units)	
For IM or IV use	
Rx only	
PL Pharmaceuticals	

PREPARATION OF SOLUTION

Diluent added	Final Concentration
8 mL	500,000 units/mL
3 mL	1,000,000 units/mL

Practice Label

Exp:

Lot:

Generic name	_____
Trade name	_____
Manufacturer	_____
National Drug Code (NDC) number	_____
Lot number (control number)	_____
Drug form	_____
Dosage strength	_____
Usual adult dose	_____
Total amount in vial, packet, box	_____
Prescription warning	_____
Expiration date	_____

3. Look at the label and provide the following information. If the information is not provided, write *not shown.*

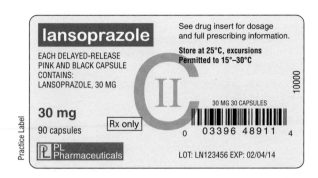

Generic name   _____

Trade name   _____

Manufacturer   _____

National Drug Code (NDC) number   _____

Lot number (control number)   _____

Drug form   _____

Dosage strength   _____

Usual adult dose   _____

Total amount in vial, packet, box   _____

Prescription warning   _____

Expiration date   _____

4. The medical assistant was asked to dispense 22 milliliters of a liquid medication. Shade the medicine cup to indicate this dosage.

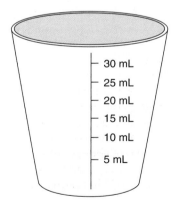

5. The physician has ordered an IM injection of 1.6 milliliters. Shade the syringe to indicate this volume of medication.

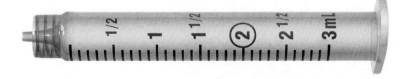

◆◆◆◆ **Unit 10** Practice Exam

Name _____

Make the following conversions:

1. 8 teaspoons = _____ milliliters

2. $12\frac{1}{2}$ quarts = _____ milliliters

3. grains 50 = _____ milligrams

4. 8 tablespoons = _____ milliliters

5. grain $\frac{1}{20}$ = _____ milligrams

6. 27 ounces = _____ tablespoons

7. fluid ounces 9 = _____ milliliters

8. $4\frac{1}{2}$ cups = _____ ounces

9. 20 teaspoons = _____ liter

10. 150 milliliters = _____ fluid ounces

11. $1\frac{1}{4}$ pints = _____ milliliters

12. $\frac{3}{4}$ cup _____ milliliters

13. 2.4 liters = _____ pints

14. 48 milliliters = _____ fluid ounces

15. $14\frac{1}{4}$ teaspoons = _____ milliliters

16. A client weighs 245 pounds. What is his weight in kilograms? _____

17. The doctor orders grain iv of medication. What is the milligram equivalent of the medication order? _____

18. The dental patient is prescribed a medicated mouth rinse. He is told to swish his mouth with $2\frac{1}{2}$ tablespoons of the mouth rinse. How many milliliters of medicated mouth rinse should the patient be given? _____

19. How many tablespoons are in fluid ounces 7 of medication? _____

20. A drug packet insert states that no more than 45 milligrams of the medication should be given in a 24-hour period. How many grains is equivalent to 45 milligrams? _____

21. The client is asked to drink at least 2400 milliliters of fluid daily. How many fluid ounces are equivalent to 2400 milliliters? _____

22. The newborn baby is drinking $1\frac{3}{4}$ ounces of milk a feeding. How many tablespoons are equivalent to $1\frac{3}{4}$ ounces? _____

23. Six and one-half ounces is _____ milliliters.

24. Three grams of medication is equivalent to gr _____.

25. The patient drinks $3\frac{1}{3}$ cups of tea each day. How many milliliters are $3\frac{1}{3}$ cups? _____

◆◆◆◆ **Unit 11** Practice Exam   Name _____

Complete the dosage calculations below using the standard conversion to find the desired dosage.

1. Ordered: Plendil 7.5 milligrams
   Have: Plendil 2.5 milligrams extended release tablets
   Desired Dose: _____

2. Ordered: Prilosec 20 milligrams
   Have: Prilosec 40 milligrams scored tablets
   Desired Dose: _____

3. Ordered: Crestor 2.5 milligrams
   Have: Crestor 5 milligrams scored tablets
   Desired Dose: _____

4. Ordered: Dilantin 100 milligrams
   Have: Dilantin 50 milligrams per tablet
   Desired Dose: _____

5. Ordered: Neurontin 500 milligrams
   Have: Neurontin 250 milligrams in 5 milliliters
   Desired Dose: _____

6. Ordered: Zocor 40 milligrams
   Have: Zocar 20 milligrams per tablet
   Desired Dose: _____

7. The doctor has ordered Zyloprim 0.25 gram orally twice a day. On hand is Zyloprim 100 milligrams scored tablets. The nurse should give _____.

8. The client receives an order for Augmentin 250 milligrams. The Augmentin is labeled 125 milligrams 5 milliliters. The client will be given _____.

9. The long-term care resident receives a medication order for albuterol sulfate liquid 4 milligrams orally three times a day. The nurse reads the albuterol sulfate liquid label and learns that each teaspoon contains 2 milligrams of the albuteral sulfate. For each dose, the resident will take _____ teaspoons.

10. The client has a drug order for Procardia 20 milligrams three times a day. The Procardia label reads Procardia 10 milligrams per tablet. The client will receive _____ tablets three times a day.

11. Doctor Smith orders Fosamax 40 milligrams once a day taken at least 30 minutes before the first meal of the day. Fosamax comes in 40 mg tablets. The client will take _____ each day.

12. The doctor orders Cozaar 75 milligrams twice a day. The Cozaar label reads 25 milligrams per tablet. The patient will take _____ tablets twice a day.

13. The doctor orders Allopurinol 0.3 gram tablets orally. Allopurinol is available in 150 milligrams per tablet. Give _____.

14. Give Benedryl 75 milligrams. The vial is labeled 3 milliliters = 25 milligrams. Give _____.

15. The physician orders 200 milligram tablets of Tagamet. On hand is 0.1 gram tablets. Give_____.

16. Give Edecrin 45 milligrams. The supply on hand is Edecrin grain $\frac{1}{4}$ tablets. Give _____.

17. The doctor orders Lanoxin 0.6 milligrams IV daily. Lanoxin is supplied in 0.4 milligrams in 2 milliliters. Give _____.

18. The patient is ordered Demerol syrup 75 milligrams orally every 4 hours as need for pain. The Demerol label reads Demerol syrup 50 milligrams in 5 milliliters. Give _____.

19. The order reads Tylenol 0.5 gram orally every 4 hours as needed for pain. The Tylenol liquid supplied is Tylenol (acetaminophen) liquid 500 milligrams in 5 milliliters. Give _____.

20. The doctor prescribed Tagamet 150 milligrams orally. The medicine label reads Tagamet liquid 300 milligrams in 5 milliliters. How many teaspoons will be given? _____

21. A label reads Compazine 10 milligrams in 2 milliliters. The doctor prescribes an order that reads Compazine 8 milligrams IM every 6 hours as needed for nausea. What is the individual dose? _____.

22. The doctor orders Codeine grain $\frac{1}{4}$ orally every day. On hand is Codeine 30 milligrams per tablet. The nurse will give _____.

23. On hand are phenobarbital 15 milligrams scored tablets. The order reads phenobarbital grain $\frac{1}{2}$ orally twice a day. Give _____.

24. On hand: Slow K potassium chloride 8 milliequivalents per milliliter. The order is for potassium chloride 24 milliequivalents orally each day for prophylaxis of hypokalemia. Give _____.

25. Digoxin is available in 0.25 milligram scored tablets. The order is for digoxin 0.5 milligram orally twice a day. Give _____.

◆◆◆◆ **Unit 12** Practice Exam   Name _____

1. The physician orders megestrol acetate 800 milligrams per day. The megestrol acetate label reads oral suspension 40 milligrams per milliliter.
   Give: _____

2. Give Dilaudid 0.5 milligram IM from a vial that is labeled 4 milligrams per milliliter.
   Give: _____

3. Ordered: Atropine sulfate 0.5 milligram IM
   Have: Atropine sulfate 0.3 milligram per milliliter
   Give: _____

4. The physician has ordered Calcitonin-Salmon 100 units IM for the client. The Calcitonin-Salmon vial reads 200 units per milliliter.
   Give: _____

5. The physician has ordered adrenalin 0.8 milligram sub-Q stat. The adrenalin label reads 1 : 1000 solution.
   Give: _____

6. Ordered: Cefotetan Sodium 200 milligrams IM every 24 hours piggy-back IV
   Have: Cefotetan Sodium 2 grams in 50 milliliters
   Give: _____

7. The physician has ordered magnesium sulfate 2 grams stat. The magnesium sulfate vial is labeled 50% solution.
   Give: _____

8. Give Butorphanol 1.75 milligrams IV for the client every three to four hours. The Butorphanol drug label reads 1 milligram per milliliter.
   Give: _____

9. The physician orders Imitrex 8 milligrams sub-Q as needed for headache for the client. The Imitrex drug label on the vial reads 12 milligrams per milliliter.
   Give: _____

10. Ordered: Zemplar 3 micrograms IM
    Have: Zemplar 5 micrograms per milliliter
    Give: _____

11. The physician has ordered Levsin 0.25 milligram IM four times a day for the client. The drug label on the vial reads 0.5 milligram hyoscyamine sulfate injection USP per milliliter.
    Give: _____

12. Ordered: Lidocaine 250 milligrams sub-Q
    Have: Lidocaine 300 milligrams in 3 milliliters
    Give: _____

13. The physician has ordered heparin 25,000 units IV from a vial that reads heparin 10,000 units per milliliter.
    Give: _____

14. Ordered: Zantac 0.75 milligram IM stat
      Have: Zantac 0.5 milligram per milliliter
      Give: _____

15. The physician has ordered Naloxone hydrochloride 1.4 milligram IV from a vial labeled 0.4 milligram per milliliter. The nurse should administer _____.

16. The supply on hand of morphine is grain $\frac{1}{4}$ per milliliter. The order is for morphine sulfate 15 milligrams IM immediately. The client will receive an injection of _____.

17. The physician orders Valium 5 milligrams IM every 6 hours as needed to calm restlessness in a client. The on-hand supply is Valium 10 milligrams in 2 milliliters. The nurse will administer _____.

18. The order is for Neostigmine methylsulfate 1 milligram IM for symptomatic control of Myasthenia Gravis. The supply is Neostigmine methylsulfate 1 : 2000. The nurse will prepare an injection of _____.

19. Ordered: Epotetin alfa 3,800 units sub-Q three times a week
      Have: Epotetin alfa 4,000 units per milliliter
      Give: _____

20. Ordered: Ceftin oral suspension 250 milligrams twice a day
      Have: Ceftin oral suspension 125 milligrams in 5 milliliters
      Give: _____

21. Ordered: E.E.S. 500 milligrams orally twice a day
      Have: E.E.S. oral suspension 200 milligrams in 5 milliliters
      Give: _____

22. A home resident is to have 15 milliliters of a medication to aid with digestion. A disposable medicine cup is not available. How can the dosage be measured accurately with the items in a residence? _____ What is the dosage? _____.

23. A patient is to receive Depo-Provera 1000 milligrams IM. The vial reads Depo-Provera 400 milligrams per milliliter. Prepare _____.

24. The physician orders Zemplar 3 micrograms IM every day. The Zemplar label reads 5 micrograms per milliliter. Give an injection of _____.

25. The Neulasta label reads Neulasta 6 milligrams in 0.6 milliliter. The doctor's order reads: Give Neulasta 6 milligrams sub-Q immediately. The nurse will prepare _____.

◆◆◆◆ **Unit 13** Practice Exam

Name _____

Complete the following calculation of IV flow rates. Round your answers to the nearest whole number.

	Amount of Fluid in Milliliters	Time in Hours	IV Set Drop Factor	Drops per Minute
1.	200	3	10	_____
2.	750	12	15	_____
3.	1250	10	60	_____
4.	650	4	20	_____
5.	2000	24	60	_____

Solve each of the following problems.

6. The physician has ordered D_5W 1000 milliliters in 12 hours using a 20 drops per milliliter infusion rate. Infuse at _____ drops per minute.

7. The registered nurse is to infuse 2 units of whole plasma (500 milliliters each) over 8 hours using a blood administration rate of 10 drops per milliliter. Infuse at _____ drops per minute.

8. The nurse reads the physician's order for 500 milliliters of $D_5\frac{1}{4}$NS over 12 hours at 15 drops per minute. Infuse at _____.

9. Infuse 550 milliliters $D_5\frac{1}{4}$NS over 4 hours. Use 60 drops per minute. Infuse at _____.

10. The nurse receives a physician's order for 250 milliliters plasma over 8 hours at 10 drops per milliliter. Infuse at _____.

11. Infuse 1000 milliliters D_5W IV in 18 hours. Infuse at _____ milliliters per hour.

12. Infuse 750 milliliters D_5 0.45% NaCl IV for 10 hours. Infuse at _____ milliliters per hour.

13. The physician orders 1000 milliliters $D_{10}W$ to infuse over 12 hours. Infuse at _____ milliliters per hour.

14. The physician's order is for D_5NS 1250 milliliters to infuse over 18 hours. Infuse at _____ milliliters per hour.

15. The nurse receives an order for 550 milliliters Normosol R over 6 hours. Infuse at _____ milliliters per hour.

16. Infuse 1000 milliliters of medication over 6 hours. Infuse at _____ milliliters per hour.

17. The nurse will administer an IV solution at 83 milliliters per hour for 8 hours. What is the total volume infused? _____

18. The patient will receive an IV therapy that runs at 150 milliliters per hour for 12 hours. What is the total volume infused? _____

19. The physician has ordered a therapeutic IV solution at 42 milliliters per hour for 18 hours. What is the total volume infused? _____

20. The nurse will administer $\frac{1}{2}$ NS IV at 75 milliliters per hour for 6 hours. What is the total volume infused? _____

21. Ordered: D_5 RL IV at 83 milliliters per hour for 4 hours. What is the total volume infused? _____

22. The nurse receives an order that reads 1500 milliliters D_5W IV at 60 milliliters per hour. Infuse for _____.

23. A baby is to receive 240 milliliters D_5NS at 35 milliliters per hour. Infuse for _____.

24. Infuse 1000 D_5W milliliters at 83 milliliters per hour. Infuse for _____.

25. The patient is to receive LR 1000 milliliters at 123 milliliters per hour. Infuse for _____.

◆◆◆◆ Unit 14 Practice Exam

Name _____

Convert the following pounds to kilograms:

Weight in Pounds and Ounces	Weight in Kilograms. Round to Hundredths Place.
1. 12 pounds 6 ounces	_____
2. 54 pounds	_____
3. 34 pounds 14 ounces	_____
4. 22 pounds 12 ounces	_____
5. 102 pounds 10 ounces	_____
6. 13 pounds 8 ounces	_____

Calculate the dosages:

Read the following client information and medication order:

    Weight: 34 pounds 6 ounces
    Dose ordered: 1.4 milligrams per kilogram per day
    Recommended dosage from drug label: 3 milligrams every 8 hours

7. What is the daily dose? _____

8. What is the individual dose? _____

9. Does the dose ordered match the recommended dosage? _____

Read the following client information and medication order:

    Weight: 26 pounds 8 ounces
    Dose ordered: 0.5 milligram/kilogram every 6 hours, prn
    Recommended dosage from drug label: dosages vary, not to exceed 45 milligrams per 24 hours.

10. What is the daily dose? _____

11. What is the individual dose? _____

12. Does the dose ordered meet the recommended dosage guidelines? _____

Read the following client information and medication order:

    Weight: 22 pounds
    Dose ordered: 0.25 microgram per kilogram every 8 hours
    Recommended dosage from drug label: no more than 5 micrograms over 24 hours

13. What is the daily dose? _____

14. What is the individual dose? _____

15. Does the dose ordered meet the recommended dosage guidelines? _____

16. The order is for theophylline 55 milligrams four times a day via nasal gastric tube. The recommended dosage is 22 milligrams per kilogram every 6 hours. The child weighs 10 kilograms. Is the doctor's dosage within the recommended dosage guidelines? _____ Yes _____ No

Cefuroxine 375 milligrams IV is ordered every 8 hours for a child whose weight is 45 pounds. The recommended dose is 50 milligrams per kilogram per day.

17. What is the ordered daily dose? _____

18. What is the ordered individual dose? _____

19. Does the dose ordered meet the recommended dosage guidelines? _____

An infant with a urinary tract infection has an order for Ampicillin IV 125 milligrams every 6 hours. The infant weighs 10 pounds. The recommended dose is 50 milligrams per kilogram every 6 hours.

20. What is the ordered daily dose? _____

21. What is the ordered individual dose? _____

22. Does the dose ordered meet the recommended dosage guidelines? _____

A 6 pound 8 ounce infant has an order for Vancomycin IV. The recommended dosage is 10 milligrams per kilogram every 12 hours for the first week of life.

23. What is the weight in kilograms? _____

24. What is the daily dose? _____

25. What is the individual dose? _____

Answer Key for Practice Exams 1–14

UNIT 1 Practice Exam Answer Key

1. 1,032
2. 3,985
3. 65 to 84 or 19
4. 912
5. 1,434
6. 1,096
7. 991
8. 946
9. 1:22 P.M.
10. $8 \times 37 = \$296.00$
11. 75 inches
12. 504
13. 6,210

14. 116 R 4
15. 418 R 8
16. 75 R 7
17. 75
18. 16
19. 84%
20. 12,890
21. $<$
22. $19\dfrac{1}{2}$
23. $4,596 \div 2 = 2,298$
24. Answers will vary. Example: $7 > 5$
25. $2^4 \times 5$

UNIT 2 Practice Exam Answer Key

1. 9
2. $\dfrac{1}{43}$
3. $\dfrac{51}{4}$
4. $26\dfrac{1}{9}$
5. $1\dfrac{7}{40}$
6. $18\dfrac{1}{6}$
7. $23\dfrac{44}{45}$
8. $27\dfrac{1}{21}$
9. $675\dfrac{8}{11}$
10. $24\dfrac{7}{12}$
11. $\dfrac{15}{56}$
12. $4\dfrac{2}{3}$

13. $18\dfrac{1}{12}$
14. 51 doses
15. $1\dfrac{1}{14}$
16. $\dfrac{57}{80}$
17. 12 grains
18. 95°F
19. 20°C
20. $2\dfrac{4}{5}$
21. $\dfrac{3}{100}$
22. $\dfrac{4}{9}, \dfrac{17}{36}, \dfrac{1}{2}, \dfrac{3}{4}$
23. $3\dfrac{1}{5}$
24. $\dfrac{9}{80}$
25. 20 minutes

UNIT 3 Practice Exam Answer Key

1. 0.07
2. Seventeen and five-thousandths
3. 25.08
4. 10.7
5. 12.51

6. 37.759
7. 49 milliliters
8. 7.028
9. 0.893
10. 9.8 kilograms

11. 1.3708
12. 1223.1
13. 2.7
14. 14.78
15. $2\dfrac{17}{20}$
16. 0.875
17. 36.9

18. 57.2
19. 112.5
20. 0.5 degrees
21. 5 ounces
22. $20.02
23. 69 gallons
24. $58.80
25. 11.2 grams

UNIT 4 Practice Exam Answer Key

1. 8 : 15
2. No
3. 72
4. $3\dfrac{1}{2}$ or 3.5
5. 2,952
6. 49
7. 45
8. $\dfrac{1}{4}$
9. $2.80
10. $196.50
11. $0.14
12. $218.75
13. 49 : 32

14. 45 : 1
15. 0.2
16. 7 sets
17. $5\dfrac{2}{3}$
18. 44.5
19. 107.8
20. $8\dfrac{1}{3}$
21. 780 milliliters
22. 5 cans
23. 405 calories
24. 6.25 grams
25. 7.5 grams

UNIT 5 Practice Exam Answer Key

1. 325%
2. 62.5%
3. 45300%
4. 40%
5. 420%
6. $0.53\dfrac{1}{3}\%$
7. 0.45
8. 0.0525 or $0.05\dfrac{1}{4}$
9. $\dfrac{3}{400}$
10. 27.96
11. 140
12. 90

13. 17.5
14. 115.2
15. 15.2
16. 300
17. 0.306
18. 4 g : 25 mL
19. 27 g : 2500 mL
20. 3 g : 125 mL
21. $6.66\dfrac{2}{3}\%$
22. 29.75 mL
23. $110.40
24. 1 g : 16 mL
25. 9 g : 100 mL

UNIT 6 Practice Exam Answer Key

1. 0.01
2. 1 : 100
3. 1%
4. $\dfrac{2}{25}$

5. 2 : 25
6. 8%
7. $\dfrac{2}{5}$

8. 0.4

9. 40%

10. $\dfrac{21}{400}$

11. 0.0525

12. 21 : 400

13. $\dfrac{1}{10}$

14. 1 : 10

15. 10%

16. $4\dfrac{1}{3}$ tablespoons

17. 18.8 inches

18. 114

19. 47.5

20. 384 ounces

21. 31.8 kilograms

22. 39

23. 6

24. 6.8

25. 6

UNIT 7 Practice Exam Answer Key

1. −30

2. +6

3. −68, −19, 9, 53

4. −34, 0, 12, 50

5. 26

6. 132

7. −5

8. −60

9. −4

10. 100

11. −2

12. 25

13. 19

14. −3

15. 7

16. 9

17. 4

18. 324

19. 37

20. 300

21. 59

22. 15

23. 8

24. 16

25. 13

UNIT 8 Practice Exam Answer Key

1. 100

2. 1000000

3. 1000

4. Mass

5. Volume

6. c

7. c

8. 0.06 mL

9. 0.2 mg

10. 93 mg

11. 0.12 kg

12. 2760

13. 250

14. 0.1208

15. 0.0047

16. 0.095

17. 12000

18. 0.00905

19. 0.01

20. 5.4

21. 500000

22. 1.2

23. 0.0238

24. 33700

25. 3.09 kg

UNIT 9 Practice Exam Answer Key

1. 175 mL

2. Generic name   penicillin G procaine

 Trade name   Not shown

 Manufacturer   PL Pharmaceuticals

 National Drug Code (NDC) number   0781-8153-94

 Lot number (control number)   Not shown

 Drug form   Liquid

 Dosage strength   Not shown

 Usual adult dose   Not shown

 Total amount in vial, packet, box   5 million units

 Prescription warning   Rx only

 Expiration date   Not shown

3. Generic name   lansoprazole

 Trade name   Not shown

 Manufacturer   PL Pharmaceuticals

 National Drug Code (NDC) number   03396 48911

 Lot number (control number)   LN 123456

 Drug form   Capsules

 Dosage strength   30 mg

 Usual adult dose   See drug insert

 Total amount in vial, packet, box   90 capsules

 Prescription warning   Rx only

 Expiration date   02/04/14

4.

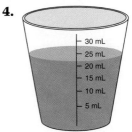

5.

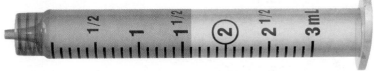

UNIT 10 Practice Exam Answer Key

1. 40

2. 12000

3. 3000 or 3250

4. 120

5. 3 or 3.25

6. 54

7. 270

8. 36

9. 0.1

10. 5

11. 600

12. 180

13. $4\frac{4}{5}$ if working from liter to pint conversion; 5 pints if using pint to cup conversion.

14. $1\frac{3}{5}$

15. 71.25

16. 111.36

17. 240

18. 37.5 mL

19. 14 tablespoons

20. grain $\frac{3}{4}$

21. fluid ounces 80

22. $3\frac{1}{2}$ tablespoons

23. 195

24. grains 50

25. 800 mL

UNIT 11 Practice Exam Answer Key

1. 3 tablets

2. $\frac{1}{2}$ tablet

3. $\frac{1}{2}$ tablet

4. 2 tablets

5. 10 mL

6. 2 tablets

7. $2\frac{1}{2}$ tablets

8. 10 mL

9. 2 teaspoons

10. 2 tablets

11. 1 tablet

12. 3 tablets twice a day

13. 2 tablets

14. 9 mL

15. 2 tablets

16. 3 tablets

17. 3 mL

18. 7.5 mL

19. 5 mL

20. $2\frac{1}{2}$ teaspoons

21. 1.6 mL

22. $\frac{1}{2}$ tablet

23. 2 tablets

24. 3 mL

25. 2 tablets

UNIT 12 Practice Exam Answer Key

1. 20 mL

2. 0.125 mL or 0.13 mL

3. 1.67 mL

4. 0.5 mL

5. 0.8 mL

6. 5 mL

7. 4 mL

8. 1.75 mL

9. 0.67 mL

10. 0.6 mL

11. 0.5 mL

12. 2.5 mL

13. 2.5 mL

14. 1.5 mL

15. 3.5 mL

16. 1 mL

17. 1 mL

18. 2 mL

19. 0.95 mL

20. 10 mL

21. 12.5 mL

22. Tablespoons or teaspoons; 1 tablespoon or 3 teaspoons

23. 2.5 mL

24. 0.6 mL

25. 0.6 mL

UNIT 13 Practice Exam Answer Key

1. 11
2. 16
3. 125
4. 54
5. 83
6. 28
7. 21
8. 10 mL/hr
9. 138 mL/hr
10. 5 gtts/min
11. 56
12. 75
13. 83

14. 69
15. 92
16. 167
17. 664 mL
18. 1800 mL
19. 756 mL
20. 450 mL
21. 332 mL
22. 25 hours
23. 6 hours 52 minutes
24. 12 hours 3 minutes
25. 8 hours 8 minutes

UNIT 14 Practice Exam Answer Key

1. 5.63 kg
2. 24.55 kg
3. 15.85 kg
4. 10.34 kg
5. 46.65 kg
6. 6.14 kg
7. 21.88 mg
8. 7.29 mg
9. No, consult physician
10. 24.12 mg
11. 6.03 mg
12. Yes
13. 7.5 mcg
14. 2.5 mcg
15. No, consult physician

16. No
17. 1125 mg/day mg/day
   $= 375$ mg/8 hours $\times$ 24 hours/day
   $= 1125$ mg/day
18. 375 mg/dose
19. No, the recommended dose is 1022.5 mg a day; the doctor's order is 1125 mg, so the ordered dosage is too high.
20. 500 mg
21. 227.5 mg
22. No, consult physician
23. 2.95 kg
24. 59 mg per day
25. 29.5 mg every 12 hours

APPENDIX C: ANSWER KEY FOR STUDENT WORK TEXT

Answers to the odd numbered questions are provided here. Answers to all problems appear in the *Instructor's Resource Manual*.

◆◆◆◆ UNIT 1
Whole Number Review

Pre-Test: pp. 1–2

1. $48 + \underline{\hspace{1cm}} + 123 = 188$ becomes $188 - 123 = 65$, then $65 - 48 = 17$
2. $2,008 - 199 = 1,809$
3. $49 \times 127 = 6,223$
4. $1,530 \div 6 = 255$
5. Draw a factor tree for 324.

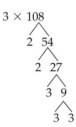

3×108

(factors trees may vary) Thus the prime factorization is $2^2 \times 3^4$

6. Round 15,875 to the nearest tens place.
   15,880
7. Round 2,893 to the nearest hundreds.
   2,900
8. Sally is a dental assistant who works a variable schedule. During the month of December, she has averaged the following weekly total hours of work: 28 hours, 32 hours, 24 hours, and 40 hours. What is the mean or the average number of hours she has worked each week during the month of December?
   31 hrs/week
9. Find the median for the chemistry data set:
   12, 37, 15, 19, 20, 42, 18, 6, 10
   Order: 6, 10, 12, 15, 18, 19, 20, 37, 42
   Then strike out 1 for 1 from each end.
   Order: 6, ~~10~~, ~~12~~, ~~15~~, 18, ~~19~~, ~~20~~, ~~37~~, ~~42~~
10. 18, 28, 47, 98, 81, 83, 87, 31, 38, 56, 76, 69.
    Subtract smallest from the largest number.
    $98 - 18 = 80$
11. $28 = $ xxviii
12. 12:23 P.M. → 1223
13. 108,273. Eight is in the thousands place $= 8,000$
14. $192 - 89 = 103$ hours
15. $13 + 3 = 16$ lost, then $198 - 16 + 7 = 189$ lbs

Practice 1: p. 3

1–10. Answers will vary: Some may be to measure medication, to weigh a patient, to count tablets, etc. Accept any reasonable answer.

Practice 2: pp. 3–4

Students circle any whole number.

Practice 3: p. 5

1. $>$
3. $>$
5. $\geq >$

7. $>$
9. $>$
11. $\leq$

Practice 4: p. 6

1–5. Answers will vary.

Practice 5: p. 6

1. 34
3. 1,494
5. 2,063

7. 488
9. 2,664

Practice 6: p. 7

1. a. 266
   b. 711
   c. 1,176
   d. 20 boxes
3. a. 300
   b. 720
   c. 75
   d. 110
   e. 1,205

Practice 7: pp. 8–9

1. 257
3. 432
5. 437

7. 1,873
9. 4,212

Practice 8: p. 9

1. 1,474

3. 3 boxes

Practice 9: p. 10

1. 464
3. 23,508
5. 99,960

7. 12,288
9. 92,656
11. 4,152

Practice 10: p. 10
1. $3,444.00
3. $525.00

Practice 11: p. 12
1. $2^2 \cdot 31$
3. $2^2 \cdot 23$

Practice 12: p. 13
1. $46\overline{)3,358}$
3. $17\overline{)49}$
5. $8\overline{)2044}$

Practice 13: p. 14
1. 116 R 4 or 116.5
3. 3,086 R 1 or 3,086.25
5. 907 R 2 or 907.3
7. 1,576 R 8 or 1,576.53…
9. 23,441
11. 12,506 R 1 or 12,506.14…

Practice 14: p. 14
1. 9 days
3. $23
5. $1,656.00
7. 9 grams

Practice 15: p. 15
1. 58
3. 18
5. 13

Practice 16: p. 15
1. 35
3. 612
5. 35

Practice 17: p. 15
1. 156
3. 58
5. 75

Practice 18: p. 16
1. 231
3. 3
5. 18

Practice 19: p. 17
1. a. 5,220
   b. 790
   c. 7,610
   d. 1,930
   e. 15,930
   f. 100
3. a. 8,000
   b. 15,000
   c. 7,000
   d. 13,000
   e. 433,000
   f. 3,000

Practice 20: p. 18
1. a. $209
   b. $581
   c. $112
   d. $2,914

Practice 21: p. 19
1. $9
3. 5
5. 7

Practice 22: pp. 20–21
1. 99
3. 26
5. 9

Practice 23: pp. 21–22
1. 14
3. #24
5. 6 & 7

Practice 24: p. 22
1. (100 − 12) or 88
3. (480 − 90) or 390
5. (99 − 12) or 87

Practice 25: p. 24
1. 13
3. 31
5. 26
7. xii
9. iss

Practice 26: p. 24
1. $9\frac{1}{2}$
3. 9
5. 99
7. xxxix
9. CCXL

Practice 27: p. 25
1. 24
3. 504
5. 39
7. 404
9. $592\frac{1}{2}$

Practice 28: p. 25
1. xxivss
5. M
7. LD
9. xvii

Practice 29: pp. 25–26
1. 91
3. 18
5. xxviii
7. CCI
9. LXVI
11. XLV
13. CCCLXII
15. IC
17. 78
19. MMDXV

Practice 30: p. 27

1. 0131
3. 0824
5. 1245

7. 1757
9. 2125

Practice 31: p. 27

1. 2:08 P.M.
3. 10:01 A.M.
5. 12:37 A.M.

7. 3:24 P.M.
9. 9:12 A.M.

Critical Thinking with Whole Numbers: pp. 28–29

1. +, −
2. ×, ÷
3. +, +, −
4. ×, −, +
5. ÷, ×
6. 14, 20, 15, 15
7. 86, 98, 38, 90
8. 89, 96, 38, 96

9. 13, 15, 5, 13
10. 87, 34, 196, 70
11. movie
12. class of drugs
13. True
14. False
15. True, this is a divisibility question.

Whole Number Post-Test: pp. 29–30

1. 724 + _____ + 48 = 1,621 becomes 1,621 − 724 − 48 = 849
2. 13 × 3 = 39 and 10 × 9 = 90 and 24 × 3 = 72 and 31 × 2 = 62. Then add 39 + 90 + 72 + 62 = 263.00, 263 dollars or $263.00
3. 263 ÷ 39 = $6.74 or $7.00
4. 432 − 184 = 248 hours
5. 16 × 3 = 48 patients and 48 ÷ 3 = 16
6. 2 × 21 = 42 + 1 × 8 = 50
7. 2 + 4 + 5 + 2 + 1 + 3 = 17
8.

	Quantity	Unit	Item	Per Unit Cost (in dollars)	Total Cost
a.	1,500	each	toothbrush	1	1,500
b.	100	each	floss (smooth)	2	200
c.	75	each	floss (glide)	2	150
d.	1,000	per 100	information booklet	10	100
e.	25	each	poster	15	375
f.				Subtotal	$2,325.00

9. 2,898 ÷ 3 = $966.00
10. 12,674 − 6,894 = 5,780
11. 16 × 7 = 112. Think 112 is closer to 110 than to 120; thus 110 is the answer.
12. 36 × 14 = $504
13. seventy thousands or 70,000
14. 10:37 + 12:00 = 2237
15. $10 + 9 + \frac{1}{2} = 19\frac{1}{2}$

◆◆◆◆ UNIT 2

Fractions

Pre-test: pp. 31–32

1. $\frac{4}{30} = \frac{2 \times 2}{2 \times 15} = \frac{2}{15}$

2. $4\frac{1}{4} + 2\frac{3}{5} = 4\frac{5}{20} + 2\frac{12}{20} = 6\frac{17}{20}$

3. $42 - 13\frac{1}{6} = 28\frac{5}{6}$

4. $3\frac{1}{2} \times 2\frac{1}{5} = \frac{7}{2} \times \frac{11}{5} = \frac{77}{10} = 7\frac{7}{10}$

5. $3\frac{1}{3} \div 5 = \frac{10}{3} \div \frac{5}{1} = \frac{10}{3} \times \frac{1}{5} = \frac{10}{15} = \frac{2 \times 5}{3 \times 5} = \frac{2}{3}$

6. $50°C \times \frac{9}{5} = 10 \times \frac{9}{1} = 90 + 32 = 122°F$

7. $\frac{7}{8}, \frac{1}{8}, \frac{3}{4}, \frac{15}{16} \rightarrow \frac{14}{16}, \frac{2}{16}, \frac{12}{16}, \frac{15}{16} \rightarrow$ order: $\frac{15}{16}, \frac{7}{8}, \frac{3}{4}, \frac{1}{8}$

8. $\frac{\frac{1}{3}}{\frac{1}{4}} \times 7 = \frac{1}{3} \div \frac{1}{4} \rightarrow \frac{1}{3} \times \frac{4}{1} = \frac{4}{3} \times \frac{7}{1} = \frac{28}{3} = 9\frac{1}{3}$

9. $\frac{\frac{1}{4}}{200} = \frac{1}{4} \div \frac{200}{1} \rightarrow \frac{1}{4} \times \frac{1}{200} = \frac{1}{800}$

10. A one-half tablet is 45 mg, which is <u>less</u> than 50 mg.

11. $14\frac{22}{66} \rightarrow 14\frac{22}{66} = 14\frac{22 \times 1}{22 \times 3} = 14\frac{1}{3}$

12. $7\frac{5}{12} \rightarrow 7 \times 12 + 5 = \frac{89}{12}$

13. 200 mg per 5 mL = $\frac{200\text{ mg}}{5\text{ mL}}$ or $\frac{40\text{ mg}}{1\text{ mL}}$

14. Think: 3,250 dollars = $\frac{1}{12}$. So 3,250 × 12 =

15. $\frac{4}{11} \times \frac{\cancel{16}}{48(12)} \times \frac{44(4)}{48(3)}$ Then this becomes $\frac{1}{1} \times \frac{1}{\cancel{12}(3)} \times \frac{4}{3}$ to become $\frac{1}{1} \times \frac{1}{3} \times \frac{1}{3} = \frac{1}{9}$

Practice 1: pp. 33–34

1. Seven parts to eight total parts
3. Three parts to five total parts

Practice 2: p. 35

1. 6
3. 8
5. 15

7. 36
9. 54

Practice 3: pp. 36–37

1. $\frac{1}{4}$
3. $\frac{1}{2}$
5. $\frac{1}{4}$

7. $\frac{1}{2}$
9. $\frac{1}{3}$

Practice 4: p. 37

1. $14\frac{1}{2}$
3. $4\frac{1}{6}$
5. $3\frac{1}{4}$

7. $2\frac{1}{9}$
9. $6\frac{1}{2}$

Practice 5: p. 38

1. $\frac{25}{43}$
3. $\frac{1}{4}$

5. $\frac{1}{8}$

Practice 6: p. 39

1. $8\frac{1}{3}$
3. $5\frac{4}{5}$

5. $9\frac{3}{7}$
7. $2\frac{3}{8}$
9. 1

Practice 7: pp. 40–41

1. $\frac{5}{6}$
3. $1\frac{3}{10}$
5. $\frac{7}{12}$
7. $\frac{7}{13}$

9. $22\frac{5}{6}$
11. $\frac{4}{5}$
13. 1
15. $140\frac{1}{4}$

Practice 8: p. 42

1. 20
3. 44
5. 25

7. 200
9. 27

Practice 9: pp. 42–43

1. $\frac{17}{20}$
3. $1\frac{1}{9}$
5. $\frac{1}{2}$
7. $\frac{13}{21}$

9. $1\frac{1}{15}$
11. $1\frac{2}{5}$
13. $106\frac{8}{9}$
15. $8\frac{7}{8}$

Practice 10: p. 44

1. 20
3. 96
5. 45

7. 36
9. 30

Practice 11: pp. 44–45

1. $9\frac{11}{12}$
3. $13\frac{1}{2}$
5. $6\frac{5}{7}$
7. $18\frac{29}{30}$
9. $18\frac{9}{10}$

11. $16\frac{17}{27}$
13. $39\frac{5}{12}$
15. $13\frac{7}{15}$
17. $4\frac{7}{16}$
19. $5\frac{1}{2}$

Practice 12: p. 45

1. $121\frac{3}{4}$
3. $1\frac{3}{16}$

5. $3\frac{5}{6}$

Practice 13: p. 46

1. $\frac{4}{12}, \frac{1}{4}, \frac{2}{9}$
3. $\frac{20}{50}, \frac{33}{100}, \frac{6}{25}$

Practice 14: pp. 47–48

1. $\frac{1}{9}$
3. $\frac{2}{11}$
5. $2\frac{1}{6}$
7. $45\frac{1}{8}$
9. $\frac{1}{2}$

11. $\frac{1}{4}$
13. $12\frac{1}{5}$
15. $31\frac{1}{9}$
17. $124\frac{1}{12}$
19. $12\frac{5}{33}$

Practice 15: p. 49

1. $10\frac{1}{6}$
3. $9\frac{3}{4}$
5. $14\frac{6}{13}$

7. $5\frac{6}{7}$
9. $10\frac{2}{5}$

Practice 16: p. 49–51

1. $7\frac{13}{20}$
3. $19\frac{17}{30}$
5. $5\frac{17}{22}$
7. $111\frac{23}{30}$

9. $31\frac{5}{8}$
11. $16\frac{5}{6}$
13. $76\frac{25}{36}$
15. $6\frac{1}{2}$

17. $13\frac{4}{7}$

19. $9\frac{8}{9}$

21. $4\frac{23}{30}$

23. $190\frac{7}{8}$

25. $44\frac{1}{16}$

Practice 17: p. 51

1. $11\frac{1}{2}$

3. $99\frac{1}{4}$

5. $3\frac{1}{2}$

Practice 18: p. 52

1. $\frac{1}{16}$

3. $\frac{28}{45}$

5. $\frac{3}{35}$

7. $\frac{4}{9}$

9. $\frac{13}{66}$

Practice 19: p. 53

1. $1\frac{1}{2}$

3. $16\frac{1}{3}$

5. $5\frac{3}{5}$

7. $11\frac{2}{3}$

9. 4

Practice 20: pp. 54–55

1. $1\frac{5}{7}$

3. $\frac{1}{4}$

5. $\frac{1}{20}$

7. $\frac{1}{4}$

9. $\frac{11}{96}$

11. $\frac{1}{24}$

Practice 21: p. 56

1. $\frac{33}{4}$

3. $\frac{88}{5}$

5. $\frac{27}{12}$

7. $\frac{32}{9}$

9. $\frac{53}{12}$

Practice 22: p. 57

1. $\frac{29}{84}$

3. $\frac{21}{40}$

5. $\frac{20}{27}$

7. $40\frac{1}{4}$

9. $3\frac{17}{20}$

Practice 23: p. 58

1. 70 doses

3. 875 milligrams

5. $18\frac{3}{4}$ cups

Practice 24: pp. 60–61

1. $\frac{5}{7}$

3. $\frac{7}{24}$

5. 8

7. $\frac{1}{45}$

9. $\frac{1}{120}$

11. $3\frac{8}{9}$

13. $2\frac{7}{9}$

15. $4\frac{8}{9}$

17. $\frac{31}{130}$

19. $1\frac{47}{105}$

Practice 25: p. 61

1. $9\frac{3}{20}$

3. $13.30

5. 10

Practice 26: p. 62

1. 68

3. 77

5. 104

7. 176

Practice 27: p. 63

1. 40

3. 10

5. 15

7. 30

Practice 28: p. 64

1. $\frac{3}{32}$

3. $\frac{1}{15,000}$

5. $1\frac{1}{5}$

7. $\frac{4}{5}$

9. $\frac{15}{16}$

Practice 29: p. 65

1. 5

3. 12

5. 1

Practice 30: pp. 66–67

1. 14 quarts

3. 124 ounces

5. 100 inches

7. $58\frac{2}{3}$ ounces

9. 162 inches

Practice 31: pp. 67–68

1. $3\frac{3}{4}$ per employee and $101\frac{1}{4}$ hours total

3. $235\frac{5}{8}$

5. 180

Critical Thinking with Fractions: pp. 68–70

1. $2\frac{1}{4}$

2. $7\frac{1}{2}$

3. $1\frac{1}{8}$

4. $3\frac{3}{4}$

5. $6\frac{5}{8}$

6. $8\frac{4}{7}$

7. $32\frac{1}{2}$

8. 11

9. 22

10. $\frac{5}{8}$

11. $\frac{3}{4}$

12. $\frac{5}{8}$

13. $5\frac{1}{3}$ ounces

14. 1 ounce

15. 18 ounces

Fraction Post-Test: pp. 71–72

1. $\frac{6}{24} = \frac{6 \times 1}{6 \times 4} = \frac{1}{4}$

2. $\frac{1}{6} = \frac{2}{12} = \frac{3}{18} = \frac{4}{24}$ and others

3. $\frac{122}{11} = 122 \div 11 = 11\frac{1}{11}$

4. $8\frac{1}{6} + 3\frac{3}{4} = 8\frac{2}{12} + 3\frac{9}{12} = 11\frac{11}{12}$

5. $52 - 12\frac{1}{5} = 51\frac{5}{5} + 12\frac{1}{5} = 39\frac{4}{5}$

6. $14\frac{1}{2} \times 2\frac{1}{8} = 14 \times 2 + 1 = \frac{29}{2}$ and

   $2 \times 8 + 1 = \frac{17}{8}$ Then $\frac{29}{2} \times \frac{17}{8} = \frac{493}{16}$, which

   reduces to $30\frac{13}{16}$.

7. $5\frac{2}{6} \div 12 = \frac{5 \times 6 + 2}{6} \div \frac{12}{1} = \frac{32}{6} \times \frac{1}{12} = \frac{32}{72}$

   $= \frac{8 \times 4}{8 \times 9} = \frac{4}{9}$

8. $77°F = $ _____ $°C \rightarrow 77 - 32 = 45 \times \frac{5}{9}$

   $= 45^5 \times \frac{5}{9} = 25°C$

9. $\frac{3}{8}, \frac{1}{3}, \frac{1}{4}, \frac{2}{12} \rightarrow \frac{9}{24}, \frac{8}{24}, \frac{6}{24}, \frac{4}{24} \rightarrow \frac{2}{12}, \frac{1}{4}, \frac{1}{3}, \frac{3}{8}$

10. $\frac{1}{4} \div \frac{1}{8} \rightarrow \frac{1}{4} \times \frac{8}{1} = \frac{8}{4} \rightarrow 2 \times 25 = 50$

11. Get a common denominator and compare:

    $\frac{1}{8} = \frac{3}{24}$ and $\frac{1}{6} = \frac{4}{24}$ The nurse will give less

    than the dose on hand.

12. $\frac{20}{60}$ reduces to $\frac{1}{3}$ of an hour.

13. $\frac{5}{8}$ becomes $\frac{15}{24}$

14. $\frac{10}{16}$ reduces to $\frac{5}{8}$

15. $7\frac{1}{3} + 6\frac{1}{2} + 6\frac{1}{2} + 5\frac{7}{8} = 7\frac{8}{24} + 6\frac{2}{24} + 6\frac{2}{24} + 5\frac{21}{24}$

    $= 26\frac{5}{24}$

◆◆◆◆ UNIT 3
Decimals

Pre-Test: pp. 73–74

1. 3.87 = three and eighty-seven hundredths

2. 32.575 → 32.5$\underline{7}$5. Notice that 5 is to the right of 7, so the answer rounds to 32.58.

3. 0.7805

4. 21.0 + 15.8 + 1.4 + 2.0 = 40.2

5. 12.00 − 0.89 = 11.11

6. 32.05 × 7.2 = 230.76

7. 749.7 ÷ 21 = 35.7

8. 32.85 × 10 = 328.5

9. 0.035 → $\frac{35}{1000}$ reduces to $\frac{7}{200}$

10. 108 − 32 = 76; then 76 ÷ 1.8 = 42.2°C

11. 0.08 × 15.2 = 1.2160; then 1.216 ÷ 0.04 = 30.4

12. 4,298.9 ÷ 1,000 = 4.2989

13. 2.2 × 14.8 = 32.56 lbs

14. $\frac{15}{60} = \frac{1}{4}$; then 1 ÷ 4 = 0.25 hours

15. 146.5 = $146\frac{5}{10}$ reduces to $146\frac{1}{2}$

Practice 1: p. 77

1. Fourteen hundredths

3. Eight hundredths

5. One hundred three and eighty-two hundredths

7. One hundred twenty-five and fourteen hundredths

9. Eighteen and eight hundredths

Practice 2: p. 77

1. 0.3

3. 600.012

5. 8.05

Practice 3: p. 78

1. 7.3

3. 1.0

5. 25.0 or 25

7. 0.1

9. 9.9

Practice 4: p. 79

1. 18.36

3. 4.29

5. 0.01

7. 35.71

9. 46.09

Practice 5: p. 80

1. 1.02

3. 4.25

5. 0.0033

Practice 6: p. 80

1. 0.89

3. 0.6

5. 0.675

Practice 7: p. 80

1. 2.5, 2.025, 0.250, 0.025
3. 5.55, 5.15, 5.05, 0.5, 0.05

Practice 8: p. 81

1. 2.6 mL
3. 0.32 mL
5. 9.2 mL

Practice 9: p. 82

1. 19.3
3. 32.3
5. 45.1092
7. 127.52
9. 214.281

Practice 10: p. 83

1. 4.5 milligrams
3. 226 milligrams
5. 124.54 centimeters

Practice 11: pp. 83–84

1. 1.88
3. 24.246
5. 5.55
7. 0.175
9. 87.436

Practice 12: p. 84

1. 0.65 liters
3. 1.5 milligrams
5. 1.8°F

Practice 13: pp. 85–86

1. 37.5
3. 40
5. 122.4
7. 0.8088
9. 0.4726
11. 0.0021
13. 151.11
15. 1.65036
17. 7.632
19. 6,942.53
21. 1,342.11
23. 10.04565

Practice 14: p. 86

1. $420.80
3. $1,618.20
5. $128.00

Practice 15: p. 87

1. 7.392
3. 0.162
5. 0.12
7. 52.4
9. 3.02

Practice 16: p. 88

1. 1,600
3. 801
5. 0.004
7. 30.66
9. 0.2099

Practice 17: p. 89

1. 6.04
3. 5.004
5. 1.04
7. 403.9

Practice 18: p. 90

1. 753
3. 2,280.5
5. 9
7. 45,070
9. 476
11. 13.45
13. 10.09
15. 23,850

Practice 19: p. 91

1. 4.85
3. 25
5. 0.0035
7. 0.254
9. 0.325
11. 10.01
13. 0.03076
15. 0.10275

Practice 20: p. 92

1. $63.25
3. 3 tablets
5. $26.24
7. 1,000
9. $71.60

Practice 21: pp. 93–94

1. $\dfrac{2}{25}$
3. $14\dfrac{1}{5}$
5. $125\dfrac{1}{20}$
7. $9\dfrac{1}{4}$
9. $9\dfrac{3}{10}$
11. $12\dfrac{3}{5}$
13. $98\dfrac{1}{5}$
15. $46\dfrac{1}{2}$

Practice 22: pp. 95–96

1. 0.5
3. 0.875
5. 0.24
7. 0.2
9. $0.83\dfrac{1}{3}$ or 0.833

Practice 23: p. 97

1. 53.6
3. 156.2
5. 8.1
7. 38
9. 53.6

Practice 24: p. 99

1. 2.2
3. 7.5
5. 0.168
7. 7.675

Critical Thinking Skills in Decimals: pp. 99–100

1. 0.249
2. Varies, but examples of possible answers are:

Sums			Differences		
> than 1	= to 1	< than 1	> than 1	= to 1	< than 1
0.9 + 0.4	0.5 + 0.5	0.25 + 0.6	2.1 − 0.8	2.0 − 1.0	1.5 − 0.9

3. Varies, but 60 × 20 = 1,200
4. 3 decimal places
5. 88 milliliters
6. 600 gallons
7. 2 tablets
8. $\dfrac{2}{5}$, 0.5, $\dfrac{2}{3}$, $\dfrac{7}{8}$
9. 7.5 milligrams
10. 5 hours and 24 minutes

11–15.

Item	Cost	Unit Price
Box of 100-count 1 milliliter syringes	$12.75	$0.13
Case of 1,000 latex-free size large gloves	$69.11	$0.07
Pack of 24 Silverlon adhesive strips	$14.25	$0.59
Pack of 200 4 × 4 sterile gauze sponges	$9.86	$0.05

Decimal Post-Test: pp. 101–102

1. $0.065 \rightarrow$ Sixty-five thousandths
2. $19 + 0.25 + 1.70 + 0.80 = 21.75$
3. $29.000 - 0.075 = 28.925$
4. $75 \times 1.8 = 135$
5. $24.02 \div 0.2 = 120.1$
6. $978.735 \rightarrow 978.74$
7. $8.018, 0.81, 0.08, 0.018$
8. $10.009 \times 100 = 1,000.9$
9. $0.5 \times 4 = 2$ milligrams
10. $2.25 \div 0.75 = 3$ tablets
11. $0.125 = \dfrac{125}{1000} = \dfrac{1}{8}$
12. $\dfrac{13}{50} \rightarrow 13 \div 50 = 0.26$
13. Separate the 3 and $\dfrac{5}{8}$. Then $5 \div 8 \rightarrow 3.625$
14. $103 - 32 = 71$. Then $71 \div 1.8 = 39.4°C$
15. $0.136 \times 2.5 = 0.3400$. Then $0.34 \div 0.2 = 1.7$

◆◆◆◆ UNIT 4
Ratio and Proportion

Pre-Test: pp. 103–104

1. $\dfrac{1 \text{ kilogram}}{2.2 \text{ pounds}} = \dfrac{24.5 \text{ kilograms}}{? \text{ pounds}} \rightarrow 2.2 \times 24.5. = 53.9$

2. $\dfrac{48}{46} = \dfrac{?}{124} \rightarrow 124 \times 48 = 5,952.$

   Then $5,952 \div 46 = 93$

3. $\dfrac{1 \text{ cup}}{8 \text{ ounces}} = \dfrac{?}{138 \text{ ounces}} \rightarrow 1 \times 138 = 138.$

   Then $138 \div 8 = 17\dfrac{1}{4}$ cups

4. $\dfrac{1}{8} : 3 = \dfrac{1}{4} : x \rightarrow \dfrac{\frac{1}{8}}{3} = \dfrac{\frac{1}{4}}{?} \rightarrow 3 \times \dfrac{1}{4} = \dfrac{3}{4}.$

   Then $\dfrac{3}{4} \div \dfrac{1}{8}$, which becomes $\dfrac{3}{4} \times \dfrac{8}{1} = \dfrac{24}{4} = 6$

5. $\dfrac{?}{225} = \dfrac{2}{5} \rightarrow 225 \times 2 = 450.$ Then $450 \div 5 = 90$

6. $\dfrac{3}{12}$ reduces to $\dfrac{1}{4}$

7. $\dfrac{73 \text{ beats}}{1 \text{ min}} = \dfrac{?}{5 \text{ min}} \rightarrow 73 \times 5 = 365$ beats

8. First $\dfrac{1 \text{ tablespoon}}{3 \text{ teaspoon}} = \dfrac{2 \text{ tablespoons}}{? \text{ teaspoons}}$

   $= 3 \times 2 = 6$ teaspoons

   Then $\dfrac{1 \text{ sandwich}}{6 \text{ teaspoons}} = \dfrac{49 \text{ sandwich}}{? \text{ teaspoons}}$

   $= 6 \times 49 = 294$ teaspoons

9. Read the label 25 mg/5 mL, which becomes

   $\dfrac{25}{5} = \dfrac{5 \times 5}{5 \times 1} = \dfrac{5}{1}$ or $5 : 1$

10. $\dfrac{2\frac{1}{2}}{6} = \dfrac{?}{15} \rightarrow 2\dfrac{1}{2} \times 15 \rightarrow \dfrac{5}{2} \times \dfrac{15}{1} = \dfrac{75}{2} \div \dfrac{6}{1}.$

    Then $\dfrac{75}{2} \times \dfrac{1}{6} = \dfrac{75}{12} = 6.25$ or $6\dfrac{1}{4}$

11. $\dfrac{4 \text{ ounces}}{1 \text{ patient}} = \dfrac{496 \text{ ounces}}{? \text{ patients}} \rightarrow 1 \times 496 = 496.$

    Then $496 \div 4 = 124$ patients

12. $\dfrac{1 \text{ tube}}{2.5 \text{ mL}} = \dfrac{4 \text{ tubes}}{? \text{ mL}} \rightarrow 2.5 \times 4 = 10$ mL

13. $\dfrac{1 \text{ day}}{62 \text{ gloves}} = \dfrac{5 \text{ days}}{? \text{ gloves}} \rightarrow 62 \times 5 = 310$ gloves

14. $\dfrac{\frac{4}{75}}{15} = \dfrac{x}{20} \rightarrow \dfrac{4}{75} \times 20 = \dfrac{80}{75} \div \dfrac{15}{1} \rightarrow \dfrac{80}{75} \times \dfrac{1}{15}$

    $= \dfrac{80}{1,125}$ reduces to $\dfrac{16}{225}$

15. $\dfrac{1 \text{ min}}{60 \text{ sec}} \times \dfrac{?}{320 \text{ sec}} \rightarrow 320 \div 60$

    $= 5$ minutes 20 seconds

Practice 1: p. 105

1. $6 : 7$
3. $8 : 15$
5. $1 : 2$

Practice 2: p. 106

1. $96 : 13$
3. $30 : 1$
5. $2 : 1$
7. $13 : 21$
9. $5 : 2$

Practice 3: pp. 107–108

1. $10,000 : 1$
3. $1 : 1$
5. $300 : 1$

Practice 4: p. 109

1. $1,394.00 cost/day
3. 8 ounces/cup
5. 39 patients/day

Practice 5: p. 110

1. No
3. Yes
5. No

Practice 6: p. 111

1. 4
3. 135
5. 27
7. 14
9. 52

Practice 7: p. 112

1. 36.1
3. 77
5. 183.7
7. 11.6
9. 98

Practice 8: pp. 114–115

1. $7\frac{2}{3}$
3. 6
5. 9
7. 4
9. 56
11. $2\frac{1}{2}$
13. 5
15. $1\frac{9}{16}$ or $1\frac{1}{2}$
17. 80
19. 5

Practice 9: p. 116

1. 3 caplets
3. 17.5 grams
5. 28 kilograms

Practice 10: p. 118

1. 3.6
3. 16
5. 1
7. $1\frac{1}{3}$
9. 2.4
11. 1.5

Practice 11: pp. 119–120

1. 9
3. 9
5. 48
7. 1,312

Practice 12: p. 120

1. 645
3. 220
5. 121.5

Practice 13: pp. 121–123

1. 840 milliliters
3. 405 calories
5. 42.9 grams
7. 240 calories
9. 40%
11. 11 grams
13. 1,200 milliliters
15. $6\frac{1}{4}$ cups

Critical Thinking with Ratio and Proportion, pp. 123–124

1. 72 mL
3. 2.8 mL
5. 150 calories per serving
7. 72 part-time employees
9. 23 calories
11. 60 mg
13. 150 mL
15. 33 grams

Ratio and Proportion Post-Test: pp. 125–126

1. Answers will vary. A proportion is two equal ratios. Examples could be milligrams to milliliters, pounds to kilograms, fat to protein, etc. Proportions can be used for mixing solutions, converting measurements, and calculating doses.

2. $\dfrac{30}{120} = \dfrac{?}{12} \rightarrow 30 \times 12 = 360.$ Then $360 \div 120 = 3$

3. $\dfrac{1\,\text{glass}}{8\,\text{ounces}} = \dfrac{?\,\text{glasses}}{78\,\text{ounces}} \rightarrow 1 \times 78 = 78.$

   Then $78 \div 8 = 9\frac{3}{4}$, but 9 full glasses

4. $\dfrac{\frac{1}{2}}{4} = \dfrac{\frac{1}{3}}{x} \rightarrow 4 \times \frac{1}{3} = \frac{4}{3} \div \frac{1}{2} \rightarrow \frac{4}{3} \times \frac{2}{1} = \frac{8}{3}$

   reduces to $2\frac{2}{3}$

5. $\dfrac{?}{625} = \dfrac{1}{5} \rightarrow 1 \times 625 = 625.$ Then $625 \div 5 = 125$

6. $\dfrac{10\,\text{milligrams}}{2\,\text{milliliters}} = \dfrac{?\,\text{milligrams}}{28\,\text{milliliters}} \rightarrow 10 \times 28 = 280.$

   Then $280 \div 2 = 140$ milligrams

7. $\dfrac{1\,\text{tablet}}{30\,\text{milligram}} = \dfrac{?\,\text{tablet}}{240\,\text{milligrams}} \rightarrow 1 \times 240 = 240.$

   Then $240 \div 30 = 8$ tablets

8. $\dfrac{100\,\text{micrograms}}{2\,\text{milliliters}} = \dfrac{15\,\text{micrograms}}{?\,\text{milliliters}} \rightarrow 2 \times 15 = 30.$

   Then $30 \div 100 = 0.3$ milliliters

9. $\dfrac{\frac{1}{100}}{6} = \dfrac{?}{8} \rightarrow \frac{1}{100} \times 8 = \frac{8}{100}.$

   Then $\dfrac{8}{100} \div \dfrac{6}{1} = \dfrac{8}{100} \times \dfrac{1}{6} = \dfrac{8}{600}$

   reduces to $\dfrac{1}{75}$

10. $\dfrac{0.04}{0.5} = \dfrac{0.12}{?} \rightarrow 0.5 \times 0.12 = 0.06.$

    Then $0.06 \div 0.04 = 1.5$

11. $\dfrac{1\,\text{min}}{60\,\text{sec}} = \dfrac{?}{130\,\text{sec}} \rightarrow 130 \div 60$

    $= 2$ minutes 10 seconds

12. $\dfrac{4}{6} = \dfrac{?}{120} \rightarrow 4 \times 120 = 480.$

    Then $480 \div 6 = 80$ patients

13. $\dfrac{1\,\text{day}}{128\,\text{covers}} = \dfrac{5\,\text{days}}{?\,\text{covers}} \rightarrow 128 \times 5 = 640.$

    Then $640 \div 1 = 640$ covers

14. $\dfrac{\frac{1}{125}}{3} = \dfrac{?}{12} \to \dfrac{1}{125} \times 12 = \dfrac{12}{125}.$

Then $\dfrac{12}{125} \div \dfrac{3}{1} \to \dfrac{12}{125} \times \dfrac{1}{3} = \dfrac{12}{375}$

reduces to $\dfrac{4}{125}$

15. $\dfrac{6 \text{ ounces} \times 4 \text{ times}}{1 \text{ day}} = \dfrac{? \text{ ounces}}{4 \text{ days}} \to 24 \times 4$

$= 96 \text{ ounces}$

◆◆◆◆▶ UNIT 5

Percents

Pre-Test: pp. 127–128

1. $35\dfrac{1}{4}\% \to 32.25 \div 100 = 0.3525$

2. $\dfrac{32}{100} = \dfrac{?}{140} \to 32 \times 140 = 4,480.$
Then $4,480 \div 100 = 44.80$

3. $\dfrac{1}{8} \to 1 \div 8 = 0.125.$ Then $0.125 \times 100 = 12.5\%$

4. $\dfrac{?}{100} = \dfrac{120}{440} \to 120 \times 100 = 12,000.$
Then $12,000 \div 440 = 27.27$ or 27.3

5. $\dfrac{15}{100} = \dfrac{75}{?} \to 75 \times 100 = 7,500.$
Then $7,500 \div 15 = 500$

6. $35:50 \to \dfrac{35}{50} = \dfrac{?}{100} \to 35 \times 100 = 3,500.$
Then $3,500 \div 50 = 70$

7. $\dfrac{?}{100} = \dfrac{11}{110} \to 11 \times 100 = 1,100 \div 110 = 10$

8. $\dfrac{15}{100} = \dfrac{?}{475} \to 15 \times 475 = 7,125.$
Then $7,125 \div 100 = 71.25.$
Subtract $\$475 - 71.25 = \$403.75$

9. $1\dfrac{1}{4} \to 1.25.$ Then $1.25 \times 100 = 125\%$

10. $2 \to 2 \times 100 = 200\%$

11. $3\dfrac{2}{3}\% \to \dfrac{11}{3} \div 100 = \dfrac{11}{3} \times \dfrac{1}{100} = \dfrac{11}{300}$

12. $\dfrac{?}{100} = \dfrac{1.15}{38} \to 100 \times 1.15 = 115.$
Then $115 \div 38 = 3.02.$ Round to the nearest whole number. So the final answer is $3\%.$

13. $36 - 16 = 20.$
Then $\dfrac{?}{100} = \dfrac{20}{36} \to 100 \times 20 = 2,000 \div 36 = 55.55\%.$

14. $\dfrac{40}{100} = \dfrac{?}{2,200} \to 2,200 \times 40 = 88,000.$
Then $88,000 \div 100 = 880$

15. $\dfrac{1}{6} \to 1 \div 6 = 0.1666.$ Then $0.1666 \times 100 = 16.66$
or 16.67% or $16\dfrac{2}{3}\%$

Practice 1: p. 129

1. 0.65

3. $0.75\dfrac{1}{2}$ or 0.755

5. $0.44\dfrac{1}{2}$ or 0.445

Practice 2: p. 130

1. 37.5%

3. 920%

5. 7.6%

Practice 3: p. 131

1. 0.825

3. 0.41

5. 7.8%

7. $125\dfrac{1}{4}\%$ or 125.25%

9. 0.015

Practice 4: pp. 132–133

1. $\dfrac{75}{100} = \dfrac{x}{200}$

3. $\dfrac{8.5}{100} = \dfrac{x}{224}$

5. $\dfrac{x}{100} = \dfrac{18}{150}$

7. $\dfrac{x}{100} = \dfrac{75}{90}$

9. $\dfrac{50}{100} = \dfrac{75}{x}$

Practice 5 : p. 134

1. 42

3. 20.16%

5. 5.88

7. 22.5%

9. 17.60

Practice 6: p. 135

1. 6.67

3. 30.3

5. 15.63

7. 1,280

9. 533.33

Practice 7: pp. 136–137

1. 20%

3. 23.5%

5. 60%

Practice 8: p. 138

1. 2 grams of pure drug to 25 milliliters of solution

3. 11 grams of pure drug to 200 milliliters of solution

5. 1 gram of pure drug to 20 milliliters of solution

Practice 9: pp. 139–140

1. **a.** 3.75 grams
   b. 5.25 grams
   c. 9.75 grams
   d. 18.75 grams

3. a. 30%

   b. 60 grams

Practice 10: pp. 140–141

1. a. 7.5 grams

   b. 100 milliliters

   c. 3 : 40

   d. 2.7 grams

   e. 6 grams

   f. 4.5 grams

3. a. 78 grams

   b. 100 milliliters

   c. 39 : 50

   d. 51.1 grams

   e. 70.2 grams

   f. 351 grams

Practice 11: p. 142

1. $2.60 $14.70   **7.** $112.68 $137.72

3. $5.74 $40.16   **9.** $63.20 $94.80

5. $88.23 $264.67

Critical Thinking in Percents, pp. 142–144

1. 66.67% or $66\frac{2}{3}$%

2. 10%

3. $266\frac{2}{3}$%

4. $1,732.14

5. $30.00

6. 66%

7. 34%

8. $800

9. 2,250

10. 60%

11. 10%

12. 5%

13. 20%

14. 75.5 pounds

15. 37.5%

Percent Post-Test: pp. 144–145

1. A percent is a part out of a hundred. A 10% discount means that one saves 10 dollars out of each 100 dollars spent. Percent is used in solutions, medical billings, insurance verification, preferred-provider plans, and other applications.

2. a. $0.66\frac{2}{3} \rightarrow 0.66\frac{2}{3} \times 100 = 66\frac{2}{3}$%

   b. $\frac{5}{6} \rightarrow 5 \div 6 = 0.833.$

      Then $0.833 \times 100 = 83.3$% or $83\frac{1}{3}$%

3. $\frac{75}{100} = \frac{?}{325} \rightarrow 75 \times 325 = 24{,}375.$

   Then $24{,}375 \div 100 = 243.75$

4. $\frac{?}{100} = \frac{8}{40} \rightarrow 100 \times 8 = 800.$

   Then $800 \div 40 = 20$

5. $\frac{14}{100} = \frac{28}{?} \rightarrow 100 \times 28 = 2{,}800.$

   Then $2{,}800 \div 14 = 200$

6. $5\frac{1}{2}$% means 5.5 grams of solvent (medication) in 100 milliliters of solution.

7. $\frac{9}{100} = \frac{?}{25} \rightarrow 9 \times 25 = 225.$

   Then $225 \div 100 = 2.25$ grams

8. 12% = 0.12. Then $129.50 \times 0.12 = 15.54.$

   Then $129.50 - 15.54 = \$113.96$

   a. $15.54

   b. $113.96

9. $\frac{?}{100} = \frac{3}{36} \rightarrow 100 \times 3 = 300.$

   Then $300 \div 36 = 8.3$% or $8\frac{1}{3}$%

10. $\frac{15}{100} = \frac{?}{326} \rightarrow 15 \times 326 = 4{,}890.$

   Then $4{,}890 \div 100 = \$48.90$

11. $\frac{?}{100} = \frac{3}{25} \rightarrow 100 \times 3 = 300.$

   Then $300 \div 25 = 12$%

12. $\frac{1}{2}$% of $500 \rightarrow \frac{0.5}{100} = \frac{?}{500} \rightarrow 0.5 \times 500 = 250.$

   Then $250 \div 100 = 2.5$

13. $8 : 125 \rightarrow \frac{8}{125}.$ Then $8 \div 125 = 0.064.$

   Then $0.064 \times 100 = 6.4$%

14. $\frac{3}{4}$% of $20 = \frac{0.75}{100} = \frac{?}{20}$

   So $0.75 \times 20 = 15.$ Then $15 \div 100 = 0.15$

15. $\frac{0.5}{100} = \frac{35}{?} \rightarrow 100 \times 35 = 3{,}500.$

   Then $3{,}500 \div 0.5 = 70{,}000$

◆◆◆◆ **UNIT 6**

Combined Applications

Pre-Test: pp. 146–147

1. $\frac{3}{18} \rightarrow 3 \div 18 = 0.166 \rightarrow 0.17$

2. $1\frac{1}{4}$% $\rightarrow \dfrac{1\frac{1}{4}}{100} \rightarrow \frac{5}{4} \div 100 = \frac{5}{400} = \frac{5 \times 1}{5 \times 80} = 1 : 80$

3. $1.05 \rightarrow 1\frac{5}{100} = \frac{5 \times 1}{5 \times 20} = 1\frac{1}{20}$

4. $2\frac{5}{6} \rightarrow 2 \times 6 + 5 = \frac{17}{6} \rightarrow 17 : 6$

5. $23\frac{3}{4} \rightarrow 3 \div 4 = 0.75$ becomes 23.75

6. $16 : 300 \rightarrow \frac{16}{300} \rightarrow 16 \div 300 = 0.0533.$

   Then $0.0533 \times 100 = 5.3$%

7. $12.325 \times 100 = 1232.5\%$

8. Think: $7\frac{1}{4} = 7.25 \rightarrow \dfrac{1 \text{ cup}}{8 \text{ ounces}} = \dfrac{7.25 \text{ cups}}{? \text{ ounces}}$.

Then $8 \times 7.25 = 58$ ounces

9. $13\frac{1}{2} = 13.5 \rightarrow \dfrac{1 \text{ ounce}}{2 \text{ tablespoons}} = \dfrac{?}{13.5 \text{ tablespoons}}$

$\rightarrow 1 \times 13.5 = 13.5$.

Then $13.5 \div 2 = 6.75$ ounces or $6\frac{3}{4}$ ounces

10. $2\frac{1}{4} \rightarrow 2.25$ Think:

$\dfrac{1 \text{ inch}}{2.54 \text{ cm}} = \dfrac{12 \text{ inches}}{?} \rightarrow 2.54 \times 12 = 30.48$ cm

Then $\dfrac{1 \text{ ft}}{30.48 \text{ cm}} = \dfrac{2.25}{?}$.

Then $30.48 \times 2.25 = 68.58$ cm

11. $\dfrac{1 \text{ hour}}{60 \text{ minutes}} = \dfrac{5.5}{?} \rightarrow 60 \times 5.5 = 330$ minutes

12. $11\frac{1}{4} \rightarrow 11.25 \rightarrow \dfrac{1 \text{ quart}}{4 \text{ cups}} = \dfrac{11.25}{?} \rightarrow 4 \times 11.25$

$= 45$ cups

13. $\dfrac{1 \text{ teaspoon}}{60 \text{ drops}} = \dfrac{8.5 \text{ teaspoons}}{?} \rightarrow 60 \times 8.5$

$= 510$ drops

14. Think: $9\frac{1}{2}\%$ means 9.5%, which as a decimal becomes 0.095. Then $0.095 \times 0.67 = 0.06365$, which rounds to 0.06.

15. $\dfrac{\frac{1}{2}\%}{5} \rightarrow \dfrac{\frac{1}{2}}{100} \rightarrow \dfrac{1}{2} \div 100 \rightarrow \dfrac{1}{2} \times \dfrac{1}{100} = \dfrac{1}{200} \div 5$

$\rightarrow \dfrac{1}{200} \times \dfrac{1}{5} = \dfrac{1}{1,000}$

Practice 1: p. 151

	Fraction	Decimal	Ratio	Percent
1.	$\frac{5}{8}$	0.625	5 : 8	62.5% or $62\frac{1}{2}\%$
3.	$\frac{1}{4}$	0.25	1 : 4	25%
5.	$\frac{1}{250}$	0.004	1 : 250	0.4%
7.	$\frac{3}{50}$	0.06	3 : 50	6%
9.	$\frac{1}{10}$	0.1	1 : 10	10%
11.	$1\frac{9}{25}$	1.36	34 : 25	136%
13.	$\frac{2}{5}$	0.4	2 : 5	40%
15.	$\frac{16}{25}$	0.64	16 : 25	64%

	Fraction	Decimal	Ratio	Percent
17.	$\frac{5}{6}$	$0.83\frac{1}{3}$	5 : 6	$83\frac{1}{3}\%$
19.	$\frac{1}{100}$	0.01	1 : 100	1%

Practice 2: pp. 152–153

1. Foot
3. Ounce
5. Pound
7. Quart
9. Drop

Practice 3: pp. 154–155

1. 3
3. 35.05
5. 3
7. 24
9. $2\frac{1}{2}$

Practice 4: pp. 156–157

1. 3
3. 36
5. 32
7. 149.6
9. 4
11. 6
13. $\frac{7}{8}$
15. 168
17. 40
19. $73\frac{1}{2}$

Practice 5: p. 157

1. 3
3. $\frac{1}{12}$
5. $\frac{1}{30}$

Practice 6: p. 158

	Fraction	Decimal	Ratio	Percent
1.	$\frac{1}{8}$	0.125	1 : 8	$12\frac{1}{2}\%$
3.	$\frac{13}{20}$	0.65	13 : 20	65%
5.	$\frac{2}{5}$	0.40	2 : 5	40%
7.	$\frac{2}{25}$	0.08	2 : 25	8%
9.	$\frac{3}{5}$	0.6	3 : 5	60%
11.	$1\frac{5}{8}$	1.625	13 : 8	162.5%
13.	$\frac{11}{50}$	0.22	11 : 50	22%
15.	$\frac{3}{25}$	0.12	3 : 25	12%
17.	$\frac{1}{6}$	$0.16\frac{2}{3}$	1 : 6	$16\frac{2}{3}\%$
19.	$\frac{1}{25}$	0.04	1 : 25	4%

Critical Thinking in Combined Applications: pp. 159–160

1. A <u>ratio</u> because it expresses a part-to-whole relationship.

2. 44.44%

3. $\dfrac{49}{300}$

4. 6

5. 32 : 225

6. 0.003

7. 0.5%

8. $\dfrac{3}{8}$

9. 1 : 200

10. 28.57%

11. $16\dfrac{2}{3}\%$

12. 48

13. 0.083%

14. Yes

15. No

Combined Application Post-Test: pp. 160–161

1. $5 \div 25 = 0.2$

2. $\dfrac{1}{4}\% = \dfrac{1}{4} \div 100 \rightarrow \dfrac{1}{4} \times \dfrac{1}{100}$, which is 1 : 400

3. $4.05 = 4\dfrac{5}{100}$, which is reduced to $4\dfrac{1}{20}$

4. $4\dfrac{1}{8}$ becomes $4 \times 8 + 1 = \dfrac{33}{8}$, which is 33 : 8

5. $27\dfrac{1}{4} \rightarrow$ Divide 1 by 4 to get 0.25. Then 27.25

6. $\dfrac{12}{200} \rightarrow$ Divide 12 by 200 to get 0.06.

   Then $0.06 \times 100 = 6\%$

7. $14\dfrac{25}{100}\% = 14\dfrac{1}{4}\%$, which is $14 \times 4 + 1 = \dfrac{57}{4}$.

   Then $\dfrac{57}{4} \div 100 = \dfrac{57}{4} \times \dfrac{1}{100} = \dfrac{57}{400} \rightarrow 57 : 400$

8. $\dfrac{1 \text{ cup}}{8 \text{ ounces}} = \dfrac{3.25 \text{ cups}}{?} \rightarrow 8 \times 3.25 = 26$

9. $\dfrac{1 \text{ ounce}}{2 \text{ tablespoons}} = \dfrac{12 \text{ ounces}}{?} \rightarrow 2 \times 12 = 24$

10. 106.68, which is 106.7 rounded to the nearest tenth.

11. 1,080

12. $\dfrac{1 \text{ quart}}{4 \text{ cups}} = \dfrac{4 \text{ quarts}}{?} \rightarrow 4 \times 4 = 16$ cups

13. Think: 1 tablespoon equals 3 teaspoons, so that equals 60 drops $\times$ 3 = 180 drops per tablespoon.

    $\dfrac{1 \text{ tablespoon}}{180 \text{ drops}} = \dfrac{2\frac{1}{3}}{?} \rightarrow$ Then $180 \times \dfrac{7}{3}$

    $= 420$ drops

14. $\dfrac{12}{100} \times 0.67 \rightarrow 12 \times 0.67 = 8.04$.

    Then $8.04 \div 100 = 0.0804$ rounded to 0.08

15. $\dfrac{15}{100} \div \dfrac{1}{2} \rightarrow \dfrac{15}{100} \times \dfrac{2}{1} = \dfrac{30}{100}$

    Reduced to 0.3 or $\dfrac{3}{10}$

◆◆◆◆ UNIT 7
Pre-Algebra Basics

Pre-Test: pp. 162–163

1. $-14 + 24 = 10$

2. $-25 - 12 = -25 + -12 = -37$

3. $3 + (2 \times 20) - 15 \div 3 = 2 \times 20 = 40$ and $15 \div 3 = 5$.
   Then $3 + 40 - 5 = 43 - 5 = 38$

4. $15 - 50 \div 5 + 13 = 50 \div 5 = 10$.
   Then $15 - 10 = 5 + 13 = 18$

5. $5^3 + 7^0 = 5 \times 5 \times 5 + 1 = 126$

6. $6^2 \times 2^3 = 6 \times 6 \times 2 \times 2 \times 2 = 36 \times 8 = 288$

7. $\sqrt{144} = 12 \times 12 = 12$ as the square root

8. $\sqrt{64} \times 2 = 8 \times 2 = 16$

9. $|-13|$ is 13

10. $20 - 4 \times 3 + 12 \div 2 = 20 - 12 + 6 = 14$

11. The coefficient of $4xf$ is 4. This is the number placed next to the variables xf.

12. Write the expression: the product of some number x and 12. $x(12)$

13. $5 \times 5 \times 5 \times 5 \times 5$ can also be written as 5^5.

14. Maria made $250.00 more than her sister. Their incomes combined equal $57,000.00. So, $x + x + 250 = 57,000$ becomes $2x - 250 = 57,000 - 250$ becomes $2x = 56,750$. Then divide 56,750 by 2 to get $x = 28,375$. Then $x + 250 = \$28,625$. Check: $\$28,625 + \$28,375 = \$57,000$.

15. $\dfrac{t}{-6} = 36$ becomes $t = -6 \times \dfrac{t}{-6} = 36(-6)$.

    Then $t = 36(-6)$ or $t = -216$

Practice 1: p. 164

1. $+18$ 7. -12

3. $+4,000$ 9. $+100$

5. -14

Practice 2: p. 164

1. Answers will vary.

Practice 3: p. 165

1. $>$ 5. $<$

3. $>$

Practice 4: p. 166

1. 12   5. 476

3. 6

Practice 5: p. 167

1. 21
3. −12
5. −66

7. +21
9. −22

Practice 6: p. 168

1. 18
3. 5
5. 6

7. −10
9. 84

Practice 7: p. 169

1. 17
3. −6
5. 20

7. 22
9. −24

Practice 8: p. 170

1. −54
3. −112
5. −230

7. −40
9. −24

Practice 9: p. 171

1. 12
3. −82
5. −6

7. −4.2
9. −6

Practice 10: p. 172

1. $5 \cdot 5 \cdot 5, 125$
3. $4^2, 4 \cdot 4$
5. $7 \cdot 7, 49$

7. 1, 1
9. 6^0 (or any equivalent exponent), 1

Practice 11: p. 173

1. 4, −4
3. 9, −9
5. 11, −11

7. 14, −14
9. 17, −17

Practice 12: p. 174

1. 240
3. 41
5. 11

7. −32
9. 9

Practice 13: p. 175

1. a^3, 12
3. x, 1.5
5. ab^2c, 12

7. bc^3, 2
9. bc, −7

Practice 14: p. 176

1. $p − 4.5$
3. $a + b$
5. $\dfrac{a + b}{6}$

7. $\dfrac{r}{3}$
9. $2(m + n)$

Practice 15: p. 176

1. some number a plus some number b decreased by some number z

3. some number x divided by some number y decreased by 15
5. the product of $7, a,$ and b decreased by 15

Practice 16: p. 177

1. 100
3. 26

5. 11

Practice 17: pp. 177–178

1. 29.75
3. $4\dfrac{1}{2}$

5. 40
7. 80
9. −1

Practice 18: p. 179

1. $x − 2$
3. $x + 500$

5. $x − 12$

Practice 19: p. 180

1. 57.5
3. 41.5
5. −12.25

7. −129.6
9. −16.4

Practice 20: pp. 181–182

1. $123 + 1,357 = x$ $x = 1,480$
3. $(2 \cdot 16.5) + 2 = x$ $x = 35$
5. $x + 7 = 18$ $x = 11$
7. $4x + 7 = 31$ $x = 6$
9. $125 + 325 + x = 625.35$ $x = 175.35$

Critical Thinking with Pre-Algebra Basics: pp. 182–183

1. $4,315.00
2. $\dfrac{x}{2} + 9$
3. $x − 5$
4. $2x + 4$
5. 7
6. 2.14
7. 240

8. $z = 4$
9. $25.80
10. 82
11. 44
12. $939.00 and $689.00
13. 28
14. 79
15. 11

Pre-Algebra Basics Post-Test: pp. 183–184

1. $−6 + 5 = −1$
2. $−12 − 12 = −12 + −12 = −24$
3. $5 + 4 \times 8 − 16 \div 4 \rightarrow 5 + 32 − 4$
   $= 37 − 4 = 33$
4. $12 − 40 \div 2 \div 5 + 2 \rightarrow 12 − 20 \div 5 + 2$
   $= 12 − 4 + 2 = 8 + 2 = 10$
5. $4^2 + 3^0 = 4 \times 4 + 1 = 17$
6. $12^3 \times 3^2 = 12 \times 12 \times 12 \times 3 \times 3 = 15,552$
7. $\sqrt{121} = 11 \times 11 = 121$
   So, the final answer is 11.
8. $\sqrt{9} \times 20 = 3 \times 20 = 60$
9. $|−68| = 68$
10. $10 − 8 \times 2 + 12 \div 3 = 10 − 16 + 4 = −2$
11. The coefficient of $4abf$ is 4.

12. The <u>quotient</u> of some number y and 5 Think: Quotient means divide by, so the expression is $\dfrac{y}{5}$

13. Solve: $\dfrac{t}{-4} = 24.4 \rightarrow \dfrac{-4}{1}$.

$\dfrac{t}{-4} = 24.4 \times \dfrac{-4}{1} = -97.6$

14. Beth has $450 more than Fred. Together they have $3,219. How much money does Fred have? $x + x + 450 = 3,219$ becomes $2x + 450 = 3,219$. Then $2x + 450 - 450 = 3,219 - 450$.
So, $2x = 2,769$. Then $2,769 \div 2 = 1,384.50$.
So $x = \$1,384.50$

15. Subtract 10 from Thanh's age and double the result, and you get Xuyen's age. Xuyen is 22. How old is Thanh? Think: The result doubled is 22 (Xuyen's age). So do two steps.

$x = \dfrac{22}{2}$. Thus, $x = 11$. Then $x - 10 = 11$.

So, $x - 10 + 10 = 11 + 10$; $x = 21$

◆◆◆◆ UNIT 8
The Metric System

Pre-Test: pp. 185–186

1. Think: Milligrams to micrograms is three places to the right ($\times$ 1000). So 25 mg = 25000 mcg.
2. Think: Milligrams to micrograms is three places to the right ($\times$ 1000). So 45 milligrams = 45000 micrograms.
3. Think: Milligrams to grams is three places to the left ($\div$ 1000). So 26 milligrams = 0.026 grams.
4. Think: Milliliters to liters is three places to the left ($\div$ 1000). So 125 mL = 0.125 liters.
5. Think: Grams to micrograms is six places to the right ($\times$ 1000000). So 0.45 g = 450000 mcg.
6. Think: Milliliters to liters is three places to the left ($\div$ 1000). So 4.9 mL = 0.0049 L.
7. Think: Milliliters to liters is three places to the left ($\div$ 1000). So 300 mL = 0.3 L.
8. Think: Micrograms to grams is six places to the left ($\div$ 1000000). So 15 mcg = 0.000015 g.
9. Think: Grams to milligrams is three places to the right ($\times$ 1000). So 45 g = 45000 mg.
10. Think: Milligrams to micrograms is three places to the right ($\times$ 1000). So 25 mg = 25000 mcg.
11. Think: Micrograms to grams is six places to the left ($\div$ 1000000). So 84 mcg = 0.000084 g.
12. Think: Kilograms to grams is three places to the right ($\times$ 1000). So 67 kg = 67000 g.
13. Think: Meters to centimeters is two places to the right ($\times$ 100). So 0.361 m = 36.1 cm.
14. $\dfrac{150 \text{ mg}}{2.5 \text{ mL}} = \dfrac{225 \text{ mg}}{?} \rightarrow 2.5 \times 225 = 562.5$.
So $562.5 \div 150 = 3.75$ mL.
15. Think: Liters to milliliters is three places to the right ($\times$ 1000). So 0.084 L = 84 mL.

Practice 1: p. 189

1. kg
3. g
5. cm
7. km
9. liter
11. kilometer
13. mcg
15. centimeter

Practice 2: pp. 189–190

1. 4.8 milligrams
3. OK
5. OK
7. 0.5 milligrams
9. 0.16 milliliters

Practice 3: p. 192

1. 0.008
3. 4250
5. 0.001
7. 0.3586
9. 0.0375

Practice 4: pp. 192–194

1. 10000
3. 0.048
5. 20500
7. 200
9. 70
11. 0.14
13. 0.25
15. 600
17. 36000
19. 7.5
21. 12500
23. 240
25. 12760
27. 235
29. 8
31. 1
33. 125
35. 125
37. 45.25
39. 0.001
41. 5.524
43. 125
45. 90
47. 100
49. 8.5

Practice 5: pp. 194–195

1. 44.53 centimeters
3. 1890 liters, 10 servings
5. 1250 milliliters
7. 123.56 centimeters, 1.2356 meters
9. Yes, 0.03 grams converts to 30 milligrams.

Practice 6: pp. 196–197

1. 23 mL
3. 29 mL
5. 20 mL
7. 132 g
9. 15 mL

Critical Thinking in the Metric System: pp. 197–198

1. mL
2. cm
3. m
4. kg
5. >
6. =
7. <
8. <
9. =
10. >
11. 9 crackers
12. 100 mg
13. 4 caplets
14. 5000
15. 40 mL

Metric System Post-Test: pp. 199–200

1. Label reads 400 mcg/mL, so that means
   $$\frac{400\,\text{mcg}}{1\,\text{mL}} = \frac{?\,\text{mcg}}{2\,\text{mL}}.$$ Then multiply $400 \times 2 = 800$,
   which is still 800 after dividing by 1. So then 800 mcg
   is converted into mg by dividing by 1000. The final
   answer is 0.8 mg.

2. Think: Micrograms to milligrams is three places to the
   left ($\div$ 1000). So 84 micrograms becomes 0.084 mg.

3. Think: Grams to kilograms is three places to the left
   ($\div$ 1000). So 24.8 grams becomes 0.0248 kg.

4. Think: Liters to milliliters is three places to the right
   ($\times$ 1000). So 2.7 liters becomes 2700 milliliters.

5. Think: Grams to micrograms is six places to the right
   ($\times$ 1000). So 0.014 grams becomes 14000 micrograms.

6. Think: Milliliters to liters is three places to the left
   ($\div$ 1000). So 1.2 milliliters becomes 0.0012 liter.

7. Think: Micrograms to grams is six places to the left
   ($\div$ 1000000). So 10 micrograms becomes 0.00001 gram.

8. Think: Milliliters to liters is three places to the left
   ($\div$ 1000). So 250 milliliters becomes 0.25 liter.

9. Think: Grams to Thinkmilligrams is three places to the
   right ($\times$ 1000). So 0.015 grams becomes 15 milligrams.

10. Think: Milligrams to micrograms is three places to the
    right ($\times$ 1000). So 30 milligrams becomes 30000 mcg.

11. Think: Micrograms to milligrams is three places to
    the left ($\div$ 1000). So 0.008 microgram becomes
    0.000008 milligram.

12. Think: Meters to centimeters is two places to the right
    ($\times$ 100). So 0.345 m = 34.5 cm.

13. $$\frac{250\,\text{mg}}{5\,\text{mL}} = \frac{375\,\text{mg}}{?} \rightarrow 5 \times 375 = 1875.$$
    Then $1875 \div 250 = 7.5$ mL

14. Think: Liters to milliliters is three places to the right
    ($\times$ 1000). So 0.24 liter becomes 240 milliliters.

15. Think: Grams to milligrams is three places to the right
    ($\times$ 1000). So 0.75 grams becomes 750 milligrams.

◆◆◆◆ **UNIT 9**

Reading Drug Labels, Medicine Cups, Syringes, and Intravenous Fluid Administration Bags

Pre-Test: pp. 202–204

1–7. Answers may vary: Trade name, Generic name,
dose, NDC, Manufacturer, drug form, preparation
of solution directions, prescription warning, storage
information, etc.

8. 9.

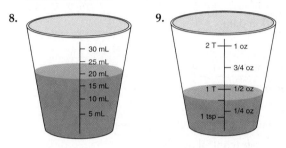

10. lansoprazole
11. 90 capsules
12. Capsule
13. 30 mg

14.

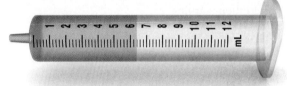

15. 200 mL

Practice 1: pp. 206–209

1.

Generic name	lorazepam
Trade name	Not shown
Manufacturer	PL Pharmaceuticals
National Drug Code (NDC) number	6077-112-81
Lot number (control number)	Not shown
Drug form	Solution
Dosage strength	4 milligrams/mL
Usual adult dose	Not shown, see accompanying information
Total amount in vial, packet, box	1 mL vial
Prescription warning	Protect from light
Expiration date	Not shown

3.

Generic name	amlodipine besylate
Trade name	Not shown
Manufacturer	PL Pharmaceuticals
National Drug Code (NDC) number	0069-1520-66
Lot number (control number)	Not shown
Drug form	Tablet
Dosage strength	2.5 milligrams
Usual adult dose	Not shown, see accompanying prescribing information
Total amount in vial, packet, box	100 tablets
Prescription warning	Federal law prohibits dispensing without prescription.
Expiration date	Not shown

5.

Generic name	erythromycin ethylsuccinate
Trade name	Not shown
Manufacturer	PL Pharmaceuticals
National Drug Code (NDC) number	0074-6302-13
Lot number (control number)	Not shown
Drug form	Oral suspension when mixed
Dosage strength	200 mg/mL when reconstituted
Usual adult dose	Not shown, see enclosure for adult dose and full prescribing information
Total amount in vial, packet, box	100 mL
Prescription warning	Rx only
Expiration date	Not shown

Practice 2: p. 209

1. 2 teaspoons or 10 milliliters
3. 2 tablespoons or 30 milliliters

Practice 3: pp. 210–211

1. 0.8 mL 5. 5.8 mL
3. 0.35 mL

Practice 4: p. 212

1. Volume infused 850 milliliters
   Volume remaining 150 milliliters
3. Volume infused 900 milliliters
   Volume remaining 100 milliliters

Critical Thinking in Reading Drug Labels, Medicine Cups, Syringes, and IV Fluid Administration Bags: pp. 213–215

1. 9 mL
2. 0.6 mL
3. 1 mL
4. 100 mg/mL
5. meperidine hydrochloride
6. Intramuscular, subcutaneous, or slow IV
7. 1 mL

8. Mark syringe to 1 mL

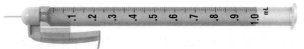

9. PL Pharmaceuticals
10. 0025-6589-82
11. IV and subcutaneous
12. Injection
13. 10000 units/mL
14. 0.5 mL
15. Yes, the label reads "Multiple Dose Vial."

Reading Drug Labels, Medicine Cups, Syringes, and IV Fluid Administration Bags Post-Test: pp. 215–217

1. Answers will vary. The generic name indicates the chemical name of the drug and includes any drug marketed under its chemical name without advertising. It is nonproprietary. The trade name is a brand name, and because these are the market names of the drug, they have advertising names.
2. Generic name fentanyl
3. Trade name Not shown
4. Manufacturer PL Pharmaceuticals

5. National Drug Code (NDC) number   10019-033-72

6. Lot number (control number)   Not shown

7. Drug form   Citrate injection

8. Dosage strength   250 mcg/5 mL or 0.05 mg/mL

9. Usual adult dose   Not shown

10. Total amount in vial, packet, box   Not shown

11. Prescription warning   C II

12. Expiration date   Not shown

13.

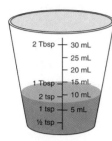

Cup showing 7.5 milliliters

14. 1.2 milliliters

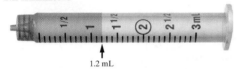

15. Volume infused   625 milliliters (may vary slightly)

     Volume remaining   375 milliliters (may vary slightly)

◆◆◆◆ UNIT 10

Apothecary Measurement and Conversion

Pre-Test: pp. 218–219

1. fifteen drops → 15 gtts

2. $\dfrac{1 \text{ ounce}}{8 \text{ tsp}} = \dfrac{2.5 \text{ ounces}}{? \text{ tsp}} \rightarrow 8 \times 2.5 = 20$ teaspoons

3. $\dfrac{1 \text{ pint}}{16 \text{ ounces}} = \dfrac{1.5 \text{ pints}}{? \text{ ounces}} \rightarrow 16 \times 1.5 = 24$ ounces

4. $\dfrac{\text{grain } 1}{60 \text{ milligrams}} = \dfrac{\text{grains } 4\frac{1}{6}}{? \text{ milligrams}} \rightarrow 60 \times 4\frac{1}{6}$

$= 60 \times \dfrac{25}{6} = 10 \times 25 = 250$ mg

5. $\dfrac{1 \text{ ounces}}{30 \text{ milliliters}} = \dfrac{8 \text{ ounces}}{? \text{ milliliters}} \rightarrow 30 \times 8 = 240$ milliliters

6. $\dfrac{1 \text{ kg}}{2.2 \text{ pounds}} = \dfrac{24 \text{ kg}}{? \text{ pounds}} \rightarrow 2.2 \times 24 = 52.8$ or $52\frac{4}{5}$

7. $\dfrac{1 \text{ ounce}}{30 \text{ milliliters}} = \dfrac{? \text{ ounces}}{78 \text{ milliliters}} \rightarrow 1 \times 78$

$= 78 \div 30 = 2\frac{3}{5}$ ounces

8. $\dfrac{\text{grain } 1}{60 \text{ milligrams}} = \dfrac{\text{grains } \frac{1}{400}}{? \text{ milligrams}} \rightarrow 60 \times \dfrac{1}{400}$

$= \dfrac{60}{400} = \dfrac{20 \times 3}{20 \times 20} = \dfrac{3}{20}$

9. $\dfrac{1 \text{ ounce}}{30 \text{ milliliters}} = \dfrac{? \text{ ounces}}{75 \text{ milliliters}} \rightarrow 1 \times 75$

$= 75 \div 30 = 2\frac{1}{2}$ ounces

10. $\dfrac{1 \text{ milliliter}}{15 \text{ drops}} = \dfrac{5.4 \text{ milliliters}}{? \text{ drops}} \rightarrow 15 \times 5.4 = 81$ drops

11. $\dfrac{1 \text{ tsp}}{5 \text{ milliliters}} = \dfrac{3.5 \text{ tsp}}{? \text{ milliliters}} \rightarrow 5 \times 3.5 = 17.5$ milliliters

12. $\dfrac{1 \text{ kg}}{2.2 \text{ pounds}} = \dfrac{? \text{ kg}}{122.25 \text{ pounds}} \rightarrow 1 \times 122.25$

$= 122.25 \div 2.2 = 55.6$ kilograms

13. $\dfrac{1 \text{ tsp}}{5 \text{ milliliters}} = \dfrac{? \text{ tsp}}{10 \text{ milliliters}} \rightarrow 10 \times 1$

$= 10 \div 5 = 2$ teaspoons

14. $\dfrac{1 \text{ ounce}}{30 \text{ milliliters}} = \dfrac{48 \text{ ounces}}{? \text{ milliliters}} \rightarrow 30 \times 48 = 1440$ milliliters

15. $\dfrac{1 \text{ cup}}{240 \text{ milliliters}} = \dfrac{4\frac{1}{3} \text{ cups}}{? \text{ milliliters}} \rightarrow 240 \times 4\frac{1}{3} \rightarrow 240 \times \dfrac{13}{3}$

$= 80 \times 13 = 1040$ milliliters

Practice 1: p. 223

1. $\dfrac{3}{4}$ 7. $\dfrac{1}{4}$

3. $1\dfrac{1}{4}$ 9. $\dfrac{1}{200}$

5. 10   11. 210

Practice 2: p. 224

1. 25   7. $23\dfrac{1}{3}$ or 23

3. $41\dfrac{2}{3}$ or 42   9. 5

5. $3\dfrac{1}{3}$ or 3

Practice 3: pp. 224–225

1. 900, 0.9   5. 15, 15000

3. $\dfrac{1}{4}$, 15   7. 90, 0.09

                  9. 510, 0.51

Practice 4: pp. 225–226

1. 6   11. 2500

3. 15   13. 5

5. 1   15. 64

7. iss   17. 75

9. 4   19. 4

Practice 5: pp. 226–228

1. 30   7. 420

3. 62.5   9. 7

5. 2250   11. 480

13. $\dfrac{1}{200}$

15. 20

17. $\dfrac{1}{2}$

19. 300

21. 0.4

23. ii

25. 420

27. 12

29. 35 or 35.56

31. v

33. 6

35. 4

37. 25

39. 36

Practice 6: pp. 228–229

1. x

3. 4

5. 75

7. 4

9. 900

11. 8

13. 4500

15. $\dfrac{1}{600}$

17. $4\dfrac{1}{2}$

19. 560

21. 120

23. 24

25. 875

Practice 7: p. 230

1. 25.9 kilograms

3. 12.5 milligrams

5. 50.5 milligrams

Practice 8: p. 230

1. $1\dfrac{3}{10}$

3. $\dfrac{1}{2}$

5. 255

7. 0.9

9. 600

11. x or 10

13. 120

15. 75

Critical Thinking in the Apothecary System: pp. 231–233

1. Not size, but potency. These are approximate measures.

2. 0.4 mg

3. 30 mm

4. 30

5. 1.4

6. 525000

7. 480

8. 44.4

9. 6.25 (using 2.54) or 6.35 (using 2.5)

10. 180

11. 7.5

12. 2 tablets (must be rounded)

13. 3125

14. 2000

15. 2 tsp, $2\dfrac{2}{3}$ tablespoons

Apothecary System Post-Test: pp. 233–234

1. 7.5 cm

2. $\dfrac{1 \text{ cup}}{240 \text{ milliliters}} = \dfrac{? \text{ cup}}{540 \text{ milliliters}} \rightarrow 1 \times 540$

$= 540 \div 240 = 2.25 \rightarrow 2\dfrac{1}{4} \text{ cups}$

3. $\dfrac{\text{grain } 1}{60 \text{ milligrams}} = \dfrac{? \text{ grain}}{0.3 \text{ milligrams}} \rightarrow \dfrac{3}{10} \div \dfrac{60}{1}$

$\rightarrow \dfrac{3}{10} \times \dfrac{1}{60} = \dfrac{3}{600} = \dfrac{3 \times 1}{3 \times 200} = \dfrac{1}{200}$

4. $2\dfrac{1}{2} = 2.5 \rightarrow \dfrac{\text{grain } 1}{60 \text{ milligrams}} = \dfrac{\text{grain } 2.5}{? \text{ milligrams}}$

$\rightarrow 60 \times 2.5 = 150 \text{ milligrams}$

5. $\dfrac{1 \text{ ounce}}{30 \text{ milliliters}} = \dfrac{4 \text{ ounces}}{? \text{ milliliters}} \rightarrow 30 \times 4 = 120 \text{ milliliters}$

6. $\dfrac{1 \text{ kg}}{2.2 \text{ lbs}} = \dfrac{48 \text{ kg}}{? \text{ lbs}} \rightarrow 2.2 \times 48 = 105.6 \text{ lbs.}$

Then $\dfrac{1 \text{ lb}}{16 \text{ ounces}} = \dfrac{105.6 \text{ lbs}}{? \text{ ounces}} \rightarrow 105.6 \times 16$

$= 1{,}689.6 \text{ ounces} \rightarrow 1{,}689\dfrac{3}{5} \text{ ounces}$

7. $\dfrac{1 \text{ tablespoon}}{15 \text{ milliliters}} = \dfrac{? \text{ tablespoons}}{95 \text{ milliliters}} \rightarrow 1 \times 95$

$= 95 \div 15 = 6\dfrac{1}{3} \text{ tablespoons}$

8. $\dfrac{\text{grain } 1}{60 \text{ milligrams}} = \dfrac{\text{grain } \frac{1}{100}}{? \text{ milligrams}} \rightarrow 60 \times \dfrac{1}{100}$

$= \dfrac{60}{100} \rightarrow 0.6 \text{ milligrams}$

9. $\dfrac{1 \text{ ounce}}{30 \text{ milliliters}} = \dfrac{? \text{ ounces}}{75 \text{ milliliters}} \rightarrow 1 \times 75 = 75 \div 30$

$= 2\dfrac{1}{2} \text{ ounces}$

10. $\dfrac{1 \text{ milliliter}}{15 \text{ gtts}} = \dfrac{1.5 \text{ milliliters}}{? \text{ gtts}} \rightarrow 15 \times 1.5 = 22.5$

becomes 23 gtts

11. $\dfrac{1 \text{ pint}}{16 \text{ ounces}} = \dfrac{? \text{ pint}}{12 \text{ ounces}} \rightarrow 12 \times 1 = 12.$

Then $12 \div 16 = \dfrac{3}{4} \text{ pint}$

12. $\dfrac{1 \text{ kg}}{2.2 \text{ pounds}} = \dfrac{? \text{ kg}}{68.5 \text{ pounds}} \rightarrow 1 \times 68 = 68.$

Then $68.5 \div 2.2 = 31.13636 \rightarrow 31.1 \text{ kg}$

13. $\dfrac{1 \text{ teaspoon}}{5 \text{ milliliters}} = \dfrac{? \text{ teaspoons}}{12 \text{ milliliters}} \rightarrow 12 \times 1 = 12.$

Then $12 \div 5 = 2\dfrac{2}{5} \text{ teaspoons}$

14. Think: 8 glasses × 8 ounces = 64 ounces. Then

$\dfrac{1 \text{ ounce}}{30 \text{ milliliters}} = \dfrac{64 \text{ ounces}}{? \text{ milliliters}} \rightarrow 30 \times 64 = 1920 \text{ milliliters}$

15. $\dfrac{1 \text{ ounce}}{30 \text{ milliliters}} = \dfrac{3 \text{ ounces}}{? \text{ milliliters}} \rightarrow 30 \times 3 = 90 \text{ milliliters.}$

Then $\dfrac{1 \text{ milliliter}}{15 \text{ gtts}} = \dfrac{90 \text{ milliliters}}{? \text{ gtts}}.$

Then $15 \times 90 = 1350 \text{ gtts}$

◆◆◆◆ UNIT 11
Dosage Calculations

Pre-Test: pp. 235–237

1. $\dfrac{20 \text{ mg}}{30 \text{ mg}} \times 5 \text{ mL} = \dfrac{100 \text{ mg}}{30 \text{ mg}} = 3.3 \text{ mL}$

2. $\dfrac{150 \text{ mg}}{100 \text{ mg}} \times 1 \text{ tablet} = \dfrac{150 \text{ mg}}{100 \text{ mg}} = 1\dfrac{1}{2} \text{ tablets}$

3. $\dfrac{0.3\text{ g}}{\text{gr v}} \times 1\text{ tablet} =$ Think: 0.3 g = 300 mg.

So, $\dfrac{\text{gr }1}{60\text{ mg}} = \dfrac{\text{gr }?}{300\text{ mg}} \rightarrow 1 \times 300 = 300.$

Then 300 ÷ 60 = 5. So the answer is grains v or 5 grains, which is 1 tablet.

4. $\dfrac{1.25\text{ mg}}{0.75\text{ mg}} \times 5\text{ mL} = \dfrac{6.25\text{ mg}}{0.75\text{ mg}} \rightarrow 6.25 \div 0.75 = 8.333.$
Rounded to 8.3 mL

5. $\dfrac{25\text{ mg}}{12.5\text{ mg}} \times 1\text{ tablet} = \dfrac{25\text{ mg}}{12.5\text{ mg}} \rightarrow 25 \div 12.5 = 2\text{ tablets}$

6. 60 mg = 20 mg + 20 mg + ? mg
Think: 60 − 40 = 20 mg

7. $\dfrac{15\text{ mg}}{5\text{ mg}} \times 1\text{ tablet} = \dfrac{15\text{ mg}}{5\text{ mg}} \rightarrow 15 \div 5 = 3\text{ tablets}$

8. $\dfrac{8\text{ mg}}{4\text{ mg}} \times 1\text{ tablet} = \dfrac{8\text{ mg}}{4\text{ mg}} \rightarrow 8 \div 4 = 2\text{ tablets}$

9. $\dfrac{200\text{ mg}}{250\text{ mg}} \times 5\text{ mL} = \dfrac{200\text{ mg}}{250\text{ mg}} \rightarrow 200 \times 5 = 1000.$
Then 1000 ÷ 250 = 4 mL

10. $\dfrac{\text{gr ii}}{60\text{ mg}} \times 1\text{ tablet} = \dfrac{\text{gr i}}{60\text{ mg}} = \dfrac{\text{gr ii}}{?\text{ mg}} \rightarrow 60 \times 2 = 120\text{ mg},$
which is 2 tablets.

11. $\dfrac{30\text{ mg}}{12.5\text{ mg}} \times 5\text{ mL} = \dfrac{150\text{ mg}}{12.5\text{ mg}} \rightarrow 150 \div 12.5 = 12\text{ mL}$

12. $\dfrac{\text{grain }\frac{1}{150}}{100\text{ mcg}} \times 1\text{ tab} =$ Think: Convert grains to mg $\dfrac{\text{gr }1}{60\text{ mg}}$

$= \dfrac{\text{grain }\frac{1}{150}}{?\text{ mg}} \rightarrow 60 \times \dfrac{1}{150} = \dfrac{60}{150} \rightarrow 60 \div 150 = 0.4\text{ mg}.$

Then convert 0.4 mg to 400 mcg
$\dfrac{400\text{ mcg}}{100\text{ mcg}} \times 1\text{ tablet} = 4\text{ tablets}$

13. $\dfrac{\text{gr v}}{\text{gr }1.25} \times 1\text{ tablet} = 5 \div 1.25 = 4\text{ tablets}$

14. $\dfrac{0.3\text{ gram}}{100\text{ mg}} \times 1\text{ tablet} = 0.3\text{ gram becomes }300\text{ mg.}$

Then $\dfrac{300\text{ mg}}{100\text{ mg}} \times 1\text{ tablet} = 3\text{ tablets}$

15. $\dfrac{15\text{ mg}}{30\text{ mg}} \times 1\text{ tablet} = 15 \div 30 = \dfrac{1}{2}\text{ tablet}$

Practice 1: p. 241

1. 3 tablets
3. 3 tablets
5. 0.5 milliliter
7. 0.5 milliliter
9. 6 tablets

Practice 2: pp. 242–243

1. 40 milliliters
3. $\dfrac{1}{2}$ caplet

5. 4 tablets
7. $1\dfrac{1}{2}$ tablets
9. 2 tablets
11. $2\dfrac{1}{2}$ tablets
13. 2 caplets
15. 2.5 tablets
17. 0.5 milliliter
19. 4 tablets

Practice 3: pp. 244–247

1. 1 tablet
3. 2 capsules
5. 1 tablet
7. 2 tablets
9. 1 tablet

Critical Thinking in Dosage Calculations: pp. 247–249

1. 47 doses
2. 94 teaspoons
3. 2 tablets
4. 1 teaspoon
5. $2\dfrac{1}{2}$ tablespoons
6. 210 milligrams
7. yes
8. 0.8
9. shade the syringe to 4 mL
10. 8 caplets/day
11. Use 15 mg
12. 1 tablet at 15 mg
13. 4 tablets
14. Think how many mg daily, so 50 mcg = 0.05 mg
15. No, because
$\dfrac{50\text{ mcg}}{25\text{ mcg}} = 2\text{ tablets a day} \times 90 = 180\text{ tablets total.}$
Vial has 100 tablets.

Dosage Calculations Post-Test: pp. 250–252

1. $\dfrac{20\text{ mg}}{10\text{ mg}} \times 5\text{ mL} = \dfrac{100}{10} = 10\text{ mL}$

2. $\dfrac{250\text{ mg}}{100\text{ mg}} \times 1\text{ tablet} = \dfrac{250}{100} = 2\dfrac{1}{2}\text{ tablet}$

3. $\dfrac{0.6\text{ g}}{\text{gr v}} \times 1\text{ tablet} =$ Think: 0.6 grams = 600 mg. Then

$\dfrac{\text{gr }1}{60\text{ mg}} = \dfrac{\text{gr }?}{600\text{ mg}} \rightarrow 1 \times 600 = 600 \div 60 = \text{grains }10.$

Then rewrite: $\dfrac{\text{gr }10}{\text{gr }5} \times 1\text{ tablet} = 2\text{ tablets}$

4. $\dfrac{1.25\text{ mg}}{0.25\text{ mg}} \times 5\text{ mL} = 6.25 \div 0.25 = 25\text{ mL}$

5. Think: Ordered is 20 mg × 10 days = 200 mg

6. $\dfrac{60\text{ mg}}{20\text{ mg}} \times 1\text{ tablet} = 60 \div 20 = 3\text{ tablets}$

7. Add the doses to equal $262\dfrac{1}{2}$; then round to 263.

8. $\dfrac{5 \text{ mg}}{2.5 \text{ mg}} \times 1 \text{ tablet} = 5 \div 2.5 = 2 \text{ tablets}$

9. $\dfrac{200 \text{ mg}}{125 \text{ mg}} \times 5 \text{ mL} = \dfrac{1000 \text{ mg}}{125 \text{ mg}} \rightarrow 1000 \div 125 = 8 \text{ mL}$

10. $\dfrac{\text{gr iii}}{60 \text{ mg}} \times 1 \text{ tab} = \dfrac{\text{gr } 1}{60 \text{ mg}} = \dfrac{\text{gr iii}}{? \text{ mg}}$.

Then $60 \times 3 = 180 \text{ mg}$

$\dfrac{180 \text{ mg}}{60 \text{ mg}} \times 1 \text{ tablet} = 3 \text{ tablets}$

11. $\dfrac{50 \text{ mg}}{12.5 \text{ mg}} \times 5 \text{ mL} = 50 \times 5 = 250$.

Then, $250 \div 12.5 = 20 \text{ mL}$

12. $\dfrac{\text{gr i}}{60 \text{ mg}} = \dfrac{\text{gr } \frac{1}{150}}{x \text{ mg}} = 60 \times \dfrac{1}{150} = \dfrac{60}{150}$.

Then $60 \div 150 = 0.4 \text{ mg}$, which becomes 400 mcg.

Set up as $\dfrac{400 \text{ mcg}}{200 \text{ mcg}} \times 1 \text{ tablet} = 2 \text{ tablets}$

13. $\dfrac{\text{gr v}}{\text{gr } 2.5} \times 1 \text{ tablet} = 5 \div 2.5 = 2 \text{ tablets}$

14. 0.2 grams becomes 200 mg. Set up as

$\dfrac{200 \text{ mg}}{100 \text{ mg}} \times 1 \text{ tablet} = 200 \div 100 = 2 \text{ tablets}$

15. $\dfrac{30 \text{ mg}}{15 \text{ mg}} \times 1 \text{ tablet} \rightarrow 30 \div 15 = 2 \text{ tablets}$

◆◆◆◆ UNIT 12
Parenteral Dosage

Pre-Test: pp. 253–255

1. $\dfrac{125 \text{ mg}}{250 \text{ mg}} \times 5 \text{ mL} = 125 \times 5 = 625$.

Then $625 \div 250 = 2.5 \text{ mL}$

2. $\dfrac{0.25 \text{ mg}}{250 \text{ mg}} \times 1 \text{ mL} \rightarrow 0.25 \div 250 = 0.125 \text{ mL}$.

Rounded to 0.13 mL

3. $\dfrac{0.4 \text{ mg}}{0.8 \text{ mg}} \times 1 \text{ mL} \rightarrow 0.4 \div 0.8 = 0.5 \text{ mL}$

4. $\dfrac{100 \text{ mg}}{200 \text{ mg}} \times 1 \text{ mL} \rightarrow 100 \div 200 = 0.5 \text{ mL}$

5. $\dfrac{0.5 \text{ mg}}{2 \text{ g}} \times 2000 \text{ mL} = \text{Think: } 0.5 \text{ mg becomes}$

0.0005 grams. Then $\dfrac{0.0005 \text{ g}}{2 \text{ g}} \times 2000 \text{ mL} = \dfrac{1 \text{ g}}{2 \text{ g}}$.

Then $1 \div 2 = 0.5 \text{ mL}$

6. $\dfrac{250 \text{ mg}}{300 \text{ mg}} \times 5 \text{ mL} = \dfrac{1250 \text{ mg}}{300 \text{ mg}}$. Then $1250 \div 300 = 4.16666$.

Rounded to 4.2 mL

7. $\dfrac{250 \text{ mg}}{20 \text{ g}} \times 100 = \text{Think: } 250 \text{ mg} = 0.25 \text{ grams}$.

So $\dfrac{0.25 \text{ g}}{20 \text{ g}} \times 100 = \dfrac{25 \text{ g}}{20 \text{ g}} = 1.25 \text{ mL}$

8. $\dfrac{0.75 \text{ mg}}{2 \text{ mg}} \times 1 = 0.75 \div 2 = 0.375 \text{ mL}$, which is rounded
to 0.38 mL

9. $\dfrac{4 \text{ mg}}{10 \text{ mg}} \times 1 = 4 \div 10 = 0.4 \text{ mL}$

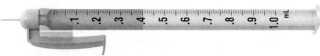

10. $\dfrac{4 \text{ mcg}}{2.5 \text{ mcg}} \times 1 = 4 \div 2.5 = 1.6 \text{ mL}$

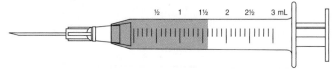

11. $\dfrac{0.75 \text{ mg}}{0.5 \text{ mg}} \times 1 = 0.75 \div 0.5 = 1.5 \text{ mL}$

12. $\dfrac{35 \text{ mg}}{5 \text{ g}} \times 100 = \text{Think: } 35 \text{ mg} = 0.035 \text{ g}$.

So $\dfrac{0.035 \text{ g}}{5 \text{ g}} \times 100 = \dfrac{3.5}{5} \rightarrow 3.5 \div 5 = 0.7 \text{ mL}$

13. $\dfrac{5000 \text{ units}}{1000 \text{ units}} \times 1 = 5000 \div 1000 = 5 \text{ mL}$

14. $\dfrac{45 \text{ mg}}{50 \text{ mg}} \times 1 = 45 \div 50 = 0.9 \text{ mL}$

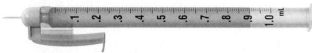

15. $\dfrac{0.01 \text{ mg}}{0.04 \text{ mg}} \times 2 = 0.01 \times 2 = 0.02$.

Then $0.02 \div 0.04 = 0.5 \text{ mL}$

Practice 1: pp. 258–260

1. 0.5 milliliter
3. 2.22 milliliters
    → 2.2 milliliters
5. 2.5 milliliters
7. 2 milliliters
9. 0.5 milliliter

11. 0.5 milliliter
13. 0.75 milliliters
    → 0.8 milliliter
15. 2 milliliters
17. 1.5 milliliters
19. 0.25 milliliter
    → 0.3 milliliters

Critical Thinking in Parenteral Dosages: pp. 261–264

1. 2 teaspoons
2. 12 mg
3. 0.002 g
4. 0.5 mL
5. 0.75 mL
6. 0.4 mg
7. 1.5 mL
8. 1.3 mL

9. 0.55 mL
10. 1 mL
11. 1.5 mL
12. 6 mL
13. 0.75 mL
14. It is ingested.
15. 60 mg

Parental Dosages Post-Test: pp. 264–266

1. $\dfrac{30 \text{ mg}}{50 \text{ mg}} \times 1 \text{ mL} \rightarrow 30 \div 50 = 0.6 \text{ mL}$

2. $\dfrac{0.5 \text{ mg}}{2 \text{ mg}} \times 1 \text{ mL} \rightarrow 0.5 \div 2 = 0.25 \text{ mL}$

3. $\dfrac{0.6 \text{ mg}}{0.8 \text{ mg}} \times 1 \text{ mL} \rightarrow 0.6 \div 0.8 = 0.75 \text{ mL}$

4. $\dfrac{100 \text{ units}}{400 \text{ units}} \times 2 \text{ mL} \rightarrow 100 \times 2 = 200.$
   Then $200 \div 400 = 0.5 \text{ mL}$

5. $\dfrac{0.5 \text{ mg}}{1 \text{ g}} \times 1000 \text{ mL} \rightarrow$ Change 0.5 to 0.0005 grams.
   Then $0.0005 \times 1000 \text{ mL} = 0.5 \text{ mL}$

6. $\dfrac{250 \text{ mg}}{500 \text{ mg}} \times 5 \text{ mL} \rightarrow 250 \times 5 = 1250.$
   Then $1250 \div 500 = 2.5 \text{ mL}$

7. $\dfrac{550 \text{ mg}}{20 \text{ g}} \times 100 \text{ mL} \rightarrow$ Change 550 mg to 0.55 grams.
   Then $0.55 \times 100 = 55$ and then $55 \div 20 = 2.75 \text{ mL}$

8. $\dfrac{0.5 \text{ mg}}{2 \text{ mg}} \times 1 \text{ mL} \rightarrow 0.5 \div 2 = 0.25 \text{ mL}$

9. $\dfrac{4 \text{ mg}}{12 \text{ mg}} \times 1 \text{ mL} \rightarrow 4 \div 12 = 0.33 \text{ mL}$

10. $\dfrac{3 \text{ mcg}}{5 \text{ mcg}} \times 1 \text{ mL} \rightarrow 3 \div 5 = 0.6 \text{ mL}$

11. $\dfrac{1 \text{ mg}}{0.5 \text{ mg}} \times 1 \text{ mL} \rightarrow 1 \div 0.5 = 2 \text{ mL}$

12. Think: 25 mg → 0.025 grams.
   Then $\dfrac{0.025 \text{ g}}{5 \text{ g}} \times 100 \text{ mL} = 0.025 \times 100 = 2.5.$
   Then $\dfrac{2.5}{5} \rightarrow 2.5 \div 5 = 0.5 \text{ mL}$

13. $\dfrac{25000}{1000} \times 1 \text{ mL} \rightarrow 25000 \div 1000 = 25 \text{ mL}$

14. $\dfrac{35 \text{ mg}}{25 \text{ mg}} \times 1 \text{ mL} \rightarrow 35 \div 25 = 1.4 \text{ mL}$

15. $\dfrac{0.01 \text{ mg}}{0.02 \text{ mg}} \times 1 \text{ mL} \rightarrow 0.01 \div 0.02 = 0.5 \text{ mL}$

◆◆◆◆◆ **UNIT 13**

The Basics of Intravenous Fluid Administration

Pre-Test: p. 268

1. $\dfrac{250 \text{ mL}}{8 \text{ hr} \times 60 \text{ min}} \times 15 \text{ mL} = \dfrac{250 \text{ mL}}{8 \text{ hr} \times \cancel{60} \, 4 \text{ min}} \times \cancel{15} \text{ mL}$
   $= \dfrac{250 \text{ mL}}{8 \times 4} = \dfrac{250 \text{ mL}}{32} = 250 \div 32 = 7.81 \text{ or } 8 \text{ gtts/min}$

2. $\dfrac{500 \text{ mL}}{6 \text{ hr} \times 60 \text{ min}} \times 15 \text{ mL} = \dfrac{500 \text{ mL}}{6 \text{ hr} \times \cancel{60} \, 3 \text{ min}} \times \cancel{20} \text{ mL}$
   $= \dfrac{500 \text{ mL}}{6 \times 3} = \dfrac{500 \text{ mL}}{18} = 500 \div 18 = 27.7 \text{ or } 28 \text{ gtts/min}$

3. $\dfrac{1200 \text{ mL}}{10 \text{ hr} \times 60 \text{ min}} \times 60 \text{ mL} = \dfrac{1200 \text{ mL}}{10 \text{ hr} \times \cancel{60} \text{ min}} \times \cancel{60} \text{ mL}$
   $= \dfrac{1200 \text{ mL}}{10 \text{ hr}} = 1200 \div 10 = 120 \text{ gtts/min}$

4. $\dfrac{125 \text{ mL}}{8 \text{ hr} \times 60 \text{ min}} \times 20 \text{ mL} = \dfrac{125 \text{ mL}}{8 \text{ hr} \times \cancel{60} \, 3 \text{ min}} \times \cancel{20} \text{ mL}$
   $= \dfrac{125 \text{ mL}}{\underset{\min}{8 \times 3}} = \dfrac{125 \text{ mL}}{24} = 125 \div 24 = 5.2 \text{ or } 5 \text{ gtts/}$

5. $\dfrac{750 \text{ mL}}{12 \text{ hr} \times 60 \text{ min}} \times 60 \text{ mL} = \dfrac{750 \text{ mL}}{12 \text{ hr} \times \cancel{60} \text{ min}} \times \cancel{60} \text{ mL}$
   $= \dfrac{750 \text{ mL}}{12 \text{ hr}} = 750 \div 12 = 62.5 \text{ or } 63 \text{ gtts/min}$

6. $\dfrac{1500 \text{ mL}}{12 \text{ hrs}} = 1500 \div 12 = 125 \text{ mL/hr}$

7. $\dfrac{550 \text{ mL}}{8 \text{ hrs}} = 550 \div 8 = 69 \text{ mL/hr}$

8. $\dfrac{1250 \text{ mL}}{12 \text{ hrs}} = 1250 \div 12 = 104 \text{ mL/hr}$

9. $\dfrac{1500 \text{ mL}}{24 \text{ hrs}} = 1500 \div 24 = 62.5 \text{ or } 63 \text{ mL/hr}$

10. $\dfrac{75 \text{ mL}}{30 \text{ min}} = \dfrac{?}{60 \text{ min}}$
    Then $75 \times 60 = 4500$. Then $4500 \div 30 = 150 \text{ mL/hr}$

11. $\dfrac{500 \text{ mL}}{83 \text{ mL}} = 500 \div 83 = 6.02.$ Then $\dfrac{1 \text{ hr}}{60 \text{ min}} = \dfrac{0.2 \text{ hr}}{? \text{ min}}$
    $\rightarrow 60 \times 0.2 = 12 \text{ min}$
    So the answer is 6 hours 12 minutes

12. $\dfrac{750 \text{ mL}}{100 \text{ mL}} = 750 \div 100 = 7.5.$ Then $\dfrac{1 \text{ hr}}{60 \text{ min}} = \dfrac{0.5 \text{ hr}}{? \text{ min}}$
    $\rightarrow 60 \times 0.5 = 30 \text{ min}$
    So the answer is 7 hours 30 minutes

13. $\dfrac{1500 \text{ mL}}{60 \text{ mL}} = 1500 \div 60 = 25 \text{ hours}$

14. $\dfrac{1000 \text{ mL}}{100 \text{ mL}} = 1000 \div 10 = 10 \text{ hours}$

15. $\dfrac{450 \text{ mL}}{33 \text{ mL}} = 450 \div 33 = 13.6363.$
    Then $\dfrac{1 \text{ hr}}{60 \text{ min}} = \dfrac{0.63 \text{ hr}}{? \text{ min}} \rightarrow 60 \times 0.63 = 37.8 \text{ or } 38 \text{ min}$
    So the answer is 13 hours 38 minutes

16. $75 \times 6 = 450 \text{ mL}$
17. $83 \times 12 = 996 \text{ mL}$
18. $75 \times 3 = 225 \text{ mL}$
19. $125 \times 8 = 1000 \text{ mL}$
20. $75 \times 2.5 = 187.5 \text{ or } 188 \text{ mL}$

Practice 1: p. 272

1. 100 drops per minute
3. 7 drops per minute
5. 104 drops per minute
7. 24 drops per minute
9. 17 drops per minute
11. 133 drops per minute
13. 25 drops per minute
15. 6 drops per minute
17. 16 drops per minute
19. 44 drops per minute

Practice 2: pp. 272–273

1. 31
3. 21 drops per minute
5. 6 drops per minute
7. 125 drops per minute
9. 10 drops per minute

Practice 3: pp. 274–275

1. 83
3. 300
5. 111
7. 125
9. 75

Practice 4: pp. 276–277

1. 10 hours
3. 16 hours
5. 4 hours 48 minutes
7. 7 hours 50 minutes
9. 9 hours 2 minutes

Practice 5: p. 278

1. 1500 milliliters
3. 498 milliliters
5. 558 milliliters
7. 268 milliliters
9. 400 milliliters

Critical Thinking in Intravenous Fluid Administration: pp. 279–280

1. 63
2. 67 gtts/min
3. True. In this case, mL and min are interchangeable, for the gtt/min is equal to mL/hr.
4. False. You should always round to the nearest whole number.
5. False; mL/min in the formula should be mL/hr
6. True
7. 1 liter
8. 15 gtts/minute
9. 42 mL
10. 31 gtts/min
11. 48 grams
12. 37.5 grams
13. 4.5 grams
14. 6 grams
15. 125 mL/hr

The Basics of Intravenous Fluid Administration Post-Test: pp. 280–281

1. $\dfrac{500 \text{ mL}}{8 \text{ hr} \times 60 \text{ min}} \times 15 \text{ mL} = \dfrac{500 \text{ mL}}{8 \text{ hr} \times \cancel{60}\,4 \text{ min}} \times \cancel{15} \text{ mL}$
   $= \dfrac{500 \text{ mL}}{8 \times 4} = \dfrac{500 \text{ mL}}{32} = 500 \div 32 = 16 \text{ gtts/min}$

2. $\dfrac{250 \text{ mL}}{6 \text{ hr} \times 60 \text{ min}} \times 20 \text{ mL} = \dfrac{250 \text{ mL}}{6 \text{ hr} \times \cancel{60}\,3 \text{ min}} \times \cancel{20} \text{ mL}$
   $= \dfrac{250 \text{ mL}}{6 \times 3} = \dfrac{250 \text{ mL}}{18} = 250 \div 18 = 14 \text{ gtts/min}$

3. $\dfrac{1500 \text{ mL}}{12 \text{ hr} \times 60 \text{ min}} \times 60 \text{ mL} = \dfrac{1500 \text{ mL}}{12 \text{ hr} \times \cancel{60} \text{ min}} \times \cancel{60} \text{ mL}$
   $= \dfrac{1500 \text{ mL}}{12 \text{ hr}} = 1500 \div 12 = 125 \text{ gtts/min}$

4. $\dfrac{125 \text{ mL}}{4 \text{ hr} \times 60 \text{ min}} \times 10 \text{ mL} = \dfrac{125 \text{ mL}}{4 \text{ hr} \times \cancel{60}\,6 \text{ min}} \times \cancel{10} \text{ mL}$
   $= \dfrac{125 \text{ mL}}{4 \times 6} = \dfrac{125 \text{ mL}}{24} = 125 \div 24 = 5.2 \text{ or } 5 \text{ gtts/min}$

5. $\dfrac{750 \text{ mL}}{8 \text{ hr} \times 60 \text{ min}} \times 60 \text{ mL} = \dfrac{750 \text{ mL}}{8 \text{ hr} \times \cancel{60} \text{ min}} \times \cancel{60} \text{ mL}$
   $= \dfrac{750 \text{ mL}}{8 \text{ hr}} = 750 \div 8 = 93.75 \text{ or } 94 \text{ gtts/min}$

6. $\dfrac{1200 \text{ mL}}{6 \text{ hrs}} = 1200 \div 6 = 200 \text{ mL/hr}$

7. $\dfrac{750 \text{ mL}}{12 \text{ hrs}} = 750 \div 12 = 62.5 \text{ or } 63 \text{ mL/hr}$

8. $\dfrac{250 \text{ mL}}{4 \text{ hrs}} = 250 \div 4 = 62.5 \text{ or } 63 \text{ mL/hr}$

9. $\dfrac{1800 \text{ mL}}{24 \text{ hrs}} = 1800 \div 24 = 75 \text{ mL/hr}$

10. Think: 30 minutes $= \dfrac{1}{2}$ hour or 0.5 hr. Then $\dfrac{100 \text{ mL}}{0.5 \text{ hr}}$
    $= 100 \div 0.5 = 200 \text{ mL/hr}$

11. $\dfrac{500 \text{ mL}}{125 \text{ mL}} = 500 \div 125 = 4 \text{ hours}$

12. $\dfrac{650 \text{ mL}}{133 \text{ mL}} = 650 \div 133 = 4.88.$ Then $\dfrac{1 \text{ hr}}{60 \text{ min}} = \dfrac{0.88 \text{ hr}}{? \text{ min}}$
    $\rightarrow 60 \times 0.88 = 53 \text{ min}$
    So the answer is 4 hours 53 minutes

13. $\dfrac{1200 \text{ mL}}{60 \text{ mL}} = 1200 \div 60 = 20 \text{ hours}$

14. $\dfrac{1000 \text{ mL}}{100 \text{ mL}} = 1000 \div 10 = 10 \text{ hours}$

15. $\dfrac{250 \text{ mL}}{83 \text{ mL}} = 250 \div 83 = 3.01.$ Then $\dfrac{1 \text{ hr}}{60 \text{ min}} = \dfrac{0.01 \text{ hr}}{? \text{ min}}$
    $\rightarrow 60 \times 0.01 = 0.6 \text{ min}.$ Rounded 1 minute. So the answer is 3 hours 1 minute.

16. $135 \times 6 = 810 \text{ mL}$
17. $83 \times 8 = 664 \text{ mL}$
18. $25 \times 3 = 75 \text{ mL}$
19. $125 \times 12 = 1500 \text{ mL}$
20. $65 \times 2.5 = 163 \text{ mL}$

◆◆◆◆ **UNIT 14**

Basic Dosage by Body Weight

Pre-Test: pp. 282–283

1. Convert 4 ounces to a decimal: $\dfrac{4}{16}$ is $\dfrac{1}{4}$ and $1 \div 4 = 0.25$.
   Then set up $\dfrac{1 \text{ kg}}{2.2 \text{ lbs}} = \dfrac{? \text{ kg}}{18.25 \text{ lbs}} \rightarrow 1 \times 18.25 = 18.25$.
   Then $18.25 \div 2.2 = 8.29545$, which is rounded to 8.30 kg or 8.3 kg

2. Set up $\dfrac{1 \text{ kg}}{2.2 \text{ lbs}} = \dfrac{? \text{ kg}}{102 \text{ lbs}} \rightarrow 1 \times 102 = 102$. Then
   $102 \div 2.2 = 46.36 \text{ kg}$

3. Convert 12 ounces to a decimal: $\frac{12}{16}$ is $\frac{3}{4}$ and $3 \div 4 = 0.75$. Then set up $\frac{1 \text{ kg}}{2.2 \text{ lbs}} = \frac{? \text{ kg}}{9.75 \text{ lbs}} \rightarrow 1 \times 9.75 = 9.75$. Then $9.75 \div 2.2 = 4.31818$, which is rounded to 4.32 kg

4. Convert 6 ounces to a decimal: $\frac{6}{16}$ is $\frac{3}{8}$ and $3 \div 8 = 0.375$. Then set up $\frac{1 \text{ kg}}{2.2 \text{ lbs}} = \frac{? \text{ kg}}{22.375 \text{ lbs}} \rightarrow 1 \times 22.375 = 22.375$. Then $22.375 \div 2.2 = 10.17$ kg

5. Convert 10 ounces to a decimal: $\frac{10}{16}$ is $\frac{5}{8}$ and $5 \div 8 = 0.625$. Then set up $\frac{1 \text{ kg}}{2.2 \text{ lbs}} = \frac{? \text{ kg}}{35.625 \text{ lbs}} \rightarrow 1 \times 35.625 = 35.625$. Then $35.625 \div 2.2 = 16.193$, which is rounded to 16.19 kg

6. Convert 5 ounces to a decimal: $\frac{4}{16}$ is $\frac{5}{16}$ and $5 \div 16 = 0.3125$. Then set up $\frac{1 \text{ kg}}{2.2 \text{ lbs}} = \frac{? \text{ kg}}{9.3125 \text{ lbs}} \rightarrow 1 \times 9.3125 = 9.3125$. Then $9.3125 \div 2.2 = 4.2329$, which is rounded to 4.23 kg

7. Convert 6 ounces to a decimal: $\frac{6}{16}$ is $\frac{3}{8}$ and $3 \div 8 = 0.375$. Then set up $\frac{1 \text{ kg}}{2.2 \text{ lbs}} = \frac{? \text{ kg}}{20.375 \text{ lbs}} \rightarrow 1 \times 20.375 = 20.375$. Then $20.375 \div 2.2 = 9.26$, which is rounded to 9.26 kg. To get the daily dose, multiply 1.5 mg by $9.26 = 13.89$ mg

8. The dosing is every 8 hours so that means divide the daily dose (24 hours) by 3 to get the answer. 13.89 mg $\div 3 = 4.63$ mg

9. No, the dose is over the recommended 3 milligrams every 8 hours, and the physician should be consulted.

10. Convert 6 ounces to a decimal: $\frac{6}{16}$ is $\frac{3}{8}$ and $3 \div 8 = 0.375$. Then set up $\frac{1 \text{ kg}}{2.2 \text{ lbs}} = \frac{? \text{ kg}}{44.5 \text{ lbs}} \rightarrow 1 \times 44.5 = 44.5$. Then $44.5 \div 2.2 = 20.227$, which is rounded to 20.23 kg. To get the daily dose, multiply 0.5 mg by $20.23 = 60.72$ mg

11. The dosing is every 4 hours so that means divide the daily dose (24 hours) by 6 to get the answer. 60.72 mg $\div 6 = 10.12$ mg

12. No, the dose is over the recommended 45 milligrams in 24 hours, and the physician should be consulted.

13. Set up $\frac{1 \text{ kg}}{2.2 \text{ lbs}} = \frac{? \text{ kg}}{25 \text{ lbs}} \rightarrow 1 \times 25 = 25$. Then $25 \div 2.2 = 11.36$ kg. Multiply 0.75 mcg by $11.36 = 25.56$ mcg, but notice that this is the dose for every 8 hours. To get the daily dose, multiply 25.56 by $3 = 76.68$ mcg

14. To get the individual dose, multiply 0.75 mcg by $11.36 = 25.56$ mcg

15. No, the dose is over the recommended 80 micrograms in 24 hours, and the physician should be consulted.

Practice 1: p. 285

1. 6.36 kilograms
3. 12.27 kilograms
5. 18.18 kilograms
7. 7.27 kilograms
9. 13.64 kilograms

Practice 2: pp. 285–286

1. 14.5, 6.59 kilograms
3. 16.25, 7.39 kilograms
5. 42.13, 19.15 kilograms
7. 12.75, 5.80 kilograms
9. 124.88, 56.76 kilograms

Practice 3: pp. 288–289

1. 3.92 kilograms, 58.8 milligrams
3. 8.18 kilograms, 2 milliliters
5. Yes, 300 milligrams, 100 milligrams
7. 19.09 kilograms, 152 milligrams, 38 milligrams
9. 12.95 kilograms, 3.9 milliliters, 1.3 milligrams

Critical Thinking with Basic Dosage by Body Weight: pp. 289–291

1. This problem comes to 0.3 (1/3) of a tablet, so contact the physician for clarification. Normally, we do not see 1/3 tablet.
2. No
3. 0.5 mL
4. 47 teaspoons
5. 7.3 kg
6. 15.5 kg
7. True
8. True
9. False. Ordered dose needs to be compared to the recommended dose.
10. 250 mg
11. 9 drops
12. $\frac{1}{3}$ tablespoons
13. 10 mL
14. 42 mL
15. 420 mL

Basic Dosage by Body Weight Post-Test: pp. 291–292

1. Convert 2 ounces to a decimal: $\frac{2}{16}$ is $\frac{1}{8}$ and $1 \div 8 = 0.125$. Then set up $\frac{1 \text{ kg}}{2.2 \text{ lbs}} = \frac{? \text{ kg}}{14.125 \text{ lbs}} \rightarrow 1 \times 14.125 = 14.125$. Then $14.125 \div 2.2 = 6.4204$, which is rounded to 6.42 kg

2. Set up $\frac{1 \text{ kg}}{2.2 \text{ lbs}} = \frac{? \text{ kg}}{82 \text{ lbs}} \rightarrow 1 \times 82 = 82$. Then $82 \div 2.2 = 37.2727$ kg, which is rounded to 37.27 kg

3. Convert 15 ounces to a decimal: $\frac{15}{16}$ and $15 \div 16 = 0.9375$. Then set up $\frac{1 \text{ kg}}{2.2 \text{ lbs}} = \frac{? \text{ kg}}{7.9375 \text{ lbs}} \rightarrow 1 \times 7.9375 = 7.9375$. Then $7.9375 \div 2.2 = 3.6068$, which is rounded to 3.61 kg

4. Convert 12 ounces to a decimal: $\frac{12}{16}$ is $\frac{3}{4}$ and $3 \div 4 = 0.75$. Then set up $\frac{1 \text{ kg}}{2.2 \text{ lbs}} = \frac{? \text{ kg}}{8.75 \text{ lbs}} \rightarrow 1 \times 8.75 = 8.75$. Then $8.75 \div 2.2 = 3.98$ kg

5. Convert 10 ounces to a decimal: $\frac{10}{16}$ is $\frac{5}{8}$ and $5 \div 8 = 0.625$.

   Then set up $\frac{1 \text{ kg}}{2.2 \text{ lbs}} = \frac{? \text{ kg}}{12.625 \text{ lbs}} \rightarrow 1 \times 12.625 = 12.625$.

   Then $12.625 \div 2.2 = 5.7386$, which is rounded to 5.74 kg

6. Convert 8 ounces to a decimal: $\frac{8}{16}$ is $\frac{1}{2}$ and $1 \div 2 = 0.5$.

   Then set up $\frac{1 \text{ kg}}{2.2 \text{ lbs}} = \frac{? \text{ kg}}{33.5 \text{ lbs}} \rightarrow 1 \times 33.5 = 33.5$.

   Then $33.5 \div 2.2 = 15.227$, which is rounded to 15.23 kg

7. Convert pounds to kilograms. 77 lbs $\div$ 2.2 = 35 kilograms. Then 1.2×35kg = 42 mg per day. This is the recommended daily dose.

8. The medication is given every 8 hours or three times a day. $42 \div 3 = 14$ milligrams each dose.

9. No, it is recommended that every 8 hours, only 3 mg be given. Consult the physician.

10. Convert pounds to kilograms. $32.5 \div 2.2 = 14.77$ kg. Then 0.5 mg $\times 14.77 = 7.39$ mg every 4 hours. So this must be multiplied by 6 to get a full daily dosage. $7.39 \times 6 = 44.31$ milligrams

11. 7.39 milligrams

12. Yes, in a full 24 hours, the patient can have up to 45 milligrams.

13. Convert pounds to kilograms. 19 lbs $\div$ 2.2 = 8.64 kilograms. Then 8.64×0.25 micrograms = 2.16 micrograms for the individual dose. If the order is for every 8 hours, to get the daily dose, you must multiply $2.16 \times 3 = 6.48$ micrograms

14. 2.16 micrograms

15. No, contact the physician for clarification.

APPENDIX D: DIMENSIONAL ANALYSIS

Medical professionals encounter real-world math problems every day. The trick to solving these problems is to report answers in the appropriate units without affecting the correct numerical value. Straight conversions as well as more complicated dosage problems will always include measurable items—that is, a number with a unit measure (the dimension) attached. **Dimensional analysis (DA)** is a mathematical system that uses **conversion factors**, or ratios, to move from one unit of measure to another. This is a modification of the proportional methods of solving for an unknown; proportions are covered in Unit 4, Ratio and Proportion. Another name for DA is the factor method or factor analysis. Don't let the term dimensional analysis unnerve you; this is just one method of using a formula to solve applied math problems.

For example: How many pounds are in 12 kilograms?

1. Place the unknown value on one side of the equation, usually the left side.

$$? \text{ pounds } =$$

2. Next, place the number being converted and the **conversion factor** on the other side of the equation, usually the right side. A *conversion factor* is used to convert *units of measure* without changing the overall numeric value. The conversion factor is actually a ratio (fraction) that has a value of 1. This ratio or conversion factor is used as a multiplier that, when applied to the starting unit, converts the starting unit into the desired unit. For example, one foot has twelve inches $\left(\dfrac{1 \text{ foot}}{12 \text{ inches}}\right)$, or twelve inches equal one foot $\left(\dfrac{12 \text{ inches}}{1 \text{ foot}}\right)$. These conversion factors are known as equivalences, and both actually have a value of 1. When multiplying by a conversion factor having a value of 1, the final answer is not altered and is expressed in the desired unit. Some problems may use more than one conversion factor, depending on how many different systems are involved.

In this example, How many pounds are in 12 kilograms?, the setup will be done as follows:

number being converted   the conversion factor/unit

$$? \text{ pounds } = 12 \text{ kg} \times \frac{2.2 \text{ pounds}}{1 \text{ kg}} \qquad\qquad 12 \times 2.2 = 26.4 \text{ pounds}$$

Dimensional analysis (DA) is a problem-solving method that multiplies the given data and its units by known conversion factors or units so that only the desired units remain as the solution to the problem. Why was the conversion factor $\left(\dfrac{2.2 \text{ pounds}}{1 \text{ kg}}\right)$ chosen as the multiplier in this problem? In this case, the numerator contained the desired unit, and the denominator contained the unit we wished to eliminate. The order of the conversion factors on the right side of the equation may vary; the order does not affect the outcome of the problem. You must always keep asking yourself: What is my desired final unit? and What unit must be eliminated?

We will use three basic facts about how numbers work when we set up equations in DA:

1. Any number multiplied by 1 is itself. In other words, 60 minutes $\times$ 1 = 60 minutes.

2. Any number divided by itself is 1. In other words, $\dfrac{60 \text{ minutes}}{60 \text{ minutes}} = 1$.

3. Conversion factors have a value of 1. $\dfrac{1 \text{ foot}}{12 \text{ inches}} = 1$ or $\dfrac{12 \text{ inches}}{1 \text{ foot}} = 1$. This is true because the measured values of both the numerator and denominator are equal.

This information may seem obvious and unnecessary to review. However, recalling these three numerical facts helps us when we begin to set up and then use cross-cancellation to solve math problems.

Let's solve another math problem using dimensional analysis:
How many minutes are there in 4 hours?

STEP 1: How many minutes are there in 4 hours? First, we need to ask, What are we solving? The answer will be how many minutes there are in 4 hours. So,? minutes is our *unknown*. This is our starting point. We place? minutes on the left side of the equation.

$$? \text{ minutes } =$$

STEP 2: Next we need to figure out what goes on the other side of the equation. We are converting 4 hours to minutes, so we place 4 hours over 1 as our first conversion factor. We use 1 so that both sides of the equation have fractions and there is no confusion about which part of the conversion to use when we are canceling like units. If the conversion factors all appear as fractions, then the visual setup looks consistent.

We know that there are 60 minutes in an hour. So we continue to write our equation:

$$? \text{ minutes } = \frac{4 \text{ hours}}{1}$$

STEP 3: Add the conversion factor for hours and minutes. Place minutes on the top because this is the unit of measure that we desire in our answer.

$$? \text{ minutes } = \frac{4 \text{ hours}}{1} \times \frac{60 \text{ minutes}}{1 \text{ hour}}$$

STEP 4: Now we will use the principles of cross-cancellation. Cross-cancellation allows us to cancel units from the top and bottom numbers, rather than from side to side. Cross-cancellation in DA helps ensure that the final answer is in the correct unit of measure.

$$? \text{ minutes } = \frac{4 \; \cancel{\text{hours}}}{1} \times \frac{60 \text{ minutes}}{1 \; \cancel{\text{hour}}}$$

STEP 5: Solve the equation.

$$\text{So ? minutes } = 4 \times 60, \text{ or } 240 \text{ minutes.}$$
$$? \text{ minutes } = 240$$

Students sometimes ask, How do I know what to put where? That is an excellent question. Use this handy model to help you know what goes where:

$$\frac{\text{units of measure of the answer go on top}}{\text{units that you are converting from go on the bottom}}$$

Remember, the denominator should be the unit that you want to disappear.

Let's see what this looks like in another problem:
How many kilograms are there in 13 pounds?

STEP 1: ? kilograms =

STEP 2: Add the first conversion factor. We will place the weight that we are converting over 1.

$$? \text{ kilogram } = \frac{13 \text{ pounds}}{1}$$

STEP 3: Add the known conversion factor for kilograms and pounds.

$$? \text{ kilogram } = \frac{13 \text{ pounds}}{1} \times \frac{1 \text{ kilogram}}{2.2 \text{ pounds}}$$

Notice that the problem is *not* written as

$$? \text{ kilogram} = \frac{13 \text{ pounds}}{1} \times \frac{2.2 \text{ pounds}}{1 \text{ kilogram}}$$

The reason this setup is incorrect is that it does not follow the model:

$$\frac{\text{units of measure of the answer go on top}}{\text{units that you are converting from go on the bottom}}$$

If we used the second setup, the final answer would not be in the correct format. The final answer must be in <u>kilograms</u>. Thus, we must follow the model and place the measure of the answer on the top.

STEP 4: Cancel like units using cross-cancellation.

$$? \text{ kilogram} = \frac{13 \, \cancel{\text{pounds}}}{1} \times \frac{1 \text{ kilogram}}{2.2 \, \cancel{\text{pounds}}}$$

$$? \text{ kilogram} = \frac{13 \times 1 \text{ kilograms}}{2.2}$$

Notice that the pounds units on the left- and right-hand sides of the equation have canceled each other out.

STEP 5: Solve the equation.

$$? \text{ kilogram} = \frac{13 \times 1 \text{ kilograms}}{2.2}$$

$$? \text{ kilogram} = \frac{13 \text{ kilograms}}{2.2}$$

$$? = 5.9 \text{ kilograms}$$

Here's another example:

A patient has an order to receive 300 milliliters of 0.9% normal saline solution over 3 hours. The tubing drop factor is 10 gtts/mL. At what rate in drops per minute should the normal saline solution be infused?

STEP 1: Establish the form for your final answer and follow it with an equal sign.

$$x \text{ gtts/min} =$$

STEP 2: Set the tubing drop rate on the other side of the equal sign.

$$x \text{ gtts/min} = \frac{10 \text{ gtts}}{1 \text{ mL}}$$

STEP 3: Add the units in mL over the time in hours.

$$x \text{ gtts/min} = \frac{10 \text{ gtts}}{1 \text{ mL}} \times \frac{300 \text{ mL}}{3 \text{ hours}}$$

STEP 4: Add the final conversion of hours over minutes since the goal is to get gtts/min.

$$x \text{ gtts/min} = \frac{10 \text{ gtts}}{1 \text{ mL}} \times \frac{300 \text{ mL}}{3 \text{ hours}} \times \frac{1 \text{ hour}}{60 \text{ minutes}}$$

STEP 5: Multiply and divide to arrive at the final answer.

$$x \text{ gtts/min} == \frac{10 \text{ gtts}}{1 \, \cancel{\text{mL}}} \times \frac{300 \, \cancel{\text{mL}}}{3 \, \cancel{\text{hours}}} \times \frac{1 \, \cancel{\text{hour}}}{60 \text{ minutes}} = \frac{3000 \text{ gtts}}{180 \text{ minutes}} \, 16.6 \text{ gtts/min} \rightarrow 17 \text{ gtts/min}$$

◆◆◆◆ Practice Using Dimensional Analysis with Converting Common Measurements

Use the following conversion table for converting among measurement systems:

1 foot = 12 inches	1 cup = 8 ounces	1 day = 24 hours
1 inch = 2.54 centimeters	1 tablespoon = 3 teaspoons	1 hour = 60 minutes
1 yard = 3 feet	1 quart = 2 pints	1 minute = 60 seconds
1 cm = 100 millimeters	1 pint = 2 cups	1 pound = 16 ounces
	1 quart = 32 ounces	1 kilogram = 2.2 pounds

◆◆◆◆ **D-1.** Solve these problems using dimensional analysis:

1. 14 pounds = _____ kilograms

2. 29 kilograms = _____ pounds

3. 26 cups = _____ pints

4. $4\frac{1}{2}$ feet = _____ inches

5. 28 ounces = _____ cups

6. $2\frac{1}{2}$ pints = _____ cups

7. 14 hours = _____ minutes

8. A patient drinks 5 cups of chicken broth. What is this intake in ounces? _____

Use the conversion table above to solve these conversions.

9. A doctor orders a mouth rinse solution of $1\frac{1}{2}$ tablespoons once a day (qd) at bedtime for 7 days. How many total ounces are needed to fill this patient's prescription? _____

10. A doctor prescribes 3 ounces of a liquid medication. How many tablespoons will the patient receive? _____

◆◆◆◆ Practice Using Dimensional Analysis with Converting Apothecary and Metric Measurements

1 quart = 1 liter	1 fluid ounce = 2 tablespoons	Add Your Own Conversions:
1 quart = 1000 milliliters	1 fluid ounce = 30 milliliters	
1 quart = 32 fluid ounces	1 tablespoon = 15 milliliters	
1 pint = 16 fluid ounces	1 teaspoon = 5 milliliters	
1 pint = 500 milliliters	1 teaspoon = 60 drops	
1 cup = 240–250 milliliters	1 gram = 1000 milligrams	
1 cup = 8 fluid ounces	1 kilogram = 1000 grams	
1 gallon = 4 quarts	1 milligram = 1000 micrograms	

◆◆◆◆ D-2. Solve these problems using dimensional analysis:

1. 1500 milliliters = _____ liters

2. $6\frac{1}{2}$ cups = _____ milliliters

3. 35 milliliters = _____ tablespoons

4. $4\frac{1}{2}$ teaspoons = _____ drops

5. 16 teaspoons = _____ milliliters

6. 2000 micrograms = _____ milligrams

7. 16 liters = _____ pints

8. An instructor asked the student to convert 148 ounces into pints. How many pints are there? _____

9. A shopper wanted to compare products. She read 60 milliliters and wondered how many ounces are in 60 milliliters. The correct answer is _____.

10. The math problem asked the student to convert 240 milliliters to ounces. The correct answer is _____.

◆◆◆◆ Practice Using Dimensional Analysis with Calculating Dosage

Dosage problems seem to be more difficult because they are often presented as story problems. Use the step-by-step approach to help you understand each problem.

Follow these steps to develop a personal discipline for solving dosage problems.

1. Read the problem at least three times before deciding what the problem is really asking you to do.

2. Determine the known information given in the problem and write that information down.

3. Determine the desired unit of measure for the answer.

4. Set up your formula using as many conversion factors as necessary. Do not worry about the numbers; instead concentrate on the elimination of unwanted units and on the desired unit of the answer.

5. Do the necessary arithmetic and write down the answer with its appropriate unit.

EXAMPLE 1:

The doctor's order reads: Give the patient 15 milligram codeine PO stat. You have 30 milligram scored tablets available.

STEP 1: Read the problem. What unit of measure should the final answer have?

The unit of measure is milligrams or tablets. The nurse will give tablets. So the final unit of measure will be in tablets.

So that is the unknown to solve for:

$$? \text{ tablets} =$$

STEP 2: Is a conversion among systems needed? No. You will give the patient the same unit of measure as you have on hand. You have a doctor's order for 15 milligrams, and your supply on hand is 30 milligrams. So, you have the correct unit of measure, milligrams. There is no need to convert among units of measure in this problem.

STEP 3: What is the desired dose? The doctor has ordered 15 milligrams of codeine. You will place this information, 15 mg, over 1 on the right side of the equation.

$$? \text{ tablets} = \frac{15 \text{ mg}}{1}$$

STEP 4: What is the conversion factor or unit?

$\dfrac{1 \text{ tablet}}{30 \text{ milligram}}$ (Note that the tablet goes on top because that is what the final dose unit should be.)

$$? \text{ tablets} = \frac{15 \text{ mg}}{1} \times \frac{1 \text{ tablet}}{30 \text{ mg}}$$

STEP 5: Cancel units:

$$? \text{ tablets} = \frac{15 \text{ \cancel{mg}}}{1} \times \frac{1 \text{ tablet}}{30 \text{ \cancel{mg}}}$$

STEP 6: Solve the equation.

$$? \text{ tablets} = \frac{15 \text{ \cancel{mg}}}{1} \times \frac{1 \text{ tablet}}{30 \text{ \cancel{mg}}} =$$

$$? \text{ tablets} = \frac{15 \times 1}{30} = \frac{15}{30} = \frac{1}{2}$$

$$? = \frac{1}{2} \text{ tablet}$$

The same method is used to calculate orders for syringes.

EXAMPLE 2:

The doctor has ordered diazepam 7.5 milligrams IM for a patient with anxiety to be given STAT. The supply on hand is a vial of diazepam that has a label reading 5 mg per 1 mL.

STEP 1: Read the problem. What unit of measure should the final answer have?

The unit of measure is milliliters. The nurse will give an injection; you know this because the route of administration is IM, or intramuscular injection. So, the final unit of measure will be in milliliters.

So that is the unknown to solve for:

$$? \text{ mL} =$$

STEP 2: Is a conversion among systems needed? No, all measures are in the metric system.

STEP 3: What is the desired dose? The doctor has ordered 7.5 milligrams. We put this over 1.

$$? \text{ mL} = \frac{7.5 \text{ mg}}{1}$$

STEP 4: What is the conversion factor or unit? Look at the information from the drug label: 5 mg per 1 mL.

$$? \text{ mL} = \frac{7.5 \text{ mg}}{1} \times \frac{1 \text{ mL}}{5 \text{ mg}}$$

STEP 5: Cancel units:

$$? \text{ mL} = \frac{7.5 \text{ mg}}{1} \times \frac{1 \text{ mL}}{5 \text{ mg}}$$

STEP 6: Solve the equation.

$$? \text{ mL} = \frac{7.5 \times 1}{1 \times 5}$$

$$? \text{ mL} = \frac{7.5}{5}$$

$$? \text{ mL} = 1.5 \text{ mL}$$

◆◆◆◆ D-3. Solve these problems using dimensional analysis:

1. The doctor has ordered 500 milligrams of Amoxicillin. You have a bottle of Amoxicillin that reads 100 mg/5 mL. How many milliliters will the patient receive? _____

2. The doctor orders 75 mg of a drug. The drug's label reads 100 mg/20 mL. How many milliliters will the patient receive? _____

3. Lorazepam 0.8 mg is prescribed. The label on the Lorazepam label reads 2 mg/mL. How many mL will the nurse give? _____

4. The doctor has ordered 0.1 grams of a medication. The medication's label reads 25 mg per 2 mL. How many milliliters of this medication will the patient receive? _____

5. The nurse receives a new order for Mr. Smith. His doctor has ordered Cardura XL 16 milligrams. The Cardura XL label reads 8 mg/tablet. How will this order be dispensed to the patient? _____

6. A patient was told to take 50 milligrams of a supplement each day. The supplement comes in the following strength: 12.5 milligrams in each 5 milliliters. How many teaspoons should the patient take each day? _____

7. The order reads lisinopril 15 mg once daily. The lisinopril label reads 5 mg/tablet. How many tablets will be given? _____

8. Simvastatin 60 milligrams are ordered each day. The Simvastatin label reads 20 mg per tablet. How many tablets are taken each day? _____

9. Dr. Wu has prescribed phenytoin 100 mg chewable tablets for a child. The label reads phenytoin 50 mg tablets. How many tablets will the child be given? _____

10. A pediatric patient is ordered 60 milligrams of a liquid cough syrup. The cough syrup has a label that reads 100 mg per 5 mL. How many milliliters will the child be given? _____

◆◆◆◆ Practice Using Dimensional Analysis with Calculating IVs

For intravenous medications, using certain equation setups will help you calculate the correct units of measure. These units are placed on the left side of the equation.

WHAT IS BEING SOLVED	WHEN TO USE IT
F mL/hr	To find the flow rate of milliliters per hour
F gtts/min	To find the flow rate of drops per minute
T h	To find the time in hours or the time in hours and minutes
V mL	To find the total volume infused in milliliters

To find the flow rate, these are the steps using dimensional analysis:

EXAMPLE 1:

Infuse 500 mg of medication in 100 mL Normal Saline solution over 30 minutes.

STEP 1: What is the unknown? It is the flow rate in mL/hr.

$$\text{F mL/hr} =$$

STEP 2: Add the first conversion factor for the time.

$$\text{F mL/hr} = \frac{60 \text{ minutes}}{1 \text{ hour}}$$

STEP 3: Add the second conversion factor; this is from the problem itself.

$$\text{F mL/hr} = \frac{60 \text{ minutes}}{1 \text{ hour}} \times \frac{100 \text{ mL}}{30 \text{ minutes}}$$

STEP 4: Cancel like units.

$$\text{F mL/hr} = \frac{60 \text{ \sout{minutes}}}{1 \text{ hour}} \times \frac{100 \text{ mL}}{30 \text{ \sout{minutes}}}$$

STEP 5: Solve the equation.

$$\text{F mL/hr} = \frac{60 \times 100 \text{ mL}}{30 \text{ hour}} = \frac{6000}{30}$$

$$\text{F mL/hr} = 200 \text{ ml/hr}$$

EXAMPLE 2:

Infuse 500 mg of medication in 100 mL Normal Saline solution over 2 hours.

STEP 1: What is the unknown? It is the flow rate in mL/hr.

$$\text{F mL/hr} =$$

STEP 2: Set up the conversion using the information from the problem.

$$\text{F mL/hr} = \frac{100 \text{ milliliters}}{2 \text{ hours}}$$

Notice in this problem that a second conversion factor is not required. The final, desired answer is mL/hr.

STEP 3: Solve the equation.

$$\text{F mL/hr} = \frac{100 \text{ milliliters}}{2 \text{ hours}}$$

$$\text{F mL/hr} = 50 \text{ mL/hr}$$

◆◆◆◆ D-4. Solve the following problems using dimensional analysis to find the gtts/min:

1. Infuse 1200 mL of medication in 12 hours. The tubing drop factor is 10 gtts/mL. Infuse at _____.

2. Infuse 1000 mL of medication in 8 hours. The tubing drop factor is 10 gtts/mL. Infuse at _____.

3. Infuse 750 mL of medication in 4 hours. The tubing drop factor is 10 gtts/mL. Infuse at _____.

4. Infuse 550 mL of medication in 5 hours. The tubing drop factor is 20 gtts/mL. Infuse at _____.

5. Infuse 800 mL of medication in 12 hours. The tubing drop factor is 20 gtts/mL. Infuse at _____.

6. Infuse 50 mL of antibiotic in D_5W in 30 minutes. The tubing drop factor is 20 gtts/mL. Infuse at _____.

7. Infuse 1500 mL Normal Saline IV in 24 hours. The tubing drop factor is 20 gtts/mL. Infuse at _____.

8. The nurse received a patient's medication order for 550 mL RL IV for 6 hours. The tubing drop factor is 60 gtts/mL. Infuse at _____.

9. The doctor writes an order for 250 mL NS IV in 3 hours. The tubing drop factor is 60 gtts/mL. Infuse at _____.

10. The physician orders 100 mL $D_{10}W$ to infuse for 75 minutes. The tubing drop factor is 60 gtts/mL. Infuse at _____.

Calculate the following order to figure out the final answer in drops per minute. For example: An order reads 1000 mL D_5W IV over 8 hours. The tubing drop factor is 20 gtts/mL.

STEP 1: Place the conversion factor for drops per minute on the left side of the equation.

$$F \text{ gtts/min } =$$

STEP 2: Place the tubing drop rate, in gtts/mL, on the right side of the equation.

$$F \text{ gtts/min } = \frac{20 \text{ gtts}}{1 \text{ mL}}$$

STEP 3: Add the milliliters/hours unit from the problem.

$$F \text{ gtts/min } = \frac{20 \text{ gtts}}{1 \text{ mL}} \times \frac{1000 \text{ mL}}{8 \text{ hours}}$$

STEP 4: Add the hours to minutes rate conversion to the equation.

$$F \text{ gtts/min } = \frac{20 \text{ gtts}}{1 \text{ mL}} \times \frac{1000 \text{ mL}}{8 \text{ hours}} \times \frac{1 \text{ hour}}{60 \text{ min}}$$

STEP 5: Cancel like units.

$$F \text{ gtts/min } = \frac{20 \text{ gtts}}{1 \text{ mL}} \times \frac{1000 \text{ mL}}{8 \text{ hours}} \times \frac{1 \text{ hour}}{60 \text{ min}}$$

STEP 6: Solve the equation.

$$F \text{ gtts/min } = \frac{1000 \times 20 \text{ gtts}}{8 \times 60 \text{ minutes}}$$

$$F \text{ gtts/min } = \frac{20000 \text{ gtts}}{480 \text{ minutes}}$$

$$F \text{ gtts/min } = 41.67 \text{ gtts/min, which is rounded to 42 gtts/min}$$

$$F \text{ gtts/min } = 42 \text{ gtts/min}$$

◆◆◆◆ D-5. Solve the following problems using dimensional analysis to find the time in drop rate in gtts/min:

1. The order reads 1000 mL in 18 hours at 15 gtts/mL. The drop rate is _____.

2. The order reads 200 mL in $1\frac{1}{2}$ hours at 20 gtts/mL. The drop rate is _____.

3. The order reads 250 mL in 8 hours at 60 gtts/mL. The drop rate is _____.

4. The order reads 750 mL in 10 hours at 20 gtts/mL. The drop rate is _____.

5. The order reads 1250 mL in 24 hours at 60 gtts/mL. The drop rate is _____.

6. The order reads 1500 mL in 12 hours at 15 gtts/mL. The drop rate is _____.

7. Infuse 325 mL 0.9% NS over 6 hours. Use 60 drops per milliliter. The drop rate is _____.

8. The physician orders 500 mL plasma over 12 hours at 10 gtts/mL. The drop rate is _____.

9. Infuse D$_5$W 150 mL in 2 hours using 10 gtts/mL. The drop rate is _____.

10. The nurse receives a physician order for 500 mL 0.9% NS over 8 hours at 20 drops/mL. The drop rate is _____.

Sometimes health care staff must calculate the duration of an IV flow in both hours and minutes. To calculate the time it will take for a specific volume at a specific rate to run, use the following conversion factor, time in hours or T h.

For example: Find the total time of infusion for 1000 mL NS at a rate of 83 mL/hr.

STEP 1: Determine what you are solving for and place the conversion factor on the left side of the equation.

$$T h =$$

STEP 2: Add the conversion factors to the right side of the equation.

$$T h = \frac{1000 \text{ mL}}{1} \times \frac{1 \text{ hour}}{83 \text{ mL}}$$

STEP 3: Cancel like units.

$$T h = \frac{1000 \text{ \cancel{mL}}}{1} \times \frac{1 \text{ hour}}{83 \text{ \cancel{mL}}}$$

STEP 4: Solve the equation.

$$T h = \frac{1000}{83} = 12.04819. \text{ Round to the hundredth}$$

$$T h = 12.05$$

STEP 5: Note that 12.05 does not mean 12 hours and 5 minutes. Another conversion is needed.

STEP 6: Set up the problem:

$$x \text{ minutes} = \frac{0.05 \text{ hour}}{1} \times \frac{60 \text{ minutes}}{1 \text{ hour}}$$

STEP 7: Cancel the like units

$$x \text{ minutes} = \frac{0.05 \text{ \cancel{hour}}}{1} \times \frac{60 \text{ minutes}}{1 \text{ \cancel{hour}}}$$

STEP 8: Solve to get the minutes.

$$x \text{ minutes} = \frac{0.05 \times 60 \text{ minutes}}{1} = 3 \text{ minutes}$$

STEP 9: Put the minutes with the hours from the first conversion.

$$T h = 12 \text{ hours } 3 \text{ minutes}$$

◆◆◆◆ **D-6.** Solve these problems using dimensional analysis to find the time the IV will infuse:

1. Infuse 500 mL D$_5$W IV at 75 mL/hr. This IV will run for _____.

2. Infuse 750 mL D$_5$W IV at 60 mL/hr. This IV will run for _____.

3. Infuse 1000 mL D$_5$W IV at 150 mL/hr. This IV will run for _____.

4. Infuse 125 mL D$_5$W IV at 75 mL/hr. This IV will run for _____.

5. Infuse 75 mL D$_5$W IV at 15 mL/hr. This IV will run for _____.

6. Infuse 1500 mL D$_5$W IV at 83 mL/hr. This IV will run for _____.

7. Infuse 1200 mL D$_5$W IV at 50 mL/hr. This IV will run for _____.

8. Ordered 850 mL NS at 83 mL/hr. This IV will run for _____.

9. Ordered 1200 mL of 0.45% NS at 75 mL/hr. This IV will run for _____.

10. Ordered 250 mL RL at 15 mL/hr. This IV will run for _____.

To calculate the volume of an infusion, use the following conversion factor:

$$V \text{ mL} \times \text{hours} = \text{total volume}$$

For example, the doctor has ordered an IV of antibiotic solution to be infused for 12 hours at a flow rate of 28 mL/hr.

STEP 1: Place the conversion factor on the left side of the equation.

$$V \text{ mL} =$$

STEP 2: Place the duration of flow in hours over 1 on the right side of the equation.

$$V \text{ mL} = \frac{12 \text{ hours}}{1}$$

STEP 3: Add the flow rate conversion from the problem.

$$V \text{ mL} = \frac{12 \text{ hours}}{1} \times \frac{28 \text{ mL}}{1 \text{ hour}}$$

STEP 4: Cancel the like units.

$$V \text{ mL} = \frac{12 \text{ \sout{hours}}}{1} \times \frac{28 \text{ mL}}{1 \text{ \sout{hour}}}$$

STEP 5: Solve the equation.

$$V \text{ mL} = \frac{12 \times 28 \text{ mL}}{1} = 336$$

$$V \text{ mL} = 336 \text{ mL infused in total.}$$

◆◆◆◆ **D-7.** Solve the following flow volumes using the conversion factor on page 370:

1. Infuse 25 mL/hr for 6 hours. How much solution will be infused in all? _____

2. Infuse 75 mL/hr for 4 hours. How much solution will be infused in all? _____

3. Infuse 125 mL/hr for 8 hours. How much solution will be infused in all? _____

4. Infuse 100 mL/hr for 7.5 hours. How much solution will be infused in all? _____

5. Infuse 75 mL/hr for 24 hours. How much solution will be infused in all? _____

6. Infuse 125 mL/hr for 12 hours. How much solution will be infused in all? _____

7. Infuse 45 mL/hr for 5 hours. How much solution will be infused in all? _____

8. The doctor prescribes an infusion of 65 mL/hr for 8 hours. How much solution will be infused in all? _____

9. The doctor orders 125 mL/hr for 12 hours. How much solution will be infused in all? _____

10. Infuse 15 mL/hr for 3.5 hours. How much solution will be infused in all? _____

Answer Key for Appendix D

D-1. Common Measurement Conversions

1. 6.4 kg or 6.36 kg
2. 63.8 lb
3. 13 pt
4. 54 in
5. $3\frac{1}{2}$ c

6. 5 c
7. 840 min
8. 40 oz
9. $5\frac{1}{4}$ oz
10. 6 T

D-2. Apothecary and Metric Measurement Conversions

1. 1.5 liters
2. 1560 mL
3. $2\frac{1}{3}$ T
4. 270 drops
5. 80 mL

6. 2 mg
7. 32 pt
8. $9\frac{1}{4}$ pt
9. 2 fl oz
10. 8 oz

D-3. Calculating Dosage

1. 25 mL
2. 15 mL
3. 0.4 mL
4. 8 mL
5. 2 T

6. 4 t
7. 3 tab
8. 3 tab
9. 2 tab
10. 3 mL

D-4. Calculating IVs—Finding gtts/min

1. 17 gtts/min
2. 21 gtts/min
3. 31 gtts/min
4. 37 gtts/min
5. 22 gtts/min

6. 33 gtts/min
7. 21 gtts/min
8. 92 gtts/min
9. 83 gtts/min
10. 80 gtts/min

D-5. Calculating IVs—Finding gtts/min

1. 14 gtts/min
2. 44 gtts/min
3. 31 gtts/min
4. 25 gtts/min
5. 52 gtts/min

6. 31 gtts/min
7. 54 gtts/min
8. 7 gtts/min
9. 13 gtts/min
10. 21 gtts/min

D-6. Calculating IVs—Finding flow time of infusion

1. 6 hr 40 min
2. 12 hr 30 min
3. 6 hr 40 min
4. 1 hr 40 min
5. 5 hr

6. 18 hr 4 min
7. 24 hr
8. 10 hr 14 min
9. 16 hr
10. 16 hr 40 min

D-7. Calculating IVs—Finding volume of flow

1. 150 mL
2. 300 mL
3. 1000 mL
4. 750 mL
5. 1800 mL

6. 1500 mL
7. 225 mL
8. 520 mL
9. 1500 mL
10. 52.5 mL or 53 mL

This appendix includes several tools to help you learn math. These tools have been used by other students who have reported that using these tools helped them learn math and streamline their learning and memorization of math concepts and formulas. The appendix includes two copies of the blank forms so that you can make your own copies and place them in a binder. The following is an explanation of how to use each tool in this appendix.

◆◆◆◆ My Glossary of Math Terms

By keeping track of the math terms you need to learn and the math terms that confuse you, you will be better able to apply the terms when you need to do so.

◆◆◆◆ Math Notetaker

When you do math by hand, you can locate your errors and track your mistakes, thus very quickly learning your error patterns. Once you identify where you tend to make errors, you can learn how to avoid making those errors.

    This tool is also very helpful when you need to ask for help because it allows you to show someone where your understanding breaks down. This will then be the route to learning the correct solving process and learning how to correct your errors.

◆◆◆◆ Think-Aloud in Math

This tool has you "think out loud" as you try to make sense of a math problem. Sometimes you can talk your way through problem solving and problem setup as you verbalize what you know and what you do not know. The idea is to make your thinking clear through talking about it. Use the prompts to get started talking about your math problems.

◆◆◆◆ Math Reading Log

Students often learn by memorizing or tracking the steps of new math rules and formulas. This reading log or notetaker is very helpful for learning new rules and also for studying for tests. Students report that by writing down this type of information in a specific and consistent way, they are better able to learn and memorize it, and can study for exams in an organized manner.

◆◆◆◆ Blank Multiplication Table

Many students come to class reliant on their calculators and rusty on their mental math. One of the first important skills to review is multiplication. Instead of referring to a filled-in chart, you can fill in this chart and brush up on this skill. This chart can also help you memorize the multiplication facts.

◆◆◆◆ Divisibility Table

Sometimes when you need to divide, the process of figuring out what number (divisor) to use to divide into the dividend (the number that is being divided into parts) is overwhelming. The divisibility table provides some guidelines to doing division quickly. These number rules can help you eliminate a lot of choices and point you to the correct number to divide by.

◆◆◆◆ Mnemonics

Mnemonics is a learning method that uses letters, words, and phrases to make it easier to remember new formulas and rules. A mnemonic associates new information with something that you already know and helps you remember that information.

◆◆◆◆ Table for Conversions among Dosing Systems

Completing this table as you read the various units on the metric, household, and apothecary systems can assist you in learning what terms are unique to each system. In addition, completing and referring to the table can help you learn the correct format of each system.

◆◆◆◆ Draw Out Truths (DOT)

This chart provides a place for you to draw pictures of system conversions to aid your memory. Once you have drawn the pictures, you may be able to "see" them in your mind when you need to remember the conversions. Here is an example of how you might use the DOT chart:

1 teaspoon	=	5 milliliters
1 teaspoon	=	60 drops
1 teaspoon	=	60 grains

◆◆◆◆ My Glossary of Math Terms

Term	Definition	Symbol	When is the term/symbol used?
Sum	The total after adding the numbers	+	Addition of whole numbers, fractions, decimals

◆◆◆◆ My Glossary of Math Terms

Term	Definition	Symbol	When is the term/symbol used?
Sum	The total after adding the numbers	+	Addition of whole numbers, fractions, decimals

◆◆◆◆ Math Notetaker

Topic/Unit _____

Page(s) _____

	Document in this column where you make your missteps in math.
Number your problems and show your work. Circle the answers.	Locate your missteps.

◆◆◆◆ Math Notetaker

Topic/Unit _____

Page(s) _____

	Document in this column where you make your missteps in math.
Number your problems and show your work. Circle the answers.	Locate your missteps.

◆◆◆◆ Think-Aloud in Math

Math always . . . _____
_____
_____

I can picture . . . _____
_____

A question I have is . . . _____
_____

My confusion starts with . . . _____
_____
_____

This is like the problem where . . . _____
_____
_____

This symbol means . . . _____
_____
_____

I'm confused about the word/term/task . . . _____
_____
_____

I'm not sure what . . . _____
_____
_____

I got stuck after I . . . (list the step or strategy) _____
_____

I need help with . . . (list a specific concept) _____
_____

   Example: I can write the equation, but I can't solve it. _____
_____
_____

When I see . . . , I get . . . _____
_____
_____

After I do . . . , I always . . . _____
_____
_____

Doing . . . is where I get lost. _____
_____

Think-Aloud in Math

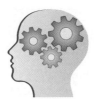

Math always . . . _____

_____

I can picture . . . _____

_____

A question I have is . . . _____

_____

My confusion starts with . . . _____

_____

This is like the problem where . . . _____

_____

This symbol means . . . _____

_____

I'm confused about the word/term/task . . . _____

_____

I'm not sure what . . . _____

_____

I got stuck after I . . . (list the step or strategy) _____

_____

I need help with . . . (list a specific concept) _____

_____

Example: I can write the equation, but I can't solve it. _____

_____

When I see . . . , I get . . . _____

_____

After I do . . . , I always . . . _____

_____

Doing . . . is where I get lost. _____

_____

◆◆◆◆ Math Reading Log

Rules or Formulas or Notes on Subject	Examples of the Rules and Applications	What aspect of the rule do I need to focus on? Where does my understanding break down or carelessness come into play and result in errors?

◆◆◆◆ Math Reading Log

Rules or Formulas or Notes on Subject	Examples of the Rules and Applications	What aspect of the rule do I need to focus on? Where does my understanding break down or carelessness come into play and result in errors?

◆◆◆◆◆ Blank Multiplication Table

×	1	2	3	4	5	6	7	8	9	10	11	12	15
1													
2													
3													
4													
5													
6													
7													
8													
9													
10													
11													
12													
15													

◆◆◆◆ Blank Multiplication Table

×	1	2	3	4	5	6	7	8	9	10	11	12	15
1													
2													
3													
4													
5													
6													
7													
8													
9													
10													
11													
12													
15													

◆◆◆◆ Divisibility Table

Divisibility of whole number	Rules for divisibility	Example
A whole number is divisible by 2	if it is an even number that has a 0, 2, 4, 6, or 8 in the ones place.	4586 is divisible by 2 because an even number, 6, is in the ones place.
A whole number is divisible by 3	if the sum of the digits is divisible by 3.	762 is divisible by 3 because 7 + 6 + 2 = 15, which is divisible by 3.
A whole number is divisible by 4	if the number formed by the last two digits is divisible by 4.	916 is divisible by 4 because the last two digits, 1 and 6, form a number that is divisible by 4.
A whole number is divisible by 5	if the number contains a 5 or a 0 in the ones place.	495 is divisible by 5 because the last digit is a 5.
A whole number is divisible by 6	if the number is divisible by 2 and by 3.	168 is divisible by 6 because it is divisible by 2 and by 3: 1 + 6 + 8 = 15, which is divisible by 3.
A whole number is divisible by 7	if, after doubling the number in the ones place and then subtracting this number from the remaining numbers, the resulting number is a multiple of 7.	574 is divisible by 7 because 4 × 2 = 8, and when 8 is subtracted from the remaining numbers of 57 (57 − 8), the result, 49, is divisible by 7.
A whole number is divisible by 8	if the number formed by the last three digits is divisible by 8.	5,120 is divisible by 8 because 120 is divisible by 8.
A whole number is divisible by 9	if the sum of the digits is divisible by 9.	945 is divisible by 9 because 9 + 4 + 5 = 18, which is divisible by 9.
A whole number is divisible by 10	if the number has a 0 in the ones place.	3,490 is divisible by 10 because the ones place has a 0.

◆◆◆◆ Mnemonics

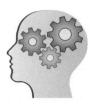

MNEMONIC	WHEN TO USE IT
DRAW: Discover the sign, Read the problem, Answer the problem, Write the answer	Any math computation problem
Box-and-add: Box the numbers and add them to ensure correct subtraction. $\frac{\begin{array}{r}200\\-19\end{array}}{181} = 181 + 19 = 200$	As a way to check whole number and decimal subtraction to ensure it is correct. Especially useful when borrowing.
Long dead monkeys smell bad: (Line up, divide, multiply, subtract, back to the top)	Steps in long division
Nice Days: Numerator on top of Denominator	Format of fractions $\frac{numerator}{denominator}$
Kentucky Fried Chicken: Keep first fraction, Flip the second fraction, Change the sign to ×	Division of fractions
PEMDAS: Please Excuse My Dear Aunt Sally Parentheses, Exponents, Multiplication, Division, Addition, and then Subtraction	The order in which algebraic equations should be solved
Lovely Cats Don't Meow: **L** = 50, **C** = 100, **D** = 500, and **M** = 1000	When working with Roman numerals
Kiss hairy dogs but drink chocolate milk, mom: kilo-, hecto-, deka-, base, deci-, centi-, milli-, x, x, micro- (the m and o in "mom" are the place holders x and x)	The order from left to right of the metric system units used in health care

◆◆◆◆◆ Mnemonics

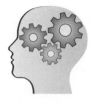

MNEMONIC	WHEN TO USE IT

◆◆◆◆ Table for Conversions among Dosing Systems

	Household	Metric	Apothecary
When is it used?			
Symbols and formatting			
Unique rules			
Questions			
Comments			
Notes			

◆◆◆◆◆ Table for Conversions among Dosing Systems

	Household	Metric	Apothecary
When is it used?			
Symbols and formatting			
Unique rules			
Questions			
Comments			
Notes			

◆◆◆◆ Draw Out Truths (DOT)

Basic unit	Equivalents in visual format

◆◆◆◆ Draw Out Truths (DOT)

Basic unit	Equivalents in visual format

INDEX

Rounding Guidelines	To the Tenth	To the Hundredth
	Temperature in Fahrenheit and Celsius	Certain medications and syringe dosages
	Pounds & Kilogram	Kilograms used for dosage by weight
		Money

Common Abbreviations IV Administration

Term for IVs	Abbreviation	Term for IVs	Abbreviation
intravenous	IV	water	H_2O, W
piggy-back	PB	5% Dextrose water	D_5W
drop/drops	gtt/gtts	10% Dextrose water	$D_{10}W$
hour	hr	Normal Saline (0.9%)	NS
minutes	min	One half Normal saline (0.45%)	$\frac{1}{2}NS$
drops per minute	gtts/min	Ringer's Lactate Solution	RL
drops per milliliter	gtts/mL	Lactated Ringer's Solution	LR
milliliters per hour	mL/hr		

Abbreviation used in Dosage

Abbreviation	Term	Abbreviation	Term
po	by mouth or orally	cap	capsule
susp	suspension	q	every
prn	as needed	bid	twice a day
tab	tablet	tid	three times a day